Sleep - Physiology, Functions, Dreaming and Disorders

Advances in Sleep Apnea

Detection, Diagnosis and Treatment

SLEEP - PHYSIOLOGY, FUNCTIONS, DREAMING AND DISORDERS

Additional books and e-books in this series can be found on Nova's website under the Series tab.

SLEEP - PHYSIOLOGY, FUNCTIONS, DREAMING AND DISORDERS

ADVANCES IN SLEEP APNEA

DETECTION, DIAGNOSIS AND TREATMENT

FRANCESCO LORUSSO
AND
SALVATORE GALLINA
EDITORS

nova
Medicine & Health
New York

NOTICE TO THE READER

Library of Congress Cataloging-in-Publication Data

ISBN: 978-1-53619-758-7

Published by Nova Science Publishers, Inc. † New York

Contents

PREFACE

Over thirty years ago my Director, Prof. Cimino, commissioned me to evaluate the upper airways of patients suffering from respiratory disorders in sleep, recruited at the Division of Pneumology directed by one of the pioneers and most accredited scholars of the aforementioned pathology: Prof. Giovanni Bonsignore.

It was the time when terms such as "Chronic Snoring" or "Obstructive Sleep Apnea Syndrome" began to take hold.

Since then, snoring complicated by sleep apnea, at the beginning almost exclusively of neurologists and pulmonologists, has involved various branches such as otolaryngology, cardiology, dentistry, internal medicine, bariatric surgery, oral medicine .

In particular, the evidence of an obstruction and a collapse of the upper airways in the determinism of the disease, has led the ENT specialist over time to develop a series of endoscopic instrumental procedures that have led to an increasingly precise diagnosis of the site of the obstruction and to an increasingly sophisticated and targeted surgical therapeutic strategy that is less and less destructive and attentive to organ function.

Our School has for decades a consolidated tradition in the study of Obstructive Sleep Apnea / Hypopneas Syndrome (OSAHS) and many of our specialists have therefore studied this pathology in depth.

Among these, Dr. Francesco Lorusso particularly distinguished himself for his great skills as a researcher and for his absolutely uncommon surgical talent.

Therefore, with particular pride and satisfaction, I present the compendium conceived and coordinated by him, in which he involved, with a view to a multidisciplinary approach, experienced and particularly qualified professionals.

All this with the aim, which I am sure will be achieved, of ensuring that the reader can find adequate answers to the many questions that this topic poses in diagnosis and therapy.

Prof. Salvatore Gallina

In: Advances in Sleep Apnea
Editors: F. Lorusso et al.
ISBN: 978-1-53619-758-7

Chapter 1

Anatomy of the Upper Airway in Obstructive Sleep Apnea (OSA)

Onofrio Guzzo, Salvatore Gallina, Rosalia Gargano and Francesco Lorusso**
Department of Otolaryngology, Head and Neck Surgery, Policlinico Paolo Giaccone University of Palermo, Palermo, Italy

Abstract

Obstructive sleep apnea syndrome (OSAS) is a sleep-related breathing disorder characterized by repetitive episodes of airflow cessation, resulting in brief arousals and intermittent hypoxemia.

The mechanism by which the upper airway collapses is not fully understood but is multifactorial and includes obesity, craniofacial changes, alteration in upper airway muscle function, pharyngeal neuropathy and fluid shift towards the neck.

It is known that collapse is a dynamic process that involves more than one area of the upper respiratory tract, the sequence of the collapse of the upper airway would present a cranio-caudal extension, from the retro-lingual to the hypopharyngeal region.

Knowledge of the upper airway anatomy including lumen, shape and length are fundamental to better understand the

* Corresponding Author's Email: dott.francescolorusso@gmail.com.

pathophysiological mechanisms underlying OSAS, in fact in these patients lumen can be reduced by congenital malformations of the mandible and/or maxilla, furthermore the shape of the upper airway in patients with OSAS have an oval conformation at the pharyngeal level, with the main axis oriented antero-posteriorly, in contrast to normal subjects in which the short axis is oriented anterior-posteriorly and finally it is known that longer airways are more collapsible compared to the shorter.

INTRODUCTION

The etiopathogenesis of OSA has not yet been fully clarified, but it has been seen that the factor that leads to the collapse of the upper airways is the generation of a critical subatmospheric pressure during inspiration, such as to exceed the capacity of the dilator muscles of the airways.

In fact, during sleep, there is a loss of the neuromuscular compensation mechanisms present during wakefulness, which combined with any anatomical anomalies of the upper airways, favors the collapse of the latter. The supine position, and especially sleep, are the crucial events in determining the reduction of muscle activity, with the consequent possibility of developing obstructive events.

Apnea will last as long as an arousal does not restore the muscle tone of wakefulness and therefore the patency of the airways.

The cycle will resume again as soon as the return to sleep occurs with 400/500 episodes per night.

Despite progress in the field, the reasons behind recurrent upper airway collapses and their timing have yet to be clearly defined.

There are two main etiopathogenetic theories:

Anatomical theory states that since the upper airways are collapsible structures, the association of anatomical anomalies contributes to increasing their collapsibility.

The neural theory states that the transition from wakefulness to sleep can result in a decrease in the activity of muscle tone such as to cause the collapse of the upper airway.

An emerging theme from the discussion of new pathogenetic theories is that upper airway collapse can be the end result of many different processes related to anatomical and functional alterations of the upper airway.

1. ANATOMY OF THE NASAL VALVE

The nasal valve is defined as the flow-limiting segment of the nasal airway, located at the triangular aperture between the upper lateral cartilage and the septum.

Nasal valve collapse is a common cause of nasal airway obstruction. In fact, nasal valvular incompetence may equal or even exceed septal deviation as the prime cause of nasal airway obstruction. The valve area may be obstructed secondary to surgical procedures (such as rhinoplasty), trauma, aging (as age progresses nasal ptosis and sagging of the sidewalls can occur) and congenital weakness of the nasal sidewalls may allow for easier collapse.

Nasal valve is composed by internal and external valve.

The internal valve is the area in which the septum articulates with the lower border of the upper lateral cartilage. The angle of this area is normally 10° to 15°. Minimal reduction in this angle can substantially restrict nasal airflow.

The external nasal valve is an area composed of the alar or lower lateral cartilage with its associated cutaneous support as a mobile alar wall. It is bordered superiorly by the caudal edge of the upper lateral cartilages, inferiorly by the nasal floor, and posteriorly by the inferior turbinate. Laterally it is supported by the pyriform aperture of the maxilla and fibrofatty tissue of the ala.

Patients may have nasal valve obstruction secondary to a deviated caudal septal position, which may nevertheless be correctable by valve suspension in selected situations. The decision to correct the valve or the septum is based on the response to the Cottle maneuver, the position of the entire septum, and whether the patient has had previous septal surgery. The Cottle maneuver consists of superolateral traction being applied to the nasofacial groove, and is considered positive when it causes improvement of the nasal airway, as perceived by the patient.

A positive Cottle maneuver is an adequate predictor of a successful outcome of nasal valve suspension for the treatment of nasal airway obstruction.

2. Anatomy of the Nasal Turbinates

Within the nasal cavity, there are three separate turbinates: superior, middle, and inferior. Turbinates are also called concha. Because the nasal cavity is symmetrical, there are technically pairs of turbinates, leading to 6 in total for an average human. These structures are on the lateral nasal wall. The inferior turbinate is independent of the superior and middle turbinates that extend from the ethmoid bones. The space between each turbinate and the nasal wall is called a meatus.

All three of the turbinates are responsible for warmth, humidification, and filtration. The inferior turbinate has respiratory and immune functions. Its structure is cartilage under soft tissue covered with respiratory epithelium. The folded structures of the turbinates increase the surface area of the cavity. The inferior turbinate has an immune response because it is the first tissue to come into contact with the outside air. Because of this, it decides pathogenicity and can trigger innate and adaptive immune reactions. The other two turbinates have similar structures in appearance, but stem from the ethmoid bone, and do not an immune function.

Inferior turbinate hypertrophy can be caused by generalized nasal mucosal diseases in allergic and vasomotor rhinitis, as well as compensatory enlargement due to a long-standing septal deviation.

3. Anatomy of the Nasal Septum

The medial wall of each nasal cavity is the nasal septum, a thin sheet of bone (posteriorly) and cartilage (anteriorly) that lies between the roof and floor of the cavity.

The nasal septum is made up of a cartilaginous septum and a bony septum.

3.1. Bony Septum

The posterosuperior part of the septum and its posterior border are formed by the vomer, which extends from the body of the sphenoid to the nasal crest of the palatine bones and maxilla. The nasopalatine nerves and vessels groove its surface.

The anterosuperior part of the septum is formed by the perpendicular plate of the ethmoid, which is continuous above with the cribriform plate and the frontal bone. Other bones that make minor contributions to the septum at the upper and lower limits of the medial wall are the nasal bones and the nasal spine of the frontal bones (anterosuperior), the rostrum and crest of the sphenoid (posterosuperior), and the nasal crests of the maxilla and palatine bones (inferior).

3.2. Cartilagineous Septum

The septal cartilage is almost quadrilateral and may extend back for some distance between the vomer and the perpendicular plate of the ethmoid.

Its anterosuperior margin is connected above to the posterior border of the internasal suture, and the distal end of its superior portion is continuous with the upper lateral cartilages.

The anteroinferior border is connected by fibrous tissue on each side to the medial crurae of the major alar cartilage. Anteroinferiorly, the cartilaginous septum is attached to the anterior nasal spine, which is formed by anterior projections of each maxillary crest, and it has a strong, tongue-in-groove attachment with the premaxilla and vomer.

The posterosuperior border joins the perpendicular plate of the ethmoid, while the posteroinferior border is attached to the vomer and, anterior to that, to the nasal crest and anterior nasal spine of the maxilla.

The anteroinferior part of the nasal septum between the nares is devoid of cartilage and is therefore called the membranous septum; it is continuous with the columella anteriorly.

4. Anatomy of Pharynx

The pharynx is a 12–14 cm long musculomembranous tube shaped like an inverted cone. It extends from the cranial base to the lower border of the cricoid cartilage (the level of the sixth or seventh cervical vertebra), where it becomes continuous with the esophagus. The width of the pharynx varies constantly because it is dependent on muscle tone, especially of the constrictors; at rest, the pharyngoesophageal junction is closed as a result of tonic closure of the upper esophageal sphincter, and during sleep, muscle tone is low and the dimensions of the pharynx are markedly decreased (which may give rise to snoring and sleep apnoea). The pharynx is limited above by the posterior part of the body of the sphenoid and the basilar part of the occipital bone, and it is continuous with the esophagus below. Behind, it is separated from the cervical part of the vertebral column and the prevertebral fascia, which covers longus colli and longus capitis, by loose connective tissue in the retropharyngeal space above and the retrovisceral space below.

The muscles of the pharynx are three circular constrictors and three longitudinal elevators. The constrictors may be thought of as three overlapping cones that arise from structures at the sides of the head and neck, and pass posteriorly to insert into a midline fibrous band, the pharyngeal raphe.

The pharynx lies behind, and communicates with, the nasal, oral and laryngeal cavities via the nasopharynx, oropharynx and laryngopharynx, respectively. Its lining mucosa is continuous with that lining the pharyngotympanic tubes, nasal cavity, mouth and larynx. The retropharyngeal and parapharyngeal spaces surround the pharynx; the retropharyngeal space lies anterior to the prevertebral and alar fascia and thus to the alar, danger space that lies between them.

4.1. Nasopharynx

The nasopharynx lies above the soft palate and behind the posterior nares, which allow free respiratory passage between the nasal cavities and the nasopharynx. The nasal septum separates the two posterior nares. Just within these openings lie the posterior ends of the inferior and middle nasal turbinates.

The nasopharynx has a roof, a posterior wall, two lateral walls and a floor. These are rigid (except for the floor, which can be raised or lowered by the soft palate), and the cavity of the nasopharynx is therefore never obliterated by muscle action, unlike the cavities of the oro and laryngopharynx.

The nasal and oral parts of the pharynx communicate through the pharyngeal isthmus, which lies between the posterior border of the soft palate and the posterior pharyngeal wall. Elevation of the soft palate and constriction of the palatopharyngeal sphincter close the isthmus during swallowing.

The lateral walls of the nasopharynx display a number of important surface features. On either side, each receives the opening of the pharyngotympanic tube (auditory or Eustachian tube). The tubal aperture is approximately triangular in shape, and is bounded above and behind by the tubal elevation that consists of mucosa overlying the protruding pharyngeal end of the cartilage of the pharyngotympanic tube. A vertical mucosal fold, the salpingopharyngeal fold, descends from the tubal elevation behind the aperture and covers salpingopharyngeus in the wall of the pharynx; a smaller salpingopalatine fold extends from the anterosuperior angle of the tubal elevation to the soft palate in front of the aperture. As levator veli palatini enters the soft palate, it produces an elevation of the mucosa immediately around the tubal opening. A small variable mass of lymphoid tissue, the tubal tonsil, lies in the mucosa immediately behind the opening of the pharyngo tympanic tube. Further behind the tubal elevation is a variable depression in the lateral wall, the lateral pharyngeal recess (fossa of Rosenmüller), located between the posterior wall of the nasopharynx and the salpingopharyngeal fold.

The pharyngeal tonsil (adenoid, nasopharyngeal tonsil) is a median mass of mucosa associated lymphoid tissue (MALT) situated in the roof and posterior wall of the nasopharynx. At its maximal size (during the early years of life), it is shaped like a truncated pyramid, often with a vertically orientated median cleft, so that its apex points towards the nasal septum and its base to the junction of the roof and posterior wall of the nasopharynx.

The free surface of the pharyngeal tonsil is marked by folds that radiate forwards and laterally from a median blind recess, the pharyngeal bursa (bursa of Luschka), which extends backwards and up.

After birth, it initially grows rapidly, but usually undergoes a degree of involution and atrophy from the age of 8–10 years (although hypoplasia may still occur in adults up to the seventh decade).

4.2. Oropharynx

The oropharynx extends from below the soft palate to the upper border of the epiglottis. It opens into the mouth through the oropharyngeal isthmus, demarcated by the palatoglossal arch, and faces the pharyngeal aspect of the tongue. Its lateral wall consists of the palatopharyngeal arch and palatine tonsil. Posteriorly, it is level with the bodies of the second, and upper part of the third, cervical vertebrae.

4.2.1. Soft Palate

The soft palate is a mobile flap suspended from the posterior border of the hard palate, sloping down and back between the oral and nasal parts of the pharynx. The boundary between the hard and soft palate is readily palpable and may be distinguished by a change in colour, the soft palate being a darker red with a yellowish tint. The soft palate is a thick fold of mucosa enclosing an aponeurosis, muscular tissue, vessels, nerves, lymphoid tissue and mucous glands; almost half its thickness is represented by numerous mucous glands that lie between the muscles and the oral surface of the soft palate. The latter is covered by a stratified squamous epithelium, while the nasal surface is covered with a ciliated columnar epithelium. Taste buds are found on the oral aspect of the soft palate.

In most individuals, two small pits, the fovea palatini, may be seen, one on each side of the midline; they represent the orifices of ducts from some of the minor mucous glands of the palate. In its usual relaxed and pendant position, the anterior (oral) surface of the soft palate is concave and has a median raphe. The posterior aspect is convex and continuous with the nasal floor, the anterosuperior border is attached to the posterior margin of the hard palate, and the sides blend with the pharyngeal wall. The inferior border is free and hangs between the mouth and pharynx. A median conical process, the uvula, projects downwards from its posterior border. It may be congenitally bifid and associated with submucous cleft palate, hypoplastic orifice of the pharyngotympanic tube and absence of the salpingo pharyngeal folds.

The anterior third of the soft palate contains little muscle and consists mainly of the palatine aponeurosis. This region is less mobile and more horizontal than the rest of the soft palate and is the chief area acted on by tensor veli palatini.

A small bony prominence, produced by the pterygoid hamulus, can be felt just behind and medial to each upper alveolar process, in the lateral part of the anterior region of the soft palate. The pterygomandibular raphe (a tendinous band between buccinator and the superior constrictor) passes downwards and outwards from the hamulus to the posterior end of the mylohyoid line. When the mouth is opened wide, this raphe raises a fold of mucosa that indicates the internal, posterior boundary of the cheek; it is an important landmark for an inferior alveolar nerve block.

4.2.2. Palatine Tonsil

The right and left palatine tonsils form part of the pharyngeal lymphoid ring. Each tonsil is an ovoid mass of lymphoid tissue situated in the lateral wall of the oropharynx. Size varies according to age, individuality and pathological status (tonsils may be hypertrophied and/or inflamed). It is therefore difficult to define the normal appearance of the palatine tonsil. For the first 5 or 6 years of life, the tonsils increase rapidly in size. They usually reach a maximum at puberty, when they average 20–25 mm in vertical, and 10–15 mm in transverse, diameters, and they project conspicuously into the oropharynx. Between the ages of 1 and 11 years, the tonsil and adenoid grow proportionally to the lower facial skeleton. Tonsillar involution begins at puberty, when the reactive lymphoid tissue begins to atrophy, and by old age only a little tonsillar lymphoid tissue remains.

The long axis of the tonsil is directed from above, downwards and backwards. Its medial, free, surface usually presents a pitted appearance. The pits, 10–20 in number, lead into a system of blind-ending, often highly branching, crypts that extend through the whole thickness of the tonsil and almost reach the connective tissue hemicapsule. In a healthy tonsil, the openings of the crypts are fissure-like and the walls of the crypt lumina are collapsed so that they are in contact with each other. The human tonsil is polycryptic. The branching crypt system reaches its maximum size and complexity during childhood. The mouth of a deep tonsillar cleft (intratonsillar cleft, recessus palatinus) opens in the upper part of the medial surface of the tonsil. It is often erroneously called the supratonsillar fossa, and yet it is not situated above the tonsil but within its substance. The mouth of the cleft is semilunar, curving parallel to the convex dorsum of the tongue in the sagittal plane. The upper wall of the recess contains lymphoid tissue that extends into the soft palate as the pars palatina of the palatine tonsil. After the age of 5 years, this embedded part of the tonsil diminishes in size. There is a tendency for the whole tonsil to involute from the age of 14 years, and for the tonsillar bed to flatten out. During young adult life, a mucosal fold, the plica triangularis, stretches back from the palatoglossal arch down to the tongue. It is infiltrated by lymphoid tissue and frequently represents the most prominent (anteroinferior) portion of the tonsil. It rarely persists into middle age.

The lateral or deep surface of the tonsil spreads downwards, upwards and forwards. Inferiorly, it invades the dorsum of the tongue; superiorly, it invades the soft palate; and, anteriorly, it may extend for some distance under the palatoglossal arch. This deep, lateral aspect is covered by a layer of fibrous tissue, the tonsillar hemicapsule. The latter is separable with ease for most of its extent from the underlying muscular wall of the pharynx, which is formed here by the superior constrictor, and sometimes by the anterior fibres of palatopharyngeus, with styloglossus on its lateral side. Anteroinferiorly, the hemicapsule adheres to the side of the tongue and to palatoglossus and palatopharyngeus. In this region, the tonsillar artery, a branch of the facial artery, pierces the superior constrictor to enter the tonsil, accompanied by venae comitantes. An important and sometimes large vein, the external palatine or paratonsillar vein, descends from the soft palate lateral to the tonsillar hemicapsule before piercing the pharyngeal wall. Hemorrhage from this vessel from the upper angle of the tonsillar fossa may complicate tonsillectomy. The muscular wall of the tonsillar fossa separates the tonsil from the ascending palatine artery, and, occasionally, from the tortuous facial artery itself, which may lie near the pharyngeal wall at the lower tonsillar level. The glossopharyngeal nerve lies immediately lateral to the muscular wall of the tonsillar fossa; it is at risk if the wall is pierced, and is commonly temporarily affected by edema following tonsillectomy. The internal carotid artery lies approximately 25 mm behind and lateral to the tonsil. In some individuals, the styloid process may be elongated and deviate towards the tonsillar bed.

4.3. Laryngopharynx

The laryngopharynx is situated behind the entire length of the larynx (known clinically as the hypopharynx) and extends from the superior border of the epiglottis, where it is delineated from the oropharynx by the lateral glossoepiglottic folds, to the inferior border of the cricoid cartilage, where it becomes continuous with the oesophagus. The laryngeal inlet lies in the upper part of its incomplete anterior wall, and the posterior surfaces of the arytenoid and cricoid cartilages lie below this opening.

4.3.1. Piriform Fossa

A small piriform fossa lies on each side of the laryngeal inlet, bounded medially by the aryepiglottic fold and laterally by the thyroid cartilage and thyrohyoid membrane. Branches of the internal laryngeal nerve lie beneath its mucous membrane. At rest, the laryngopharynx extends posteriorly from the lower part of the third cervical vertebral body to the upper part of the sixth. During deglutition, it may be elevated considerably by the hyoid elevators.

4.3.2. Inlet of Larynx

The obliquely sloping inlet of the larynx lies in the anterior part of the laryngopharynx and is bounded above by the epiglottis, below by the arytenoid cartilages of the larynx, and laterally by the aryepiglottic folds. Below the inlet, the anterior wall of the laryngopharynx is formed by the posterior surface of the cricoid cartilage.

4.4. Pharyngeal Tissue Spaces

Pharyngeal tissue spaces can be subdivided into peripharyngeal and intrapharyngeal spaces. The anterior part of the peripharyngeal space is formed by the submandibular and submental spaces, posteriorly by the retropharyngeal space and laterally by the parapharyngeal spaces. The retropharyngeal space is an area of loose connective tissue that lies behind the pharynx and anterior to the prevertebral fascia, extending upwards to the base of the skull and downwards to the retrovisceral space in the infrahyoid part of the neck. Each parapharyngeal space passes laterally around the pharynx and is continuous with the retropharyngeal space. However, unlike the retropharyngeal space, it is a space that is restricted to the suprahyoid region. It is bounded medially by the pharynx, laterally by the pterygoid muscles (where it is part of the infratemporal fossa) and by the sheath of the parotid gland, superiorly by the base of the skull, and inferiorly by suprahyoid structures, particularly the sheath of the submandibular gland; it may be helpful to think of it as shaped like an inverted pyramid extending from the base of the skull to the greater cornu of the hyoid bone. The parapharyngeal space is divided into an anterior, or prestyloid, compartment and a posterior, or retrostyloid, compartment. The prestyloid compartment contains the retromandibular portion of the parotid gland, fat and lymph nodes. The retrostyloid compartment contains the internal carotid artery, the internal jugular vein, the glossopharyngeal, vagus, accessory and hypoglossal nerves, the sympathetic chain, fat and lymph nodes.

Lumen of Upper Airway

The patency of the upper airway lumen is a function of the encumbrance created by the soft tissues (tongue, pharynx walls, adipose tissue), which occupy the space constituted by the bone structure of the skull.

The size of the bone structure can be reduced by hypoplasia or by the retroposition of some cranial structures, among which the reduction in the length of the jaw is an important factor.

Congenital malformations of the mandible and/or maxilla are present in over 50 syndromes, such as that of Treacher Collins or that of Pierre Robin, which are predisposing syndromes to OSAS, precisely because of the crowding that develops at the level of the VAS due to the presence of soft tissues housed in a reduced bony compartment. Cephalometric studies have shown subtle anomalies in patients with OSAS, such as a shorter jaw with greater retroposition, medialization of the branches of the lower jaw and displacement of the hyoid bone. The position of the mandible also influences the patency of the lumen of the upper airways, with the mouth open it favors the collapse of the upper airway by reducing the size of the containing bone structure. Furthermore, an increase in the soft tissue surrounding the airways will result in a reduction in the lumen of the upper airway, in obese subjects a greater amount of adipose tissue has been documented at the level of the uvula, tongue, soft palate, and walls. lateral pharynx. Finally, a combination of both factors, for example, as evidenced in acromegaly, certainly results in a reduction in lumen.

Studies by Immaging have shown that during wakefulness the main site of upper airway collapse is at the retropalatal level. Subsequently, many authors, using different techniques such as computed tomography (CT), cephalometry, acoustic reflection, and magnetic resonance imaging (MRI), have shown that both the section and the volume of the upper airway are reduced in patients with DRS compared to normal subjects.

Oral breathing is often reported in association with snoring, especially in children with severe nasal obstruction caused by adenoid hypertrophy often in association with chronic nasal congestion from allergic rhinitis or exposure to ambient smoke. Oral breathing can lead to secondary impairment of maxillomandibular growth during the first 4 years of age. Orthodontic data have demonstrated the impact of adenoid hypertrophy on orofacial growth in children, thus leading to alterations in maxillomandibular relationships which further contribute to the obstruction of the upper airway.

Soft Tissue of Upper Airway

Schwab and coll. have highlighted the importance of evaluating the soft tissues surrounding the upper airway, in order to understand the cause of the narrowing and collapse of the latter. Using volumetric magnetic resonance and other imaging techniques they have shown that the volume of soft tissue at the level of the upper airway is greater in subjects with OSA than in normal subjects. In particular, the greater volume of the lateral walls of the pharynx and tongue significantly increases the risk of sleep apnea. As described by Schwab, the lateral oropharyngeal structures, including the walls, are composed of the oropharyngeal muscles (ioglossus, styloglossus, stylohyoid, stylopharyngeal, palatoglossus, and palato-pharyngeal), the superior, medium, and inferior pharyngeal constrictor muscles, and the adipose tissue consisting of parapharyngeal fat pads and lymphatic tissue (adenoids, palatine and lingual tonsils).

Above all, adenotonsillar hypertrophy can contribute to the development of sleep apnea through narrowing of the lumen of the OSA, especially in children, where adenotonsillectomy is an effective and usually decisive treatment.

Finally, the presence of elevated jugular pressures associated with distension of these veins has also been proposed as a possible compression mechanism on the upper airway.

Shape of Upper Airway

The shape of the upper respiratory tract can contribute to their collapse. Studies with volumetric MRI have suggested that the upper airway in patients with OSA have an oval conformation at the pharyngeal level, with the main axis oriented antero-posteriorly, in contrast to normal subjects in which the short axis is oriented anterior-posteriorly. Leiter theorized that this orientation places the dilator muscles of the upper airway in a mechanical difficulty in maintaining their patency. Schwab and coll. based on the results obtained with volumetric MRI, they hypothesized that the narrowing and collapse of the upper airway may be due to compression by the lateral walls of the pharynx, with relative saving of the A-P diameter. This is associated with the evidence that lateral decubitus can promote the reduction of the lateral diameter of the upper airway. While, the obstruction at the retrolingual level is favored by the supine decubitus due to the retroglossoptosis favored by the action of the force of gravity and by the lower muscle tone during sleep in patients with OSA. Kim and coll. reported a higher AHI in patients with lateral-type occlusion, the cause of which is not clear, but the deposition of fat in the lateral pharyngeal walls certainly plays an important role. Cisacar and coll. confirmed these results, and also demonstrated that patients with OSAS can also have a circular type occlusion, underlining the importance of the increase in volume of the lateral pharyngeal walls in the pathogenesis of the obstruction, associating it with a hypertrophy of the parapharyngeal muscles rather than to a real deposit of fat at the parapharyngeal level. However, these results remain controversial and contrast with the conclusions of other works, which highlight the collapse of the A-P plan.

Length of Upper Airway

In addition to the size of the lumen, the shape and the influence of adjacent structures, the length of the upper airway can also affect their collapse. Often, the oropharynx is relatively long and therefore tends to have greater resistance, being more prone to collapse. Malhotra and coll. using magnetic resonance imaging, they observed that male subjects in a waking state have a greater length of the upper airway (measured from the upper edge of the hard palate to the base of the epiglottis) than female subjects. Longer airways are more collapsible, this has led Malhotra et al. to suggest that the greater length of the upper airway in men may be one of the determining factors in the predisposition to pharyngeal collapse in men.

Collapse Sites of Upper Airway

Endoscopic pressure recording and other diagnostic modalities were used to locate the sites and dynamics of upper airway collapse in OSA. These studies have shown that the level of collapse varies from individual to individual, just as in the same subject it can vary according to the phase of sleep. The retropalatal region is the most common site of collapse, followed by the retrolingual region. Through upper airway endoscopy, Morrison et al. observed in a cohort of 64 patients with OSAS that the retropalatal region was the main site of collapse in 81% of patients. In addition to retropalatal narrowing > 75% retrolingual and hypopharyngeal narrowing was observed in 38% and 22% of patients, respectively. They also highlighted secondary shrinkage sites (25 - 75% diameter reduction) present in a maximum of one third of the subjects. Some studies have shown that collapse is a dynamic process that involves more than one area of the upper respiratory tract, the sequence of the collapse of the upper airway would present a cranio-caudal extension, from the retro-lingual to the hypopharyngeal region. Further observations have shown that the reopening of the upper airway proceeds instead with a caudo-cranial sequence. Watanabe and coll. have shown that the shrinkage sites vary according to the body habitus (presence of obesity) and craniofacial anatomical anomalies. Collapse at the velopalatine level has been associated with obesity and, the association between that at the velopalatine level and that at the oropharyngeal level, has been related to craniofacial anomalies.

Conclusion

The deep knowledge of the anatomy of the upper airways, including the shape, length, characteristics of its lumen and surrounding structures is fundamental to better understand the pathophysiological processes that underlie OSA and related therapies.

REFERENCES

Bruno, A; Di Sano, C; Lorusso, F; Dino, P; Russo, D; Ballacchino, A; Gallina, S; Modica, DM; Chiappara, G; Simon, HU; Pace, E. Notch-1 decreased expression contributes to leptin receptor downregulation in nasal epithelium from allergic turbinates. *Biochim Biophys Acta Mol Basis Dis.*, 2019 Jun 1, 1865(6), 1642-1650.

Ciscar, MA; Juan, G; Martinez, V; et al. Magnetic resonance imaging of the pharynx in OSA patients and healthy subjects. *Eur Respir J*, 2001, 17, 79e86.

Ciscar, MA; Juan, G; Martinez, V; et al. Magnetic resonance imaging of the pharynx in osa patients and healthy subjects. *Eur respir j*, 2001, 17(1), 79–86.

Cistulli, PA. Craniofacial abnormalities in obstructive sleep apnoea: implications for treatment. *Respirology*, 1996, 1(3), 167–174.

Constantian, M; Clardy, R. The relative importance of septal and nasal valvular surgery in correcting airway obstruction in primary and secondary rhinoplasty. *Plast Reconstr Surg*, 1996, 98, 38–54. discussion 55–8.

Galvin, JR; Rooholamini, SA; Stanford, W. Obstructive sleep apnea: diagnosis with ultrafast CT. *Radiology*, 1989, 171(3), 775–778.

Georgakopoulos, B; Le, PH. Anatomy, Head and Neck, Nasal Concha. 2020 Aug 31. In: *StatPearls* [Internet]. Treasure Island (FL): StatPearls Publishing, 2020 Jan–. PMID: 31536243.

Gray's Anatomy. The Anatomical Basis of Clinical Practice (45th ed.)

Haponik, EF; Smith, PL; Bohlman, ME; Allen, RP; Goldman, SM; Bleecker, ER. Computerized tomography in obstructive sleep apnea. Correlation of airway size with physiology during sleep and wakefulness. *Am Rev Respir Dis*, 1983, 127(2), 221–226.

Horner, RL; Shea, SA; Mcivor, J; Guz, A. Pharyngeal size and shape during wakefulness and sleep in patients with obstructive sleep apnoea. *Q j med*, 1989, 72(268), 719–735.

Horner, RR; Mohiaddin, D; Lowell, S; et al. Sites and sizes of fat deposits around thepharynx in obese patients with obstructive sleep apnea and weight matched controls. *Eur Respir J*, 1989, 2, 613–622.

Huang, Y; White, DP; Malhotra, A. The impact of anatomic manipulations on pharyngeal collapse: results from a computational model of the normal human upper airway. *Chest*, 2005, 128(3), 1324–1330.

Hudgel, DW. Variable site of airway narrowing among obstructive sleep apnea patients. *J Appl Physiol*, 1986, 61(4), 1403–1409.

Hyo Yeol Kim, Kwon Hyo Bok, Hun-Jong Dhong, Seung-Kyu Chung. The correlation between pharyngeal narrowing and the severity of sleep-disordered breathing. Seoul, Korea. *Otolaryngology–Head and Neck Surgery*, (2008), 138, 289-293.

Isono, S; Tanaka, A; Tagaito, Y; Ishikawa, T; Nishino, T. Influences of head positions and bite opening on collapsibility of the passive pharynx. *J Appl Physiol*, 2004, 97(1), 339–346.

Jamieson, A; Guilleminault, C; Partinen, M; Quera-Salva, MA. Obstructive sleep apneic patients have craniomandibular abnormalities. *Sleep*, 1986, 9(4), 469–477.

Katsantonis, GP; Moss, K; Miyazaki, S; Walsh, J. Determining the site of airway collapse in obstructive sleep apnea with airway pressure monitoring . *Laryngoscope*, 993, 103(10), 1126–1131.

Koenig, J; Thach, B. Effects of mass loading on the upper airway. *J Appl Physiol*, 1988, 64, 2294–2299.

Kuna, S; Remmers, JE. Anatomy and physiology of upper airway obstruction. In: kryger mh, roth t, dement wc, eds. *Principles and practice of sleep medicine*, 3rd ed. Philadelphia: w.b. saunders company, 2000, 840–858.

Leiter, JC. Upper airway shape: Is it important in the pathogenesis of obstructive sleep apnea? *Am J Respir Crit Care Med*, 1996, 153(3), 894–898.

Lorusso, F; Dispenza, F; Modica, DM; Gallina, S. The Role of Modified Expansion Sphincter Pharyngoplasty in Multilevel Obstructive Sleep Apnea Syndrome Surgery. *Int Arch Otorhinolaryngol.*, 2018 Oct, 22(4), 432-436.

Lorusso, F; Dispenza, F; Saraniti, C; Sireci, F; Modica, DM; Gallina, S. Sleep disordered breathing: evaluation of dynamic patterns of the upper airways in obese subjects. *Otorinolaringologia*, 2014, 64, 57–64

Lorusso, F; Gallina, S; Modica, DM; Di Salvo, N; Riggio, F. Bipolar Quantum Molecular Resonance versus Blunt Dissection tonsillectomy. *B-ENT*, 2015, 11(02), 101–108.

Lorusso, F; Dispenza, F; Martinciglio, G; Battaglia, A; Gallina, S. Postural changes in patients undergoing hyoid surgery for OSAS. *EuroMediterranean Biomedical Journal*, 2017, 12(29), 140-143.

Lorusso, F; Martines, F; Mistretta, A; Dispenza, F; Gallina, S. Effects of adenotonsillectomy on neurocognitive and behavioural function in pediatric obstructive sleep apnea syndrome. *B-ENT*, 2018, 14, 113-118.

Malhotra, A; Huang, Y; Fogel, RB; et al. The male predisposition to pharyngeal collapse: importance of airway length. *Am j respir crit care med*, 2002, 166(10), 1388–1395.

Miles, PG; Vig, PS; Weyant, RJ; Forrest, TD; Rockette, HE. Jr. Craniofacial structure and obstructive sleep apnea syndrome a qualitative analysis and meta-analysis of the literature. *Am J Orthod Dentofacial Orthop*, 1996, 109(2), 163–172.

Modica, DM; Lorusso, F; Presti, G; Fasola, S; Gallina, S. Our Assessment Using Palate Postoperative Problems Score (PPOPS): Tool for the Evaluation of Results in Palatal Surgery Techniques. *Indian J Otolaryngol Head Neck Surg.*, 2019 Oct, 71(Suppl 1), 766-770

Modica, DM; Marchese, D; Lorusso, F; Speciale, R; Saraniti, C; Gallina, S. Functional Nasal Surgery and Use of CPAP in OSAS Patients: Our Experience. *Indian J Otolaryngol Head Neck Surg.*, 2018 Dec, 70(4), 559-565.

Morrison, DL; Launois, SH; Isono, S; Feroah, TR; Whitelaw, WA; Remmers, JE. Pharyngeal narrowing and closing pressures in patients with obstructive sleep apnea. *Am Rev Respir Dis*, 1993, 148(3), 606–611.

O'ryan, FS; Gallagher, DM; Labanc, JP; et al. The relation between nasorespiratory function and dentofacial morphology: a Review. *Am J Orthod.*, 1982, 82, 403–10.

Own, GO; Canter, RJ; Robinson A. Overnight pulse oximetry in snoring and non snoring children. *Clin Otolaryngol.*, 1995, 20, 402–6.

Redline, S. Genetics of obstructive sleep apnea. In: Kryger MH, Roth T, Dement WC, eds. *Principles and Practice of Sleep Medicine*. Philadelphia: Elsevier Saunders, 2005, 1013–1022.

Ryan, CM; Bradley, TD. Pathogenesis of obstructive sleep apnea. *J Appl Physiol*, 2005, 99 (6), 2440–2450.

Schwab, RJ; Gupta, KB; Gefter, WB; Metzger, LJ; Hoffman, EA; Pack, AI. Upper airway and soft tissue anatomy in normal subjects and patients with sleep-disordered breathing. Significance of the lateral pharyngeal walls. *Am J Respir Crit Care Med*, 1995, 152(5 Pt1), 1673–1689.

Schwab, RJ. Pro: sleep apnea is an anatomic disorder. *Am J Respir Crit Care Med*, 2003, 168(3), 270–271. discussion 273.

Schwab, RJ. Pro: sleep apnea is an anatomic disorder. *Am J Respir Crit Care Med*, 2003, 168(3), 270–271. discussion 273.

Shelton, KE; Gay, SB; Woodson, H; Surratt, PM. Pharyngeal fat in obstructive sleep apnea. *Am Rev Respir Dis*, 1993, 148, 462–466.

Shepard, JW; Jr. Pevernagie, DA; Stanson, AW; Daniels, BK; Sheedy, PF. Effects of changes in central venous pressure on upper airway size in patients with obstructive sleep apnea. *Am J Respir Crit Care Med*, 1996, 153(1), 250–254.

Shepard, JW; Jr. Thawley, SE. Evaluation of the upper airway by computerized tomography in patients undergoing uvulopalatopharyngoplasty for obstructive sleep apnea. *Am Rev Respir Dis*, 1989, 140(3), 711–716.

Shepard, JW; Jr. Thawley, SE. Localization of upper airway collapse during sleep in patients with obstructive sleep apnea. *Am Rev Respir Dis*, 1990, 141(5 Pt 1), 1350–1355.

Strohl, KP. CON: sleep apnea is not an anatomic disorder. *Am J Respir Crit Care Med*, 2003, 168(3), 271–272. discussion 272–273.

Watanabe, T; Isono, S; Tanaka, A; Tanzawa, H; Nishino, T. Contribution of body habitus and craniofacial characteristics to segmental closing pressures of the passive pharynx in patients with sleep-disordered breathing. *Am J Respir Crit Care Med*, 2002, 165(2), 260–265.

Watanabe, T; Isono, S; Tanaka, A; Tanzawa, H; Nishino, T. Contribution of body habitus and craniofacial characteristics to segmental closing pressures of the passive pharynx in patients with sleep-disordered breathing. *Am J Respir Crit Care Med*, 2002, 165(2), 260–265.

Young, T; Shahar, E; Nieto, FJ; et al. Predictors of sleep-disordered breathing in community dwelling adults: the Sleep Heart Health Study. *Arch Intern Med*, 2002, 162, 893–900.

In: Advances in Sleep Apnea
Editors: F. Lorusso et al.
ISBN: 978-1-53619-758-7

Chapter 2

PATHOPHYSIOLOGY OF OBSTRUCTIVE SLEEP APNEA (OSA)

Maria R. Bonsignore*

PROMISE Department, University of Palermo, Palermo, Italy
and Institute for Biomedical Research and Innovation (IRIB),
National Research Council (CNR), Palermo, italy

ABSTRACT

Obstructive sleep apnea (OSA) is a complex disorder characterized by total or partial collapse of the upper airways (UA) during sleep, causing obstructive apneas or hypopneas, respectively. During respiratory events, respiratory efforts occur against the restricted or collapsed upper airway, hypoxia and hypercapnia develop, and sympathetic activation increases. The main symptoms of OSA are intermittent snoring and excessive daytime sleepiness. OSA is often associated with obesity, hypertension, and increased cardiovascular risk. Pathophysiological aspects include: anatomical and physiological determinants of UA closure, and immediate and long-term consequences of chronic intermittent hypoxia (CIH), which is believed to be the most relevant alteration induced by OSA. This

* Corresponding Author's Email: mariarosaria.bonsignore@unipa.it.

chapter will briefly review OSA pathophysiology, with special attention to physiological phenotypes of OSA, and the role of intermittent hypoxia in the pathogenesis of cardiometabolic abnormalities.

INTRODUCTION

Obstructive sleep apnea (OSA) is frequent in the general population, and its prevalence is higher in men and increases with age and body mass index (BMI) (Senaratna et al. 2016). Almost a billion of people are estimated to be affected by OSA worldwide, and about half of them with moderate-severe OSA would require treatment (Benjafield et al. 2019).

Upper airway (UA) collapse during sleep, and subsequent partial or complete closure of the airways, is associated with respiratory efforts and changes in intrathoracic pressure and progressive hypoxemia and hypercapnia. Respiratory events often terminate with an arousal, causing sleep fragmentation. Sympathetic activation occurs during apnea, and causes hypertensive blood pressure peaks during the ventilation period. OSA patients are prone to develop cardiovascular complications, also secondary to several intermediate pathophysiological mechanisms activated in OSA (Levy et al. 2015).

OSA is a complex disorder, characterized by variability of respiratory events, for example according to sleep stage or body position. The usual metric to define OSA severity is the apnea-hypopnea index, i.e., the mean number of events/hour of sleep, derived from full polysomnography. OSA is defined as AHI>5/h, with mild, moderate, and severe OSA being defined as AHI 5-<15/h, 15-<30/h, and >30/h, respectively. This definition has been criticized because it poorly reflects the impact of OSA on clinical symptoms or outcomes (Pevernagie et al. 2020). Additional markers of OSA severity commonly used in clinical practice include oxygen saturation (SpO2) variables, such as lowest SpO2 or time spent at SpO2 < 90%. More recently, the hypoxic burden has been proposed, which takes into account the degree and the duration of SpO2 falls during sleep, and could predict cardiovascular mortality (Azarbarzin et al. 2019) or incident heart failure (Azarbarzin et al. 2020).

The most common treatment modality of OSA is the application of continuous positive airway pressure (CPAP) during sleep (Sullivan, 2018). Although highly effective, this treatment is often refused, especially by patients with no or minor symptoms. Good adherence is defined as use of CPAP for at least 4 h/night during 70% of the nights, or more. Intense research is ongoing to define clinical phenotypes of OSA which may be treated with measures alternative to CPAP, including drugs, positional treatment or surgery. In this context, pathophysiological studies have regained interest, in order to identify personalized treatment approaches.

This chapter will briefly review OSA pathophysiology, with special attention to the recently described physiological phenotypes of OSA, and the role of intermittent hypoxia in the pathogenesis of cardiometabolic abnormalities.

PHYSIOLOGICAL PHENOTYPES OF OSA

The upper airway behaves like a collapsible tube, i.e., a Starling resistor (Gold and Schwartz, 1996). In such a model, the collapsible airway is inside a rigid box with a constant pressure (P_{out}), and no flow can occur if P_{out} is higher than intraluminal pressure. Conversely, when intraluminal pressure is higher than P_{out}, flow depends on the pressure and resistance inside the lumen. In the intermediate situation, pressure upstream of the collapsible segment is higher than P_{out}, while pressure downstream is lower, generating intermittent flow and snoring (Gold and Schwartz, 1996).

The concept of critical closing pressure, or P_{crit}, corresponding to the P_{out} of the model, has been very useful to conduct clinical research on human OSA patients, in order to assess which factors determine or contribute to increased UA collapsibility. Mean P_{crit} in normal subjects is on average -14 cmH_2O, meaning that a very negative pressure must be applied to obtain collapse of UA under normal circumstances. Conversely, P_{crit} is supra-atmospheric (2-3 cmH_2O) in severe OSA patients, with intermediate values found in snorers (-6 cmH_2O)

(Schwartz et al. 1994). Treatment with CPAP normalizes airflow by increasing intraluminal airway pressure and preventing UA collapse (Gold and Schwartz, 1996). However, therapeutic pressure has to be determined in each patient, given the variability of P_{crit}.

P_{crit} is influenced by age, obesity and sex. Aging increases passive UA collapsibility (Kirkness et al. 2008). Women show a lower P_{crit}, and their UA are less affected by obesity, than men (Kirkness et al. 2008), possibly because of peripheral distribution of adipose tissue in women. OSA in women is generally less severe than in men (Bonsignore et al. 2019).

Several factors can modify P_{crit}, and different physiological phenotypes of OSA have been described (Eckert 2018). This approach is important in clinical practice since it may guide treatment by addressing one or more of the mechanisms responsible for UA collapse, especially in consideration of the poor adherence to CPAP treatment in a significant proportion of patients. The primary cause of OSA remains "impaired anatomy" but in about 20% of OSA patients "non-anatomical factors" occur in the absence of a narrow collapsible airway (Eckert, 2018). Such factors include: impaired function of UA dilator muscles, a low respiratory arousal threshold, and respiratory control instability.

Impaired UA anatomy in OSA is very common. The main cause is represented by obesity, with deposition of fat around the airways and in the tongue (Wang et al. 2020), increased UA length (Malhotra et al. 2002), or craniofacial abnormalities. In children, adenotonsillar hypertrophy is the major cause of OSA (McGinley et al. 2016).

The activity of UA dilator muscles during sleep is relevant, because it reduces upper airway collapsibility and counteracts airway closure. UA dilator muscle activity decreases during sleep due to reduced neural drive, especially in REM sleep. Airway collapse is especially common in the supine position, when functional residual capacity of the lungs physiologically decreases, and the UA becomes less stable due to a low level of traction exerted by the lungs. Subjects with higher active responses of UA dilator muscles may not develop respiratory events during NREM sleep because of their compensatory capability. However in REM sleep respiratory events may occur, due to the absent muscle tone typical of this sleep phase. Women show more active UA responses than men (Kirkness et al. 2008), and the prevalence of isolated REM OSA is more common in women (O'Connor et al. 2000). Conversely, insufficient UA muscle responsiveness or effectiveness will reinforce the UA collapse promoted by anatomical factors. The issue of the UA dilator muscles during sleep is further complicated by the type of their activity, for example the genioglossus muscle shows both tonic and phasic activity, whereas the tensor palatini muscle mainly shows tonic activity during sleep. The interested reader is referred to comprehensive reviews on this topic (Horner, 2012; Eckert, 2018).

Respiratory events are often terminated with arousals, causing sleep fragmentation. Arousal are short periods in which wakefulness is re-established, usually without a full awakening of the subject. The interplay between respiratory drive, arousals and OSA is highly complex, and arousal threshold appears as a distinct pathophysiological trait in OSA (Amatoury et al. 2016). Arousal intensity may also vary, and higher arousal intensity causes greater ventilatory responses. Arousal intensity does not appear to correlate with the magnitude of the preceding respiratory stimuli. More intense arousals were positively associated with arousal duration, time to arousal, rate of change in epiglottic pressure, and negatively associated with BMI (Amatoury et al. 2016). Negative effects of a low arousal threshold include prevention of UA dilator muscle activation, decreased amount of deep sleep, and the increase in ventilation which can be followed by a period of decreased respiratory drive (Eckert, 2018).

Finally, respiratory control instability is recognized as a factor contributing to the perpetuation of respiratory events during sleep. Since chemical control of ventilation is active in non-REM sleep, hyperventilation following apneas or hypopneas may decrease $PaCO_2$ level below the apneic threshold, thus favoring the establishment of the subsequent cycle. A high "loop gain" occurs when the ventilatory response is larger than the disturbance causing it. About 35% of OSA patients show increased loop gain and post-apneic hyperventilation (Eckert et al. 2013).

To better describe the different physiological traits in OSA patients, the PALM scale has been proposed to define the physiological phenotype, accounting for the following factors:

- Pcrit (P) as a marker of anatomical abnormalities
- Arousal threshold (A)
- Loop gain (L)
- Muscle responsiveness (M)

The PALM scale includes 3 levels (Eckert, 2018):

- PALM scale 1, defined as severe anatomical impairment (Pcrit > +2 cmH2O), affecting 23% of patients;
- PALM scale 2, defined as moderate anatomical impairment: (Pcrit -2 to +2 cmH2O), affecting 58% of patients;
- PALM scale 3, defined as minor anatomical impairment (Pcrit <-2 cmH2O), affecting 19% of patients, with all of them presenting functional abnormalities.

Over 60% of patients classified as PALM 1 or PALM 2 also show some functional abnormality, underlying the complexity of UA abnormalities in OSA (Eckert, 2018).

The advantage of this classification is that while OSA patients with significant anatomical abnormalities are good candidates to CPAP or mandibular advancement devices (MAD), other patients with predominant "functional" abnormalities can be managed differently, i.e., with pharmacological treatment or other therapeutic approaches addressing specific problems, such as hypoglossal nerve stimulation to improve UA muscle function, hypnotics to increase arousal threshold, or O_2 to blunt high loop gain (Eckert, 2018). The current disadvantage is that identification of physiological phenotypes requires full polysomnography, limiting its practical applicability. However, ongoing research aims at assessing the usefulness of simplified methods to be applicable in clinical practice, especially when cardiorespiratory polygraphy is used for diagnosis. Nevertheless, the concepts at the basis of the PALM have already gained the clinical arena, especially in consideration of the poor performance of AHI for prognosis or prediction of CPAP adherence (Pevernagie et al. 2020), even though evidence from large samples is not yet available.

Intermittent Hypoxia in the Pathogenesis of Cardiometabolic Abnormalities

The high prevalence of cardiovascular and metabolic comorbidities in OSA patients has been investigated in the last 20 years by using animal models (Farré et al. 2008) and in clinical studies (Bonsignore et al. 2019). Many observational studies indicate that OSA increases cardiovascular mortality (Fu et al. 2017), and a bidirectional relationship may occur between OSA and diabetes (Aurora and Punjabi, 2013). The frequent occurrence of obesity in OSA patients complicates the assessment of the independent role of OSA; on the other hand, it indicates that the increased cardiometabolic risk in OSA is likely multifactorial.

Studies on the effects of chronic intermittent hypoxia (CIH) during sleep in rodent models have been important to define intermediate mechanisms associated with increased cardiometabolic risk, in the presence or absence of obesity (Drager et al. 2015). However, they show some limitations, since CIH does not reproduce all aspects of human OSA: for example, CIH stimulates ventilation and hypocapnia, and no respiratory efforts occur during CIH.

At the cardiovascular level, CIH evokes activation of the sympathetic nervous system, endothelial cell dysfunction, and inflammation (Ryan et al. 2005, Drager et al. 2015), and may contribute to the pathogenesis of atherosclerosis (Song et al. 2012). CIH is a major factor in the pathogenesis of blood pressure elevation in OSA models during sleep (Drager et al. 2015), and may contribute to daytime hypertension in OSA patients (Tkacova et al. 2014).

CIH causes dysfunction of the carotid body, the main sensor of oxygen, which in turn causes prolonged activation of ventilatory and pressor responses to hypoxia, known as long-term facilitation (Peng et al, 2003) and sympathetic hyperactivity (Mansukhani et al. 2014; Prabakhar and Semenza, 2016). Obesity is also known to be associated with sympathetic activation (Grassi et al. 2019).

The high sympathetic activation state induced by CIH may explain why reversal of autonomic disturbance in OSA requires prolonged CPAP treatment (Waradekar 1996). Conversely, acute or short-term

CPAP exerts minor effects on systemic blood pressure, while its effects on nocturnal blood pressure variability become evident within a shorter time course because hypertensive peaks caused by apneas do not occur during CPAP (Marrone and Bonsignore, 2018). However, prevention of OSA is not sufficient to normalize blood pressure in hypertensive patients, and CPAP treatment decreases blood pressure by only a few mmHg (Green et al., 2020). This finding can be explained by several factors, including the multiple pathogenetic factors involved in systemic hypertension, and the possible detrimental effects of chronic hypertension on vascular remodeling. Nevertheless, in patients with hypertension resistant or refractory to treatment, i.e., not normalized by treatment with at least three or five anti-hypertensive drugs respectively, OSA could contribute to the poor control of blood pressure, and in such cases CPAP treatment is associated with significant decrease in blood pressure (Oscullo et al. 2019). OSA is also a major cause of masked hypertension, with high blood pressure values recorded during the night or at awakening, and normal values during wakefulness (Baguet et al. 2008). Ambulatory blood pressure monitoring is indicated in OSA patients to evaluate the impact of OSA on the cardiovascular system, and a rise in nocturnal blood pressure is a major contributor to high cardiovascular risk (Kario et al. 2020).

CIH also affects metabolism, especially in the adipose tissue. Although the effects of CIH are clinically difficult to assess in the presence of obesity, as it commonly occurs in OSA patients, several animal studies have shown that CIH worsens insulin resistance and adipose tissue inflammation (Bonsignore et al. 2012a, Ryan et al. 2019). OSA is commonly associated with visceral obesity, evaluated clinically as the occurrence of the metabolic syndrome, i.e., a cluster of cardiometabolic risk factors including waist circumference, triglyceride and HDL-cholesterol levels, blood pressure and fasting blood glycemia (Bonsignore et al. 2012b). As such, OSA could favor the development of type 2 diabetes. Indeed, not only OSA but sleep disturbances in general could be considered as risk factors for incident type 2 diabetes (Anothaisintawee et al. 2016). Altered glucose metabolism during CIH occurs in non-diabetic OSA patients and shows a dose-response relationship with OSA severity (Michalek-Zrabkowska et al., 2021), whereas the contribution of OSA in diabetic patients is still controversial since CPAP treatment at best slightly improves glycemic control (Shan et al., 2021). Interestingly, experimental studies suggest that changes in intestinal microbiome during CIH may be involved in the pathogenesis of both hypertension (Durgan et al., 2016; Ganesh et al., 2018) and insulin resistance (Badran et al., 2020; Khalyfa et al., 2021) in OSA. CIH is also a major factor with regard to prevalence of kidney dysfunction at baseline (Marrone et al., 2016), and its progression during follow-up, which appear blunted bt CPAP treatment (Marrone et al., 2018). Finally, incidence of cancer in OSA patients may be promoted by intermittent hypoxia, as underlined by recent studies (Marrone and Bonsignore 2020).

Conclusion

Figure 1 summarizes the current state of knowledge regarding OSA pathophysiology, which is highly complex, encompassing anatomical and functional aspects of upper airways and increasingly recognized effects of OSA on cardio-metabolic derangements. Chronic intermittent hypoxia is the single factor best explored in OSA pathophysiology, but the less studied role of sleep fragmentation is likely important as well, especially as cardiovascular risk, sympathetic activation and cognitive derangement are concerned. This chapter summarized our current understanding of the main aspects of OSA pathophysiology, but more work to better define the emerging clinical phenotypes of the disease is still necessary (Bonsignore et al., 2017; Randerath et al., 2018). A major limitation of the current literature is the definition of OSA severity based on the frequency of respiratory events, which poses several problems due to its lack of relationship with OSA symptoms and outcomes (Pevernagie 2020). The degree of hypoxemia induced by OSA could be a good alternative, but no conclusion can be drawn yet since research is ongoing.

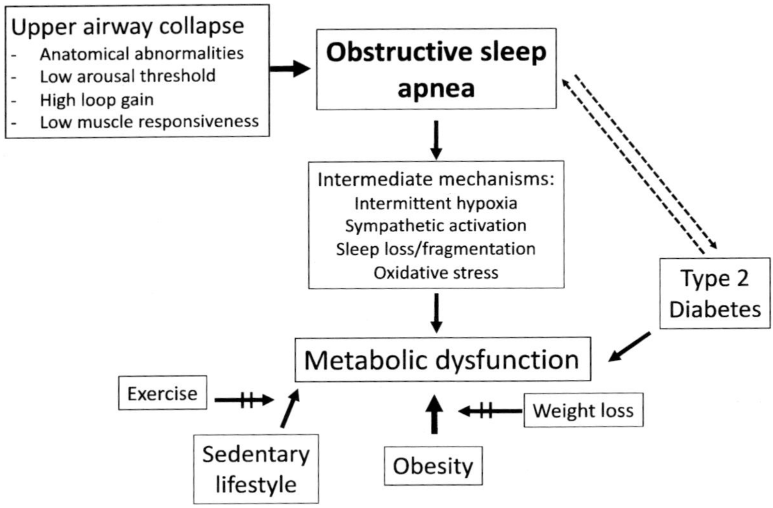

Figure 1. Summary of the different pathophysiological factors in obstructive sleep apnea (OSA). Dashed lines indicate the bidirectional relationship between OSA and diabetes. Interruped arrows indicate inhibitory effects.

REFERENCES

Amatoury, J., Azarbarzin, A., Younes, M., Jordan, A. S., Wellman, A. & Eckert, D. J. (2016). Arousal intensity is a distinct pathophysiological trait in obstructive sleep apnea. *Sleep*, 39(12), 2091–2100.

Anothaisintawee, T., Reutrakul, S., Van Cauter, E. & Thakkinstian, A. (2016). Sleep disturbances compared to traditional risk factors for diabetes development: Systematic review and meta-analysis. *Sleep Med Rev*, 30, 11-24.

Aurora, R. N. & Punjabi, N. M. (2013). Obstructive sleep apnoea and type 2 diabetes mellitus: a bidirectional association. *Lancet Respir Med*, 1(4), 329-338.

Azarbarzin, A., Sands, S. A., Stone, K. L., Taranto-Montemurro, L., Messineo, L., Terrill, P. I., Ancoli-Israel, S., Ensrud, K., Purcell, S., White, D. P., Redline, S. & Wellman, A. (2019). The hypoxic burden of sleep apnoea predicts cardiovascular disease-related mortality:

the Osteoporotic Fractures in Men Study and the Sleep Heart Health Study. *Eur Heart J*, 40(14), 1149-1157.

Azarbarzin, A., Sands, S. A., Taranto-Montemurro, L., Vena, D., Sofer, T., Kim, S. W., Stone, K. L., White, D. P., Wellman, A. & Redline, S. (2020). The sleep apnea-specific hypoxic burden predicts incident heart failure. *Chest*, 158(2), 739-750.

Badran, M., Mashaqi, S. & Gozal, D. (2020). The gut microbiome as a target for adjuvant therapy in obstructive sleep apnea. *Expert Opin Ther Targets*, 24(12), 1263-1282.

Baguet, J. P., Lévy, P., Barone-Rochette, G., Tamisier, R., Pierre, H., Peeters, M., Mallion, J. M. & Pépin, J. L. (2008). Masked hypertension in obstructive sleep apnea syndrome. *J Hypertens*, 26, 885-892.

Benjafield, A. V., Ayas, N. T., Eastwood, P. R., Heinzer, R., Ip, M. S. M., Morrell, M. J., Nunez, C. M., Patel, S. R., Penzel, T., Pépin, J. L., Peppard, P. E., Sinha, S., Tufik, S., Valentine, K. & Malhotra, A. (2019). Estimation of the global prevalence and burden of obstructive sleep apnoea: a literature-based analysis. *Lancet Respir Med*, 7(8), 687-698.

Bonsignore, M. R., McNicholas, W. T., Montserrat, J. M. & Eckel, J. (2012a). The adipose tissue in obesity and obstructive sleep apnea. *Eur Respir J*, 39, 746-767.

Bonsignore, M. R., Esquinas, C., Barcelo´, A., Sanchez-de-la-Torre, M., Paterno´, A., Duran-Cantolla, J., Marin, J. M. & Barbé, F. (2012b). Metabolic syndrome, insulin resistance and sleepiness in real-life obstructive sleep apnoea. *Eur Respir J*, 39, 1136–1143.

Bonsignore, M. R., Suarez Giron, M. C., Marrone, O., Castrogiovanni, A. & Montserrat, J. M. (2017). Personalised medicine in sleep respiratory disorders: focus on obstructive sleep apnoea diagnosis and treatment. *Eur Respir Rev*, 26(146), 170069.

Bonsignore, M. R., Saaresranta, T. & Riha, R. L. (2019). Sex differences in obstructive sleep apnoea. *Eur Respir Rev*, 28(154), 190030.

Bonsignore, M. R., Baiamonte, P., Mazzuca, E., Castrogiovanni, A. & Marrone, O. (2019). Obstructive sleep apnea and comorbidities: a dangerous liaison. *Multidiscip Respir Med*, 14, 8. doi: 10.1186/s40248-019-0172-9.

Drager, L. F., Polotsky, V. Y., O'Donnell, C. P., Cravo, S. L., Lorenzi-Filho, G. & Machado, B. H. (2015). Translational approaches to understanding metabolic dysfunction and cardiovascular consequences of obstructive sleep apnea. *Am J Physiol Heart Circ Physiol*, 309(7), H1101-H1111.

Durgan, D. J., Ganesh, B. P., Cope, J. L., Ajami, N. J., Phillips, S. C., Petrosino, J. F., Hollister, E. B. & Bryan, R. M. Jr. (2016). Role of the gut microbiome in obstructive sleep apnea-Induced hypertension. *Hypertension*, 67(2), 469-474.

Eckert, D. J., White, D. P., Jordan, A. S., Malhotra, A. & Wellman, A. (2013). Defining phenotypic causes of obstructive sleep apnea. Identification of novel therapeutic targets. *Am J Respir Crit Care Med*, 188, 996e1004.

Eckert, D. J. (2018). Phenotypic approaches to obstructive sleep apnoea - New pathways for targeted therapy. *Sleep Med Rev*, 2018, 37, 45-59.

Farré, R., Montserrat, J. M. & Navajas, D. (2008). Morbidity due to obstructive sleep apnea: insights from animal models. *Curr Opin Pulm Med*, 14, 530–536.

Fu, Y., Xia, Y., Yi, H., Xu, H., Guan, J. & Yin, S. (2017). Meta-analysis of all-cause and cardiovascular mortality in obstructive sleep apnea with or without continuous positive airway pressure treatment. *Sleep Breath*, 21(1), 181-189.

Ganesh, B. P., Nelson, J. W., Eskew, J. R., Ganesan, A., Ajami, N. J., Petrosino, J. F., Bryan, R. M. Jr. & Durgan, D. J. (2018). Prebiotics, probiotics, and acetate supplementation prevent hypertension in a model of obstructive sleep apnea. *Hypertension*, 72(5), 1141-1150.

Gold, A. R. & Schwartz, A. R. (1996). The pharyngeal critical pressure. The whys and hows of using nasal continuous positive airway pressure diagnostically. *Chest*, 110(4), 1077-1088.

Green, M., Ken-Dror, G., Fluck, D., Sada, C., Sharma, P., Fry, C. H. & Han, T. S. (2020). Meta-analysis of changes in the levels of catecholamines and blood pressure with continuous positive airway pressure therapy in obstructive sleep apnea. *J Clin Hypertens*, 2020, Sep 24. doi: 10.1111/jch.14061. Epub ahead of print.

Grassi, G., Biffi, A., Seravalle, G., Trevano, F. Q., Dell'Oro, R., Corrao, G. & Mancia, G. (2019). Sympathetic neural overdrive in the obese and overweight state. *Hypertension*, 74(2), 349-358.

Horner, R. L. (2012). Neural control of the upper airway: integrative physiological mechanisms and relevance for sleep disordered breathing. *Compr Physiol*, 2(1), 479-535.

Kario, K., Hoshide, S., Mizuno, H., Kabutoya, T., Nishizawa, M., Yoshida, T., Abe, H., Katsuya, T., Fujita, Y., Okazaki, O., Yano, Y., Tomitani, N., Kanegae, H. & JAMP Study Group. (2020). Nighttime blood pressure phenotype and cardiovascular prognosis: practitioner-based nationwide JAMP Study. *Circulation*, 142(19), 1810-1820.

Khalyfa, A., Ericsson, A., Qiao, Z.. Almendros, I., Farré, R. & Gozal, D. (2021). Circulating exosomes and gut microbiome induced insulin resistance in mice exposed to intermittent hypoxia: Effects of physical activity. *EBioMedicine*, e-pub ahead of print, doi: 10.1016/ j.ebiom.2021.103208.

Kirkness, J. P., Schwartz, A. R., Schneider, H., Punjabi, N. M., Maly, J. J., Laffan, A. M., McGinley, B. M., Magnuson, T., Schweitzer, M., Smith, P. L. & Patil, S. P. (2008). Contribution of male sex, age, and obesity to mechanical instability of the upper airway during sleep. *J Appl Physiol*, 104, 1618–1624.

Lévy, P., Kohler, M., McNicholas, W. T., Barbé, F., McEvoy, R. D., Somers, V. K., Lavie, L. & Pépin, J. L. (2015). Obstructive sleep apnoea syndrome. *Nat Rev Dis Primers*, 1, 15015.

Lorusso, F., Dispenza, F., Saraniti, C., Sireci, F., Modica, D. M. & Gallina, S. (2014). Sleep disordered breathing: evaluation of dynamic patterns of the upper airways in obese subjects. *Otorinolaringologia*, 64, 57–64

Malhotra, A., Huang, Y., Fogel, R. B., Pillar, G., Edwards, J. K., Kikinis, R., Loring, S. H. & White, D. P. (2002). The male predisposition to pharyngeal collapse: importance of airway length. *Am J Respir Crit Care Med*, 166(10), 1388-1395.

Mansukhani, M. P., Kara, T., Caples, S. M. & Somers, V. K. (2014). Chemoreflexes, sleep apnea, and sympathetic dysregulation. *Curr Hypertens Rep*, 16, 476.

Marrone, O., Battaglia, S., Steiropoulos, P., Basoglu, O. K., Kvamme, J. A., Ryan, S., Pepin, J. L., Verbraecken, J., Grote, L., Hedner, J., Bonsignore, M. R. & ESADA study group. (2016). Chronic kidney disease in European patients with obstructive sleep apnea: the ESADA cohort study. *J Sleep Res*, 25(6), 739-745.

Marrone, O., Cibella, F., Pépin, J. L., Grote, L., Verbraecken, J., Saaresranta, T., Kvamme, J. A., Basoglu, O. K., Lombardi, C., McNicholas, W. T., Hedner, J., Bonsignore, M. R. & ESADA Network. (2018). Fixed but not autoadjusting positive airway pressure attenuates the time-dependent decline in glomerular filtration rate in patients with OSA. *Chest*, 154(2), 326-334.

Marrone, O. & Bonsignore, M. R. (2018). Blood-pressure variability in patients with obstructive sleep apnea: current perspectives. *Nat Sci Sleep*, 10, 229-242.

Marrone, O. & Bonsignore, M. R. (2020). Obstructive sleep apnea and cancer: a complex relationship. *Curr Opin Pulm Med*, 26(6), 657-667.

McGinley, B. M., Kirkness, J. P., Schneider, H., Lenka, A., Smith, P. L. & Schwartz, A. R. (2016). Utilizing inspiratory airflows during standard polysomnography to assess pharyngeal function in children during sleep. *Pediatr Pulmonol*, 51(4), 431-438.

Michalek-Zrabkowska, M., Macek, P., Martynowicz, H., Gac, P., Mazur, G., Grzeda, M. & Poreba, R. (2021). Obstructive sleep apnea as a risk factor of insulin resistance in nondiabetic adults. *Life*, 11, 50. doi: 10.3390/life11010050

Modica, D. M., Marchese, D., Lorusso, F., Speciale, R., Saraniti, C. & Gallina, S. Functional Nasal Surgery and Use of CPAP in OSAS Patients: Our Experience. *Indian J Otolaryngol Head Neck Surg.*, 2018 Dec, 70(4), 559-565.

O'Connor, C., Thornley, K. S. & Hanly, P. J. (2000). Gender differences in the polysomnographic features of obstructive sleep apnea. *Am J Respir Crit Care Med*, 161(5), 1465-1472.

Oscullo, G., Torres, G., Campos-Rodriguez, F., Posadas, T., Reina-González, A., Sapiña-Beltrán, E., Barbé, F. & Martinez-Garcia, M. A. (2019). Resistant/refractory hypertension and sleep apnoea: current knowledge and future challenges. *J Clin Med*, 8(11), 1872.

Peng, Y. J., Overholt, J. L., Kline, D., Kumar, G. K. & Prabhakar, N. R. (2003). Induction of sensory long-term facilitation in the carotid body by intermittent hypoxia: Implications for recurrent apneas. *Proc Natl Acad Sci*, 100, 10073-10078.

Pevernagie, D. A., Gnidovec-Strazisar, B., Grote, L., Heinzer, R., McNicholas, W. T., Penzel, T., Randerath, W., Schiza, S., Verbraecken, J. & Arnardottir, E. S. (2020). On the rise and fall of the apnea-hypopnea index: A historical review and critical appraisal. *J Sleep Res*, 29(4), e13066.

Prabakhar, N. R. & Semenza, G. L. (2016). Regulation of carotid body oxygen sensing by hypoxia-inducible factors. *Pflugers Arch - Eur J Physiol*, 468, 71-75.

Randerath, W., Bassetti, C. L., Bonsignore, M. R., Farre, R., Ferini-Strambi, L., Grote, L., Hedner, J., Kohler, M., Martinez-Garcia, M. A., Mihaicuta, S., Montserrat, J., Pepin, J. L., Pevernagie, D., Pizza, F., Polo, O., Riha, R., Ryan, S., Verbraecken, J. & McNicholas, W. T. (2018). Challenges and perspectives in obstructive sleep apnoea: Report by an *ad hoc* working group of the Sleep Disordered Breathing Group of the European Respiratory Society and the European Sleep Research Society. *Eur Respir J*, 52(3), 1702616.

Ryan, S., Taylor, C. T. & McNicholas, W. T. (2005). Selective activation of inflammatory pathways by intermittent hypoxia in obstructive sleep apnea syndrome. *Circulation*, 112(17), 2660-2667.

Ryan, S., Cummins, E. P., Farré, R., Gileles-Hillel, A., Jun, J. C., Oster, H., Pepin, J. L., Ray, D. W., Reutrakul, S., Sanchez-de-la-Torre, M., Tamisier, R. & Almendros, I. (2020). Understanding the pathophysiological mechanisms of cardiometabolic complications in obstructive sleep apnoea: towards personalised treatment approaches. *Eur Respir J*, 56, 1902295.

Schwartz, A. R., Smith, P. L., Kashima, H. K., et al. (1994). Respiratory function of the upper airways. In: Murray JF, Nadel JA, eds. *Textbook of Respiratory Medicine*. 2nd ed. Philadelphia: WB Saunders, 1451-1470.

Senaratna, C. V., Perret J. L., Lodge, C. J., Lowe, A. J., Campbell, B. E., Matheson, M. C., Hamilton, G. S. & Dharmage, S. C. (2017).

Prevalence of obstructive sleep apnea in the general population: A systematic review. *Sleep Med Rev*, 34, 70-81.

Shang, W., Zhang, Y., Wang, G. & Han, D. (2021). Benefits of continuous positive airway pressure on glycaemic control and insulin resistance in patients with type 2 diabetes and obstructive sleep apnoea: A meta-analysis. *Diabetes Obes Metab*, 23(2), 540-548.

Song, D., Fang, G., Mao, S. Z., Ye, X., Liu, G., Gong, Y. & Liu, S. F. (2012). Chronic intermittent hypoxia induces atherosclerosis by NF-κB-dependent mechanisms. *Biochim Biophys Acta*, 1822(11), 1650-1659.

Sullivan, C. E. Nasal positive airway pressure and sleep apnea. (2018). Reflections on an experimental method that became a therapy. *Am J Respir Crit Care Med*, 198, 581-587.

Tkacova, R., McNicholas, W. T., Javorsky, M., Fietze, I., Sliwinski, P., Parati, G., Grote, L., Hedner, J. & European Sleep Apnoea Database study collaborators. (2014). Nocturnal intermittent hypoxia predicts prevalent hypertension in the European Sleep Apnoea Database cohort study. *Eur Respir J*, 44(4), 931-941.

Wang, S. H., Keenan, B. T., Wiemken, A., Zang, Y., Staley, B., Sarwer, D. B., Torigian, D. A., Williams, N., Pack, A. I. & Schwab, R. J. (2020). Effect of weight loss on upper airway anatomy and the apnea-hypopnea index. The importance of tongue fat. *Am J Respir Crit Care Med.*, 201(6), 718-727.

Waradekar, N. V., Sinoway, L. I., Zwillich, C. W. & Leuenberger, U. A. (1996). Influence of treatment on muscle sympathetic nerve activity in sleep apnea. *Am J Respir Crit Care Med*, 153, 1333-1338.

In: Advances in Sleep Apnea
Editors: F. Lorusso et al.
ISBN: 978-1-53619-758-7

Chapter 3

ADVANCES IN ADULTS OSAS DIAGNOSIS

Donatella Marchese*, Salvatore Gallina and Francesco Lorusso

Department of Otolaryngology, Head and Neck Surgery,
Policlinico Paolo Giaccone University of Palermo, Palermo, Italy

ABSTRACT

Obstructive sleep apnea syndrome (OSAS) is a chronic systemic illness, characterized by recurrent episodes of cessation (apnea) and reduction (hypopnea) of oronasal airflow during sleep and excessive daytime sleepiness. The major risk factor is represented by obesity: about 70% of those with OSA are obese and, at the same time, the prevalence of OSA in obese adults is about 40%.

The first guidelines for the diagnosis of OSAS were elaborated by American Academy of Sleep Medicine in 2005 and it defines the nocturnal polysomnography as the gold standard; but it is a time-consuming and costly procedure and moreover it requires the expertise of sleep medicine specialists. Hence new studies have been employed such as specific questionnaires and different instruments like sleep endoscopy and radiologic ones. The

---

* Corresponding Author's Email: marchesedonatella@hotmail.com.

alternative exams proposed have been demonstrated a lot of limits in order to make diagnosis of OSAS and they can be used only upon completion of a correct diagnosis.

INTRODUCTION/DEFINITION

Obstructive sleep apnea syndrome (OSAS) is a highly sleep-related breathing disorder characterized by recurrent episodes of cessation (apnea) and reduction (hypopnea) of oronasal airflow during sleep and excessive daytime sleepiness. This breathing disorder is a result of abnormal anatomy superimposed on physiological or excessive reduction of muscle tone during sleep.

The history of sleep disorders and its identification started with Burwell, Robin, Waley and Bickelmann (1956), rather of the Pickwickian Syndrome, in homage to the English writer Charles Dickens, which described an obese, sleepy and snoring boy. During the 60's, when polysomnography (PSG) became available, European authors started to investigate the Pickwickian syndrome as a sleep respiratory disorder.

We have to thanks to Guilleminault in Italy in 1972 for the terminology: Obstructive Sleep Apnea Syndrome. He described a clinical illness characterized by excessive day-time sleepiness and apnea episodes detected by PSG.

The signs, symptoms and consequences of OSA are a direct result of the derangements that occur due to repetitive collapse of the upper airway: sleep fragmentation, hypoxemia, hypercapnia, marked swings in intrathoracic pressure, and increased sympathetic activity.

OSAS is still an underdiagnosed chronic illness and it represents an independent risk factor for cardiovascular, metabolic, neurological diseases, and motor vehicle accidents. This risk can be reduced with effective treatment. Therefore, the diagnosis and effective treatment of OSA in adults is an urgent health priority.

The first guidelines for the diagnosis of OSAS were elaborated by American Academy of Sleep Medicine (AASM): "Practice Parameters for the Indications for Polysomnography and Related Procedures: An

Update for 2005" the first and "Clinical Guidelines for the Use of Unattended Portable Monitors in the Diagnosis of Obstructive Sleep Apnea in Adult Patients (2007)" later.

Concerning the definition of apnea, the American Academy of Sleep Medicine (AASM) states that it corresponds to a cessation in airflow lasting at least 10 sec. instead of hypopnea is defined as a recognizable transient reduction (but not complete cessation) of breathing for at least10 sec. 46, heach events can occur during sleep, many times per hour.

Concerning hypopnea definition, the literature's data show large differences: a hypopnea event is only considered to be clinically significant if there is a 30% or more reduction in flow with a 3% oxygen desaturation or a cortical arousal, alternatively an association with a 4% oxygen desaturation without consideration of cortical arousals.25–27, that introduces complexity in the evaluation of evidence regarding the diagnosis of OSA.

The Apnea-Hypopnea Index (AHI) is an index used to assess the severity of sleep apnea based on the total number of apneas and hypopneas occurring per hour of sleep. A diagnosis of OSA syndrome (OSAS) is established when a patient has an apnea–hypopnea index (AHI; number of apneas and hypopneas per hour of sleep) >5 and associated symptoms (e.g., excessive daytime sleepiness, fatigue or impaired cognition) or an AHI ≥ 15 regardless of associated symptoms. The AHI index is also employed to stratify the population where normal is AHI <5, mild OSA defined as an AHI of 5–14, moderate as 15–29 and severe as ≥30.

To better define the complexity of this syndrome we have to introduce another respiratory event that cause sleep disruption, but not correspond to a narrow definition of apnea or hypopnea: respiratory event related arousals (RERAs). These events are measured in the Respiratory Disturbance Index (RDI), including apneas and hypopneas. Some research studies have found that 30% of symptomatic patients would have been left untreated if the AHI were used rather the RDI.

DIAGNOSIS

The guidelines elaborated by AIPO (Italian Association of Hospital Pneumologist) in association with AIMS (Italian Association of sleep medicine) in 2011 predicted a modulation in OSAS diagnosis based on clinical presentation. The same idea has been elaborated in the American Academy of Sleep Medicine (AASM) guidelines. The modulation of the employed instruments is function of the AHI value. Indeed in case of AHI≥15 no more clinical evaluation is necessary. The presence of symptoms and signs are essentials in case of 5≥AHI≤15.

Obstructive Sleep Apnea Syndrome (OSAS) is the most frequent sleep breathing disorder in the general population. To reach a correct diagnosis, the clinical work-up requires the association of comprehensive clinical evaluation throughout anamnesis, rating of risk factors and physical examination, as well as a nocturnal polysomnography (PSG) or a portable home based test (PHBT).

Polysomnography (PSG) is the gold standard for the diagnosis of OSAS, providing information about the severity of OSAS and the degree of sleep fragmentation, but it does not provide any information for the level or the degree of upper airway obstruction. To date, various methods have been used to investigate the site of upper airway obstruction in patients with OSAS including magnetic resonance imaging, computerized tomography, lateral cephalometry and nasopharyngoscopy.

Despite, in-laboratory polysomnography is the worldwide accepted standard for diagnosing OSA, it is a time-consuming and costly procedure, requires the expertise of sleep medicine specialists and furthermore it is not sufficient to detect borderline cases.

For the reasons above, a number of screening questionnaires and clinical screening models have been developed and therewith many alternative household diagnostic tools were proposed to help identify patients with OSA.

Although individual clinical features are an important part of the diagnosis of OSA, such as the acknowledgement of snoring and excessive daytime sleepiness increase the suspicion of OSA, at the same time, their absence cannot be used to exclude OSA with any degree of certainty. In an effort to deal with this issue, a number of screening tests were developed to identify high-risk patients. However, because of the lack of awareness by the public and healthcare professionals, the vast majority remain undiagnosed and untreated.

EPIDEMIOLOGY

OSAS is a worldwide chronic potentially lethal pathology. Its diffusion is increased during the last years, involving not only adults but also children. The prevalence of OSAS is different in the studies published, because of various criteria employed to define the illness. For example in a population-based study utilizing an AHI cutoff of ≥ 5 events/h (hypopneas associated with 4% oxygen desaturations) combined with clinical symptoms, the prevalence of OSA has been estimated to be 14% of men and 5% of women. When the prevalence is stratified based on an AHI > 15 events/h, the prevalence rate is about 10% to 20%. Concerning the different prevalence of OSAS amongst male and female, the ratio is about 3:1 prior to menopause, and become equal after that. Presumably it depends on body fat distribution and sex hormones, that play a role in the modulation of upper airway musculature. To support this theory no differences in prevalence are recorded between males and females prior to puberty. Besides, age represents a risk factor: the prevalence triple in individuals greater than 65 years of age compared with individuals aged 30-64 years. In terms of ethnicity, African American individuals appear to be more predisposed to OSA than Caucasians, with an odds ratio of 3 in children younger than 14 and 2 in adults greater than 25. Individuals of Asian descent, particularly Chinese individuals, have a more crowded upper airway and retrognathia compared with Caucasians. OSA has a prevalence rate similar in the Asian population sample to those in Caucasians despite a lower obesity rate. Asians have an increased risk of developing OSA, regardless of weight or neck circumference, as well as greater disease severity.

High Risk Screening (Risk Factors and Questionnaire)

a) Obesity
b) Male
c) Age > 40
d) Neck circumferences (>43 cm in men; >40.5 in women)
e) Structural Abnormalities
f) Family History
g) Positive Questionnaires

The employment of a screening tool is necessary in order to identify individuals at high risks of OSA in general population to submit to PSG and provide them a treatment. To screen the population, first of all it is necessary to collect history and carry out a physical examination. The sleep history is focused on the presence of risk factors for OSA and on the other hand to investigate related symptoms of obstructive sleep apnea. Primary risk factors to detect OSA patients include: male gender, those over age 40, obese persons or recent weight gain, and patients with a large neck size or small chin/jaw. The increase of body mass index (BMI ≥ 30 kg/m2) is the strongest risk factor for OSA: about 70% of those with OSA are obese and, at the same time, the prevalence of OSA in obese men and women is about 40%. Indeed, the twenty-six percent of patients with a BMI greater than 30 and 33% of those with a BMI greater than 40 have moderate OSA. Regarding neck circumference, a size >43 cm in men, >40 cm in women, may have a greater sensitivity and specificity than BMI in predicting OSA, regardless of the person's sex.

Questions to be asked during a routine health maintenance evaluation should include an evaluation for snoring, witnessed apneas, gasping/choking episodes, excessive sleepiness not explained by other factors, total sleep amount, nocturia, morning headaches, sleep fragmentation/sleep maintenance insomnia, and decreased concentration and memory.

Features to be evaluated that may suggest the presence of OSA include body abnormalities, evaluated during ENT visit: a modified

Mallampati score of 3 or 4, the presence of retrognathia, lateral peritonsillar narrowing, macroglossia, tonsillar hypertrophy, elongated/enlarged uvula, high arched/narrow hard palate, nasal abnormalities (polyps, deviation, valve abnormalities, turbinate hypertrophy) and/or overjet. The clinical examination is supported by video examinations (nasal endoscopy, laryn-goscopy, nasofibrolaryngoscopy), cephalometry, computedtomography, and magnetic resonance imaging. The otorhinolaryngologist thanks to nasoendoscopy may investigate dynamic pattern of collapse of naso-, oro-, and hypopharynx during forced inspiration against closed mouth and nose. This examination is called Muller's maneuver (MM), first described in 1983, and it's performed when the patient was in sitting position, following topical nasal anesthesia achieved with 4% lidocaine and 0.5% ephedrine spray. A flexible endoscope is inserted through the anesthetized nasal cavity into the nasopharynx and then advanced to oro, hypopharynx and larynx. The degree of obstruction is evaluated in a semi-quantitative manner (no obstruction = 0;25% obstruction = 1; 50% obstruction = 2; 75% obstruction = 3 and 100% obstruction = 4).

Positive Questionnaires

Berlin Questionnaire

The Berlin questionnaire consists of eleven questions address snoring behaviour, fatigue, and history of obesity or hypertension that predict the risk of OSA as high or low.

The Berlin Questionnaire produced a large number of false negative results. The sensitivity of the Berlin questionnaire with regards to high-risk patients having sleep apnea was 86%. Specifically, in the revision carried out by AASM in 2017 in subjects with a AHI cutoff of ≥ 5, the pooled sensitivity is 0.76 (95% CI: 0.72 to 0.80), while the pooled specificity is 0.45 (95% CI: 0.34 to 0.56). Furthermore, the questionnaire had suboptimal accuracy, ranging from 56% to 70%; accuracy became progressively more compromised with consideration of higher OSA severity thresholds.

Epworth Sleepiness Scale

The Epworth sleepiness scale (ESS) has been universally adopted as an effective screening method to monitor for clinical symptoms of sleep: it is easy to understand and to fill in. It is a self-reported questionnaire involving eight questions to assess how frequently the patient is likely to doze. Unfortunately, the ESS has a large number of false negative results limiting its utility for the diagnosis of OSA. The AASM reported revealed a range of sensitivity of 0.27–0.72 and specificity of 0.50–0.76 in case of an AHI of ≥ 5.

After all, the ESS is a subjective self assessment measure and may be inaccurate for this reason, indeed if a patient has multiple risk factors for sleep apnea, the individual should be sent for further evaluation if there is a suspicion of sleep apnea despite a low ESS.

Stop-Bang Questionnaire

Another screening tool called the *STOP BANG* questionnaire was developed to screen for the most common risk factors seen specifically in OSA. It is an OSA screening tool consisting of four yes/no questions and four clinical attributes.

The term refers to a mnemonic that represents 8 factors: Snoring, Tiredness, Observed apneas, elevated blood Pressure, BMI (greater than 35 kg/m2), Age (greater than 50), Neck circumference (greater than 40cm), and Gender (male). Patients receive a point for each positive risk factor, and those whose scores are equal to or greater than 3 have a higher likelihood of having OSA. The sensitivities of the STOP BANG questionnaire for mild, moderate, and severe sleep apnea were 83.6%, 92.9%, and 100%, respectively.

For the American Academy of Sleep Medicine the STOP BANG has got an high sensitivity, but low specificity for the detection of OSA.

For moderate to severe OSA (AHI > 15), the sensitivity and specificity of the STOP questionnaire are 74% and 53%, respectively. For severe OSA (AHI > 30), sensitivity is 80% and specificity is 49%. The STOP-Bang questionnaire includes the four questions used in the STOP questionnaire plus four additional demographic queries. For each question, answering "yes" scores 1, a "no" response scores 0, and the total score ranges from 0 to 8.

The questionnaire can be completed quickly and easily (usually within 1-2 min), and overall response rates are typically high (90%-100%). If patients score 0 to 2 on the STOP-Bang questionnaire, they are considered to be at low risk of OSA, those with a STOP-Bang score of 5 to 8 can be classified as being at high risk for moderate to severe OSA. In patients with a STOP-Bang score of 3 or 4, the specific combinations of positive items should be examined further to ensure proper classification and the possibility of those patients having moderate to severe sleep apnea can be confidently ruled out.

Although its high sensibility, the modest specificity (43% to detect moderate to severe sleep apnea) will yield a high false positive rate, limiting the employment of this questionnaire during OSAS screening.

STOP Questionnaire

The STOP questionnaire showed moderate to high sensitivity, low specificity, and moderate accuracy, indeed in case of AHI≥ 5, the accuracy in a high-risk population ranged from 74% to 86%. The quality of evidence for the use of the STOP questionnaire ranged from low to moderate across different diagnostic cutoffs and risk groups after being downgraded due to heterogeneity or imprecision.

OSA50 Questionnaire

The OSA50 questionnaire involves four components including age ≥50, snoring, witnessed apneas and waist circumference.

The OSA50 in the primary care setting81 showed a sensitivity ranging from 0.49–0.98 and a specificity of 0.82.

OSAS Score

The OSAS score involves assessment of the Friedman tongue position, tonsil size, and body mass index. In a sample of individuals suspected to have OSA, the sensitivity of the OSAS score was 0.86 (95% CI: 0.80 to 0.91) against PSG at an AHI > 5 cut = off, however; specificity was lower at 0.47 (95% CI: 0.34 to 0.56) with a high number of false positives in the low-risk group.

Kushida Index

One study evaluating the performance of the Kushida Index against PSG showed a high sensitivity of 0.98 (95% CI: 0.95 to 0.99) and high specificity of 1.00 (95% CI: 0.92 to 1.00) to detect AHI ≥ 5.

Instrumental Diagnosis

Sleep Endoscopy

The technique of Drug Induced Sedation Endoscopy DISE, developed by Croft and Pringle in 1991, is aimed at exploring the upper airways during pharmacologically-induced sleep using a flexible fibro-optic endoscope. The European Position Paper On Drug-Induced Sleep Endoscopy of 2017, changed the name of the technique put in "sleep" in place of "sedation."

During the exam, the patient is in a drug-induced sleep state using propofol administrated by an anesthetist while monitoring ECG, blood pressure, oxygen saturation and pulse. Endoscopy is often equipped with a suction channel which is useful to advance through the nose.

The most used drugs (for sedation) to perform DISE are midazolam and propofol, as single agents or together. Some authors combine them with remifentanil or ketamine. Another drug that can be used is Dexmedetomidine, an alpha 2 adrenergic drug that produces sedation plus analgesia by inhibiting the locus ceruleus. A review of 2013 compared the efficacy of Propofol vs Dexmedetomidine among 220 studies, pointing out how they're both effective. Dexmedetomidine ensures cardiopulmonary system stability; propofol has a rapid onset and half-life.

According to the Position Paper the ideal observation window lasts at least two cycles or one minute but it may take longer both for each segment of upper airway and during the maneuvers. A cycle is a complete and stable sequence of snoring–obstructing hypopnea/apnea–oxygen desaturation–breathing with good observation of levels.

The indications to perform the exam are: patients affected by disturbing snoring and OSAHS, in whom non-CPAP therapy is considered, patients who have failed or don't tolerate CPAP therapy, patients already submitted at a previous surgery but failed. Absolute contraindications to DISE are ASA 4, pregnancy, and patients with an allergy to DISE drugs. Relative contraindications may include morbid obesity. The technique is valid, dynamic, safe, and easy to perform.

The enhanced advantage of this exam is the direct visualization of obstruction sites and patterns of collapse and can be useful in discriminating subjects who would benefit from surgical management from those who would not. Moreover, odontologists can test mandibular advancement devices (MAD) in patients during DISE, in order to set them in the most effective shape to prevent sleep apneas/ hypopneas.

In the literature, many authors have developed different grading systems to describe the anatomical structures involved in upper airway collapse in OSAS patients.

The VOTE classification encompasses the most commonly involved structures and the configuration of obstruction. It can be described as anteroposterior (typically anterior structures moving posteriorly against the posterior pharyngeal wall), lateral (laterally located structures moving towards the center of the airway), or concentric (combination of the former two). The sites described are: Velum, Oropharyngeal lateral walls, Tongue base, Epiglottis. The degrees of severity are: none, partial, complete. Another option is the employment of NOHL classification published by Vicini in 2012. According to the NOHL classification, grading and pattern of obstruction can be evaluated at four different anatomic levels: N (Nasopharynx cavity and walls), O (Oropharynx – retro-palatal space), H (Hypopharynx - tongue base) and L (Larynx - epiglottis). Grading of obstruction for nasopharynx cavities and pharyngeal walls can be classified as follows: • Grade 1: 0-25% collapse; • Grade 2: 25-50% collapse; • Grade 3: 50-75% collapse; • Grade 4: total collapse during Muller manoeuvre (100%). furthermore, it is possible to define the pattern of pharyngeal collapse (for O and H), as transversal (t), antero-posterior (ap) or concentric (c). The presence of any laryngeal (L) obstruction could be reported as p (positive) or n (negative), and if a consistent grade of palatine tonsillar hypertrophy is observed, it can be noted in the final report as TS (grade 3 or 4).

Polysomnography

The gold-standard to detect OSAS patients is represented by polysomnography that, however requires specialized personnel and devoted setting which limits a wide use of the tool and compels to screen the population to refer to the specialist. Questionnaires are validated screening tools, however up to 45% of patients referred with the suspicion of OSAS are not confirmed by PSG. Likewise no clinical model is recommended to predict severity of obstructive sleep apnea therefore objective testing such as PSG is required.

The severity of OSA must be established in order to make an appropriate treatment decision.

An overnight polysomnography is recorded during the normal sleeping hours of a patient. Patients sleep 6 to 8 hours before either awakening spontaneously or being awakened. The goal of the PSG is to quantify the amount of time spent in various stages of sleep during the night and to document clinically relevant events such as cardiopulmonary abnormalities and/or changes in sleep stages. The standard PSG includes limited multi-channel recording of an individual's electroencephalography (EEG) to assess for sleep architecture, sleep stages and arousals.

Electro-oculogram, airflow, pulse oximetry, respiratory effort, electrocardiographic (ECG) tracings, body position, and snoring are all accumulated. Additional recommended parameters include body position and leg EMG derivations. Anterior tibialis EMG is useful to assist in detecting movement arousals and may have the added benefit of assessing periodic limb movements, which coexist with sleep related breathing disorders (SRBD) in many patients. Apneas are classified as obstructive, central or mixed, according to the presence or absence of respiratory efforts.

The limites of PSG are: inconvenient, resource-intensive with limited availability, and not representative test of a typical night's sleep (particularly the first night the test is given). Furthermore, there are variations across laboratories in the definitions of OSA (using different thresholds of AHI, from 5 to 15 events/hr) and in the way that the PSG results are read and interpreted. Moreover, AHI, which is used as the single metric to define OSA, can vary from night to night and does not take into account symptoms, comorbidities, or response to treatment.

Home Sleep Testing

HST is considered a cost-effective alternative for OSAS diagnosis in selected patients. American Academy Sleep Medicine (AASM) and the American Thoracic Society (ATS) recommend the management of OSAS by HST in pre-test subjects with high OSAS suspicion without notorious morbidity or suspicion of neurological disorders, as stated in their guidelines for the use of portable monitors.

The HST is useful because there also many limited accesses to in laboratory testing in some areas. There are potential disadvantages to using HST, relative to PSG, because of the differences in the physiologic parameters being collected and the availability of personnel to adjust sensors when needed. The sensor technology used by HST devices varies considerably by the number and type of sensors that are utilized. Measurement error is inevitable in HST, compared against PSG, as standard sleep staging channels are not typically monitored in HST (electroencephalography (EEG), electrooculography (EOG) or electromyography (EMG)) monitoring are not typically performed HST devices that use conventional sensors are unable to detect hypopneas only associated with cortical arousals, which are included in the recommended AHI scoring rule in the AASM Scoring Manual. Sensor dislodgement and poor quality signal during HST are additional contributors to the measurement error. Due to these limitations, an HST may underestimate the severity of OSA.

Although it is less sensitive than polysomnography in the detection of OSA, an HST may be used in the unattended setting as an alternative to PSG for the diagnosis of OSA in patients with a high pretest probability of moderate to severe OSA and no comorbid sleep disorder or major comorbid medical disorders when all of the previous parameters are met. Therefore, it is essential for the raw HST data to be reviewed and interpreted by a physician who is either board-certified in sleep medicine or overseen by a board-certified sleep medicine physician and it should be performed only in conjunction with a comprehensive sleep evaluation.

The Pulse Transit Time (PTT) represents an exam that may be overlooked in HST group. It is a non-invasive indirect marker of sleep fragmentation in subjects with OSAS and refers to the time taken for the arterial pulse pressure wave to travel from between 2 separate sites, usually the aortic valve to a peripheral site such as the finger. In case of OSAS patients, the obstruction of the upper airway results in a fall in blood pressure: this is associated with a longer time for the Pulse wave to reach the periphery, and results in an "increment" in the PTT. In the opposite, during the arousal from sleep there is an increase in blood pressure, the stiffening of the arterial wall and the increase in vascular tone leading to a "decrement" in the PTT. Therefore, changes in PTT have been demonstrated to correlate with changes in oxygen saturation, oesophageal pressure swings, inspiratory effort and EEG arousals in the setting of OSAS and have also been shown to be useful in detecting obstructive non-apnoeic respiratory event.

WatchPAT (Peripheral Arterial Tonometer) -200 is a wrist-worn portable device that detects obstructive events by identifying the changes in sympathetic activity associated with the termination of the events. It has two finger probes and a main body. One of the probes contains a sensor that detects the PAT signal and the other probe measures arterial oxygen saturation. The main body of the device differentiates sleep time from wake time, carries out signal processing, provides the power supply and stores data. WatchPAT-200 measures AHI, respiratory disturbance index (RDI), total sleep time and sleep stages by using PAT signal.

Cephalometric Radiography

Lateral cephalography is useful to analyze skeletal and soft tissue characteristics of patients with OSAS and has the advantage of being available in most clinics, easy to perform, and less expensive than a polysomnographic examination. It provides information on the morphology of the upper airway, does not allow dynamic evaluation. Cephalometric radiography is usually performed in the upright posture and is increasingly being used as an adjunctive diagnostic tool for the assessment of OSAS patients. In addition to provide quantitative assessment of bony tissue landmarks, cephalometric radiography may be also useful to evaluate soft tissue structures in the oropharyngeal passage.

The evidences often showed in OSAS patients, are shorter dimension of the cranial base and maxillary length, maxillo-mandibular retrognathia, and increased anterior lower facial height and mandibular plane angle.

OSAS patients often have reduced midface length, and this finding may cause a reduction of space available for the air way. The hyoid bone is more inferiorly placed and considering its relationship with tongue position, there is a reduction of upper airway space. The tongue mass concentrated in the hypopharyngeal area may therefore be a poor prognostic indicator for the successful use of mandibular advancement splints.

Furthermore, some studies describe more protrusive upper incisors in OSAS patients, but others did not find any such difference.

Magnetic Resonance Imaging

Magnetic resonance imaging (MRI) allows to study upper airway and its site of collapses. There are two type of studies already known: with magnetic resonance in a classic way and with the employment of ultrafast MRI, that obtains multiple images in different subsites of upper airway with sufficient quality and temporal resolution to allow a dynamic and tridimensional assessment of the pharyngeal musculature. The exam is obtained in supine position, during wakefulness and during sleep, obtained with sedation or in a natural way. The information detected in OSAS patients show a circular oropharynx instead of the more frequent elliptical shape (lateral narrowing), for the adipose tissue deposition, suggested as one of the mechanisms of airway compression in obese apneic patients, with or without an increase neck size. Moreover the acknowledgement of the thickness of lateral pharyngeal walls varied inversely to the airway lumen, probably indicates that lateral pharyngeal walls are compressed or stretched as a result of a changes in the airway caliber.

Exhaled Nitric Oxid (FeNO)

Nitric oxide (NO) is a gaseous molecule produced by nitric oxide synthase (NOS) enzymes from L-arginine and oxygen. There are three isoforms of NOS, two are constitutively produced (endothelial NOS–eNOS– and neuronal NOS–nNOS–) and one is inducible (iNOS), increasing during inflammation. Therefore FeNO is a non invasive marker of airway inflammation. Only few studies declare that OSAS patients have an overnight increase in the concentration of nitric oxide exhaled by the nose (nasal nitric oxide–nNO–) and by the mouth (orale nitrix oxide–oNO–), others failed to confirm this evidence, or they found an overnight increase limited to subgroups of OSAS, such as obese OSAS patients or children with mild OSAS but not moderate/severe. A possible explanation is that the inflammation is located in the upper airway and not close to alveoli where NO is produced- Therefore other flogosi's markers will be employed such as pro-inflammatory cytokines detected in the exhaled breath condensated (EBC) of the OSAS patients and the study of volatile organic compounds. The breath analysis seem more promising than FeNO for a clinical use, but others studies are necessary to confirm it.

References

Ceylan T, Fırat H, Kuran G, Ardıç S, Bilgin E, Çelenk F. *Quick Diagnosis in Obstructive Sleep Apnea Syndrome: WatchPAT-200 Iran Red Crescent Med J.* 2012; 14(8): 475-478.

Chang ET, Certal V, Song SA, Zaghi S, Carrasco-Llatas M, Torre C, Capasso R, Camacho M. Dexmedetomidine versus propofol during drug-induced sleep endoscopy and sedation: a systematic review. *Sleep and Breathing*, 2017, Volume 21, Number 3, Page 727.

Chung F, Abdullah HR, Liao P. STOP-Bang Questionnaire: A Practical Approach to Screen for Obstructive Sleep Apnea. *Chest.* 2016 Mar; 149(3):631-8.

Ciscar MA, Juan G, Martínez V, Ramón M, Lloret T, Mínguez J, Armengot M, Marín J, Basterra J. Magnetic resonance imaging of the pharynx in OSA patients and healthy subjects. *Eur Respir J.* 2001 Jan; 17(1):79-86.

Da Cunha Viana Jr A, Thuler LCS, de Araújo-Melo MH Drug-induced sleep endoscopy in the identification of obstruction sites in patients with obstructive sleep apnea: a systematic review 2015. *Braz J Otorhinolaryngol.* Jul-Aug 2015; 81(4):439-46.

De Stefano, A., Di Giovanni, P., Kulamarva, G., Gennachi, S., Di Fonzo, F., Sallustio, V., Patrocinio, D., Candido, S., Lamarca, G., Dispenza, F. Oropharyngeal dysphagia in elderly population suffering from mild cognitive impairment and mild dementia: Understanding the link (2020) *American Journal of Otolaryngology - Head and Neck Medicine and Surgery*, 41 (4), art. no. 102501.

De Stefano, A., Dispenza, F., Kulamarva, G., Lamarca, G., Faita, A., Merico, A., Sardanelli, G., Gabellone, S., Antonaci, A. Predictive factors of severity and persistence of oropharyngeal dysphagia in sub-acute stroke (2020) *European Archives of Oto-Rhino-Laryngology*, doi: 10.1007/s00405-020-06429-2.

Epstein LJ, Kristo D, Strollo Jr PJ, Friedman N, Malhotra A, Patil SP, Ramar K, Rogers R, Schwab RJ, Weaver EM, Weinstein MD. Clinical guideline for the evaluation, management and long-term care of obstructive sleep apnea in adults. *J Clin Sleep Med.* 2009 Jun 15; 5(3):263-76.

Finamore P, Scarlata S, Cardaci V, Antonelli Incalzi R. Exhaled Breath Analysis in Obstructive Sleep Apnea Syndrome: A Review of the Literature2019 *Medicina* (Kaunas). 2019 Aug 27; 55(9):538.

Ho ML, Brass SD. Obstructive sleep apnea *Neurol Int.* 2011 Nov 29; 3(3): e15.

Hoogeveen RC, Sanderink GC, Berkhout WE. Effect of head position on cephalometric evaluation of the soft-tissue facial profile. *Dentomaxillofac Radiol.* 2013; 42(6):20120423.

Kapur VK, Auckley DH, Chowdhuri S, et al. Clinical Practice Guideline: Diagnostic Testing OSA *Journal of Clinical Sleep Medicine*, Vol. 13, No. 3, 2017.

Kezirian EJ, Hohenhorst W, de Vries N. Drug-induced sleep endoscopy: the VOTE classification *Eur Arch Otorhinolaryngol.* 2011 Aug; 268(8):1233-1236.

Kum RO, Ozcan M, Yılmaz YF, Gungor V, Kum NY, Unal A. The Relation of the Obstruction Site on Muller's Maneuver with BMI, Neck Circumference and PSG Findings in OSAS 2014 *Indian J Otolaryngol Head Neck Surg* 2014 Jun; 66(2):167-72.

Lorusso F, Dispenza F, Martinciglio G, Battaglia A, Gallina S. Postural changes in patients undergoing hyoid surgery for OSAS. *EuroMediterranean Biomedical Journal*, 2017; 12(29):140-143.

Lorusso F, Dispenza F, Modica DM, Gallina S. The Role of Modified Expansion Sphincter Pharyngoplasty in Multilevel Obstructive Sleep Apnea Syndrome Surgery. *Int Arch Otorhinolaryngol.* 2018 Oct; 22(4):432-436.

Lorusso F, Dispenza F, Saraniti C, Sireci F, Modica DM, Gallina S. Sleep disordered breathing: evaluation of dynamic patterns of the upper airways in obese subjects. *Otorinolaringologia* 2014; 64:57–64.

Mattos Soares MC, Raposo Sallum AC, Themis Moraes Gonçalves M, Martinho Haddad FL, Gregório LC Use of Muller's maneuver in the evaluation of patients with sleep apnea - literature review 2009 *Braz J Otorhinolaryngol.* May-Jun 2009; 75(3):463-6.

Mistretta A, Battaglia A, Gallina S, Lorusso F. Chapter *the Role of Drug-Induced Sleep/Sedation Endoscopy (DISE) in the Detection of OSAHS.*

Modica DM, Lorusso F, Presti G, Fasola S, Gallina S. Our Assessment Using Palate Postoperative Problems Score (PPOPS): Tool for the Evaluation of Results in Palatal Surgery Techniques. *Indian J Otolaryngol Head Neck Surg.* 2019 Oct; 71(Suppl 1):766-770.

Modica DM, Marchese D, Lorusso F, Speciale R, Saraniti C, Gallina S. Functional Nasal Surgery and Use of CPAP in OSAS Patients: Our Experience. *Indian J Otolaryngol Head Neck Surg.* 2018 Dec; 70(4): 559-565.

Raccomandazioni per la diagnosi e cura dei disturbi respiratori nel sonno AIPO Associazione italiana pneumologi ospedalieri [*Recommendations for the diagnosis and treatment of respiratory disorders in sleep AIPO Italian association of hospital pulmonologists*].

Riley R, Guilleminault C, Herran T, Powell N. Cephalometric analyses and flow-volume loops in obstructive sleep apnea patients *Sleep.* 1983; 6(4):303-11.

Rosen IM, Kirsch DB, Carden KA, Malhotra RK, Ramar K, Aurora RN, Kristo DA, Martin JL, Olson EJ, Rosen CL, Rowley JA, Shelgikar AV. Clinical Use of a Home Sleep Apnea Test: An Updated

American Academy of Sleep Medicine Position Statement 2018. *J Clin Sleep Med*. 2018 Dec 15; 14(12): 2075–2077.

Steinhart H, Kuhn-Lohmann J, Gewalt K, Constantinidis J, Mertzlufft F, Iro H Upper Airway Collapsibility in Habitual Snorers and Sleep Apneics: Evaluation with Drug-induced Sleep Endoscopy. *Acta Otolaryngol* 2000; 120: 990±994.

Toraldo DM, Passali D, Sanna A, De Nuccio F, Conte L, De Benedetto M. Cost-effectiveness strategies in OSAS management: a short review *Acta Otorhinolaryngol Ital*. 2017 Dec; 37(6):447-453.

Vavougios GD, George GD, Pastaka C, Zarogiannis SG, Gourgoulianis KI Phenotypes of comorbidity in OSAS patients: combining categorical principal component analysis with cluster analysis *J Sleep Res*. 2016 Feb; 25(1):31-8.

Vicini C, Colabianchi V, Marrano GG, Barbanti F, Spedicato GA, Lombardo L, Siciliani G Description of the relationship between NOHL classification in drug-induced sleep endoscopy and initial AHI in patients with moderate to severe OSAS, and evaluation of the results obtained with oral appliance therapy *Acta Otorhinolaryngol Ital*. 2020 Feb; 40(1):50-56.

In: Advances in Sleep Apnea
Editors: F. Lorusso et al.
ISBN: 978-1-53619-758-7

Chapter 4

ADVANCES IN PAEDIATRIC OSAS DIAGNOSIS

Donatella Marchese**, Salvatore Gallina and Francesco Lorusso

Department of Otolaryngology, Head and Neck Surgery,
Policlinico Paolo Giaccone University of Palermo, Palermo, Italy

ABSTRACT

The incidence of Obstructive sleep apnea syndrome (OSAS) in the pediatric population is about 2%. The diagnosis is based on the employment of questionnaires, but they are unable to differentiate OSAS from primary snoring, and polysomnography (PSG) that is the gold standard also among children. The PSG allows to classify OSAS as mild in case of 1 < Apnea Hypopnea Index (AHI) ≤ 5, moderate if 5 < AHI ≤ 10 and severe OSAS when the AHI is > 10. If polysomnography is not available, we need alternative diagnostic tests such as nocturnal oximetry studies and respiratory polygraphy. The risk factors identified are different from adults, first tonsillar hypertrophy wins over others.

The symptoms and signs described are similar to adult population, but sleep enuresis, neurocognitive impairment and

* Corresponding Author's Email: marchesedonatella@hotmail.com.

behavioral problems (attention-deficit/hyperactivity disorder, learning problems) are typical of pediatric OSAS.

Definition

Pediatric OSAS is defined as a "Disorder of breathing during sleep characterized by prolonged partial upper airway obstruction and/or intermittent complete obstruction (obstructive apnea) that disrupts normal ventilation during sleep and normal sleep patterns," accompanied by symptoms or signs, listed below. Such as the adults, also for children the classification of severity is based on the Apnea hypopnea index, but in case of obstructive $1 < AHI \leq 5$ is already defined as mild OSA, $5 < AHI \leq 10$ is a moderate OSA, and an $AHI > 10$ correspond to a severe OSA.

Epidemiology

The incidence of OSAS in the pediatric population is about 2% according to the pediatric OSAS guidelines[4]. It occurs equally in both sexes, although a male predominance may be seen as the children approach puberty. The syndrome is widespread among children of 2–8 years age, in consideration of the adeno tonsillar hypertrophy5. Others risk factors are African Americans and obese children. Allergic Rhinitis, Inflammatory Factors and Biomarkers, craniofacial anomalies, and neuromuscular disorders.

Diagnosis

The diagnosis of OSAS in children is based on clinical history, analyzing risk factors and nocturnal and diurnal symptoms, physical examination and polysomnogram to confirm it.

The first question is whether the child or adolescent snores. In case of affirmative answer or if the patient complains signs or symptoms typical for OSAS, it is necessary to perform a polysomnogram for a more extensive evaluation. The symptoms and signs have been described among these: frequent snoring (≥ 3 nights/wk), labored breathing during sleep, gasps or snoring noises, episodes of apnea, sleep enuresis (especially secondary enuresis), sleeping in a seated position or with the neck hyperextended, cyanosis, headaches on awakening, neurocognitive impairment and behavioral problems (attention-deficit/hyperactivity disorder, learning problems). Daytime sleepiness may occur, but is uncommon in young children. OSAS is besides associated with, failure to thrive, hypertension, cardiac dysfunction, and systemic inflammation. At the physical examination, the patients appear underweighted or overweighted, with tonsillar hypertrophy, and adenoidal facies, micrognathia/retrognathia and high-arched palate. Several genetic syndromes may affect breathing during sleep, particularly those that cause micrognathia (Robin sequence, Treacher Collins syndrome), midface hypoplasia (achondroplasia, Crouzon, Apert, and Pfeiffer syndromes), disorders of respiratory control (Arnold-Chiari malformation, Prader- Willi syndrome), as well as miscellaneous and multifactorial disorders (Mucopolysaccharidoses, Down syndrome, sickle cell anaemia).

Risk Factors

Obesity: in the upper airway of the OSAS obese children occur a reduction of the pharyngeal lumen and a collapse of the structures themselves, in correspondence of thorax and abdomen, a reduction of respiratory function. All described above is justified for the increased fat in soft tissue. Each increment in body mass index (BMI) above the 50th percentile is associated with around a 10% increased risk for OSAS.

Adenotonsillar hypertrophy: Adenoid and/or tonsil hypertrophy are the most common causes of upper airway lumen reduction in children, evaluated by the Friedman Grading Scale; after all, the lymphoid tissue of the Waldeyer ring is more developed aged 3- 6, according to the peak incidence of OSAS. The mechanism that leads to the nocturnal apneas is the obstruction caused by narrowing of the retro-palatal area, which has the smallest cross-sectional area. Therefore, in case of adenotonsillar hypertrophy there is an increased expression of various mediators of inflammatory, that play a role in case of OSAS.

Allergic Rhinitis: this is considered a risk factor for two kinds of problem, firstly for the nasal congestion, secondly for the inflammatory mediators of the allergic process.

Craniofacial Abnormalities and Genetics Craniofacial abnormalities can also be a cause of upper airway obstruction syndrome. Alterations of the size, position, and geometry of the mandible and of the tongue can lead to the thickening of the retro-palatal region which, as already mentioned above, is the most frequent site of obstruction in pediatric patients.

Inflammatory Factors and Biomarkers: Several studies have highlighted the role of oxidative stress in the genesis of endothelial damage in both adult and pediatric OSAS patients. Intermittent hypoxemia leads to anoxia and re-oxygenation, which triggers the production of oxygen radicals and consequently local and systemic inflammation. Indeed in OSAS patients there is an up regulation of the expression of pro-inflammatory mediators and cytokines.

Diagnostic Methods

There have been many attempts to diagnose OSA in children by clinical criteria. A recent review of the biomedical literature concluded that "clinical history and physical examination are not reliable for diagnosing OSAHS."

Less than half of the children referred to sleep centres because of a clinical suspicion of OSA meet polysomnographic criteria for the disorder.

Questionnaires alone have been unable to differentiate OSA from primary snoring. The Sleep Related Breathing Disorder Scale of the validated Pediatric Sleep Questionnaire was shown to predict polysomnography (PSG) results "to an extent useful for research but not reliable enough for most individual patients."

Clinical scores that include factors such as difficulty breathing during sleep, observed apnoeas, and snoring have been suggested to differentiate children with OSA but these have not been helpful in diagnosing polysomnographically proven OSA in children who have been referred to a paediatric sleep centre.

Studies in the home have the advantage of a more natural sleeping environment, but fewer channels make for less precision of measurement. In addition, there is no technologist available to solve technical problems, so some percentage of home studies will need to be repeated.

Polysomnography

PSG includes monitoring of frontal, central, and occipital electroencephalograph (EEG) and submental electromyograph (EMG) activity to determine sleep architecture. Pneumotachography is the most accurate way to measure airflow, but the facemask required can be bulky and disturbing to the child. Surrogate measurements such as thermisters are inexpensive, easy to use and sensitive, but the signal is non-linear and only qualitative. Nasal pressure sensors can be helpful in discerning hypopnoeas since flow limitation may result in a flattening of the waveform, but it can be challenging to maintain a good quality signal in children. End-tidal CO_2 measurements can also help to assess gas exchange. This is particularly important in children with obesity, neuromuscular weakness, or other factors that may place them at higher risk for hypoventilation. Inductance plethysmography provides a semiquantitative estimate of chest wall and abdominal movement. Strain gauges, usually with piezoelectric crystals, are less accurate. Serious dysrhythmias are less common in children than adults, but sinus bradycardia is often seen in association with respiratory events. Tibial EMG is used to assess leg movements and is essential to quantitate periodic limb movements during sleep. The child is under the constant video observation of a trained technologist who is available to replace sensors if necessary, insures a quality recording, and assists the patient should he or she develop difficulties that require intervention.

There are unique challenges to performing and interpreting PSG in children compared to a cooperative adult. The décor of the laboratory should be friendly and comfortable to the child, while not too juvenile to discourage adolescents. Technologists need to be comfortable in dealing with children and their families. It is helpful to have an extra bed or cot in the room so a parent can sleep with the child. It is usually better if the parent does not share the same bed, since movements and other activity by the parent can either disturb or be misinterpreted as originating from the child.

Children tend to have shorter and fewer respiratory events than adults, and a high proportion of hypopnoeas, so the studies must be scored and reviewed with great care. In adults, obstructive apnoeas 10 s or longer are scored, but in children, with a faster respiratory rate, a respiratory event of 2 missed breaths is scored.

PSG remains the "gold standard" for diagnosing OSA in children. If polysomnography is not available, we need alternative diagnostic tests:

1. Nocturnal oximetry studies: oximetry studies have a high specificity but low sensitivity in the diagnosis of paediatric OSA.[32] Three or more clusters of desaturation events $\geq 4\%$ and at least three desaturations to $< 90\%$ are considered abnormal (McGill criteria). However, the rate of false negative or inconclusive results is high. Nocturnal oximetry studies could help in the prioritization of treatment in resource poor countries where PSGs are not available;
2. Respiratory polygraphy (RP) studies: respiratory polygraphies are essentially PSGs without the EEG, EMG, and EOG sensors. They are performed commonly in Europe and are quicker to set up and score than PSGs. Some centers have reported good agreement with in-lab PSGs, but there is the possibility that the AHI may be underestimated due to missed hypopnoeas resulting in arousals but not desaturation.
3. Ambulatory RP or PSG: there has been a recent drive towards performing ambulatory PSG or RP studies, not only because they are seen as a less expensive alternative to in-lab PSGs, but also because the results may be more representative of the child's typical night's sleep at home. Data on direct comparison with in-lab PSG are still limited but a recent study by Alonso-Álvarez *et al.,* compared home RP with in-lab PSG in 50 children clinically suspected to have OSA and showed that all

the home RP studies were successful and the area under the curve was consistently > 90% when various PSG cut-off values OAHI ≥ 1, 3 and 5 were used. This would suggest the validity of home RP for the diagnosis of OSA in children with a high pre-test probability of having OSA. However, more research is required to further optimize the sensitivity and specificity of home RP testing for the diagnosis of children with mild OSA;

4. Paediatric sleep questionnaire: this parent-filled questionnaire assesses symptoms of SDB, such as snoring, excessive daytime sleepiness, attention problems, and hyperactive behaviour in children aged 2–18 years. Its sensitivity and specificity for diagnosing OSA in otherwise healthy children are 78% and 72%, respectively, but it may be useful in predicting OSA-related neurobehavioural morbidity and its improvement after adenotonsillectomy;
5. Sleep clinical record: this is a diagnostic tool composed of physical examination, subjective symptoms and clinical history of behavioural and cognitive problems. These items are used to determine the sleep clinical score (SCS). A SCS of ≥ 6.5 is considered positive for OSA, with a sensitivity of 96.05% and specificity of 67.00%. This may potentially be a useful tool to screen patients for suspected OSA.

Whilst these investigations may be less sensitive and specific than PSGs, they can still be valuable in assessing SDB as long as clinicians are aware of their limitations.

References

Alonso Alvarez M. L., Terán Santos J., Cordero Guevara J. A., et al. Reliability of respiratory polygraphy for the diagnosis of sleep apnea-hypopnea syndrome in children. *Arch. Bronconeumol.* 2008; 44:318-23.

Alonso-Álvarez M. L., Terán-Santos J., Ordax Carbajo E., et al. Reliability of home respiratory polygraphy for the diagnosis of sleep apnea in children. *Chest* 2015;147:1020-8.

Arens, R., Sin, S., Nandalike, K., Rieder, J., Khan, U. I., Freeman, K., Wylie-Rosett, J., Lipton, M. L., Wootton, D. M., McDonough, J. M., et al. Upper airway structure and body fat composition in obese children with obstructive sleep apnea syndrome. *Am. J. Respir. Crit. Care Med.* 2011, 183, 782–787.

Brooks L. J. Genetic syndromes affecting breathing during sleep in children. In: Lee-Chiong T., Sateia M. J., Carskadon M. A., editors. *Sleep Medicine*. Philadelphia: Hanley & Belfus, 2002:305-14.

Brouillette R., Hanson D., David R., Klemka L., Szatkowski A., Fernbach S., et al. A diagnostic approach to suspected obstructive sleep apnea in children. *J. Pediatr.* 1984; 105:10-4.

Chervin R. D., Weatherly R. A., Garetz S. L., Ruzicka D. L., Giordani B. J., Hodges E. K., et al. Pediatric sleep questionnaire: prediction of sleep apnea and outcomes. *Arch. Otolaryngol. Head Neck. Surg.* 2007; 133:216-22.

Ciccone, M. M., Scicchitano, P., Mitacchione, G., Zito, A., Gesualdo, M., Caputo, P., Damiani, M. F., Sassara, M., Favale, S., Resta, O., et al. Is there a correlation between OSAS duration/severity and carotid intima-media thickness? *Respir. Med.* 2012, 106, 740–746.

Dehlink E., Tan H. L. Update on paediatric obstructive sleep apnoea *J. Thorac. Dis.* 2016; 8(2):224-235.

Griffiths A., Maul J., Wilson A., Stick S. Improved detection of obstructive events in childhood sleep apnoea with the use of the nasal cannula and the differentiated sum signal. *J. Sleep Res.* 2005;14:431-6.

Gulotta G., Giannicola I., Vicini C., Polimeni A., Greco A., de Vincentiis M., Visconti I. C. Risk Factors for Obstructive Sleep Apnea Syndrome in Children: State of the Art *Int. J. Environ. Res. Public Health* 2019, 16, 3235.

Gut G., Tauman R., Greenfeld M., et al. Nasal nitric oxide in sleep-disordered breathing in children. *Sleep Breath* 2015.

Hannon, T. S., Rofey, D. L., Ryan, C. M., Clapper, D. A., Chakravorty, S., Arslanian, S. A. Relationships among obstructive sleep apnea, anthropometric measures, and neurocognitive functioning in adolescents with severe obesity. *J. Pediatr.* 2012, 160, 732–735.

Heitzman S. J., Atkar R. S., Hajduk E. A., Wanner R. A., Flemons W. W. Validation of nasal pressure for the identification of apneas/hypopneas during sleep. *Am. J. Respir. Crit. Care Med.* 2002; 166:386-91.

Jeans, W. D., Fernando, D. C., Maw, A. R., Leighton, B. C. A longitudinal study of the growth of the nasopharynx and its contents in normal children. *Br. J. Radiol.* 1981, 54, 117–121.

Kimple, A., Ishman, S. Allergy and sleep-disordered breathing. *Curr. Opin. Otolaryngol. Head Neck Surg.* 2013, 21, 277–281.

Lee J. Brooks. Diagnosis and Management of Childhood Obstructive Sleep Apnea Syndrome *Ann. Acad. Med. Singapore* 2008; 37:701-5.

Lorusso F., Gallina S., Modica D. M, Di Salvo N, Riggio F. Bipolar Quantum Molecular Resonance versus Blunt Dissection tonsillectomy. *B-ENT* 2015; 11(02):101–108.

Lorusso, F., Martines, F., Mistretta, A., Dispenza, F., Gallina, S. Effects of adenotonsillectomy on neurocognitive and behavioural function in pediatric obstructive sleep apnea syndrome. *B-ENT* 2018; 14:113-118.

Loube D. I., Andrada T., Howard R. S. Accuracy of respiratory inductive plethysmography for the diagnosis of upper airway resistance syndrome. *Chest* 1999;115:1333-7.

Lu, D., Li, N., Yao, X., Zhou, L. Potential inflammatory markers in obstructive sleep apnea-hypopnea syndrome. *Bosn. J. Basic Med. Sci.* 2017, 17, 47–53.

Lumeng J. C., Chervin R. D. Epidemiology of pediatric obstructive sleep apnea. *Proc. Am. Thorac. Soc.* 2008; 5:242.

Manczur T., Greenough A., Hooper R., Allen K., Latham S., Price J. F., et al. Tidal breathing parameters in young children: comparison of measurement by respiratory inductance plethysmography to a facemask pneumotachograph system. *Pediatr. Pulmonol.* 1999; 28: 436-44.

Marcus C. L., Brooks L. J, Draper K. A., Gozal D., Halbower A. C., Jones J., Schechter M. S., Ward S. D., Sheldon S. H., Shi_man R. N., et al. Diagnosis and Management of Childhood Obstructive Sleep Apnea Syndrome. *Pediatrics* 2012, 130, 576–584.

Marcus, C. L. Pathophysiology of childhood obstructive sleep apnea: Current concepts. *Respir. Physiol.* 2000, 119, 143–154.

Myer, C. M., 3rd, Reed, J. M., Cotton, R. T., Willging, J. P., Shott, S. R. Airway management in Pierre Robin sequence. *Otolaryngol. Head Neck Surg.* 1998, 118, 630–635.

Nieminien P., Tolonen U., Lopponen H., Lopponen T., Luotonen J., Jokinen K. Snoring children: factors predicting sleep apnea. *Acta Otolaryngol* (Stockh) 1997;Suppl 529:190-4.

Nixon G. M., Brouillette R. T. Diagnostic techniques for obstructive sleep apnoea: is polysomnography necessary? *Paediatr. Respir. Rev.* 2002;3:18-24.

Redline S., Budhiraja R., Kapur V., Marcus C. L., Mateika J. H., Mehra R., et al. The scoring of respiratory events in sleep: reliability and validity. *J. Clin. Sleep Med.* 2007; 3:169-200.

Russell R. I. R., Helms P. J. Evaluation of three different techniques used to measure chest wall movements in children. *Eur. Resp. J.* 1994; 7: 2073-6.

Scott, A. R., Tibesar, R. J., Sidman, J. D. Pierre Robin sequence: Evaluation, management, indications for surgery, and pit-falls. *Otolaryngol. Clin. North Am.* 2012, 45, 695–710.

Spruyt K., Sans Capdevila O., Serpero L. D., et al. Dietary and physical activity patterns in children with obstructive sleep apnea. *J. Pediatr.* 2010; 156:724-30, 730.e1-730.e3.

Tan H. L, Gozal D., Ramirez H. M., et al. Overnight polysomnography versus respiratory polygraphy in the diagnosis of pediatric obstructive sleep apnea. *Sleep* 2014; 37:255-60.

Tan, H. L., Gozal, D., Kheirandish-Gozal, L. Obstructive sleep apnea in children: A critical update. *Nat. Sci. Sleep* 2013, 5, 109–123.

Tarasiuk A., Greenberg-Dotan S., Simon-Tuval T., et al. Elevated morbidity and health care use in children with obstructive sleep apnea syndrome. *Am. J. Respir. Crit. Care Med.* 2007; 175:55-61.

Tarasiuk A., Simon T., Tal A., et al. Adenotonsillectomy in children with obstructive sleep apnea syndrome reduces health care utilization. *Pediatrics* 2004; 113:351-6.

Tauman R., Gozal D. Obesity and obstructive sleep apnea in children. *Paediatr. Respir. Rev.* 2006; 7:247-59.

Van de Graa_, W. B. Thoracic traction on the trachea: Mechanisms and magnitude. *J. Appl. Physiol.* 1991, 70, 1328–1336.

Villa M. P., Paolino M. C., Castaldo R., et al. Sleep clinical record: an aid to rapid and accurate diagnosis of paediatric sleep disordered breathing. *Eur. Respir. J.* 2013; 41:1355-61.

In: Advances in Sleep Apnea
Editors: F. Lorusso et al.
ISBN: 978-1-53619-758-7

Chapter 5

ADVANCES IN MANAGEMENT OF CENTRAL APNEA

Angelo Torrente[1,*], MD, Laura Pilati[2], MD, Roberta Priola[1], MD and Salvatore Di Marco[2], MD

[1]Department of Biomedicine, Neurosciences and Advanced Diagnostics (Bi.N.D.), University of Palermo, Italy
[2]Neurology and Stroke Unit, Sant'Antonio-Abate Hospital of Trapani, Italy

ABSTRACT

Central sleep apnea (CSA) is a condition characterized by cyclic or intermittent transient reduction or interruption of airflow during sleep, in absence of any concomitant respiratory effort to contrast such event. The central causative mechanism is represented by a reduction of the upper ponto-medullary ventilatory drive, due to various conditions. CSA is in contrast with obstructive sleep apnea (OSA), in which respiratory effort is observed, even if the two conditions often coexist in the same

* Corresponding Author's Email: angelotorrente92@gmail.com.

patient. In this chapter, we will discuss the main CSA syndromes and their general or specific management, based on the most recent literature. We will then mention even other sleep breathing disorders constituted by hypoventilation syndromes.

INTRODUCTION

CSA is a common condition, though by far less frequent than OSA. A large community-based study that included 5804 over-40-years-old-adults showed how CSA was found in 0.9% of the population studied. CSA is defined as the presence at polysomnography (PSG) of a central apnea hypopnea index (AHI) ≥ 5 with central apneas/hypopneas accounting for more than 50% of all apneas/hypopneas, as from the International Classification of Sleep Disorders, 3rd ed. (ICSD-3).

It is worth to note that a central apnea is not always a pathologic event, but may be even the result of a physiologic mechanism, for example during the transition from wakefulness to the superficial stages of sleep (i.e., N1, N2). Such form of CSA is attributable to respiratory control system high sensitivity to $PaCO_2$ levels; during sleep $PaCO_2$ eucapnic level is set 2-6 mmHg above the wakefulness one, so, when falling asleep, the initial $PaCO_2$ results to be too low and a physiologic central apnea occurs. Another situation able to trigger CSA is represented by cortical arousals. When cortical arousals occur, the chemoreceptor threshold is set back to wakefulness levels and this will trigger an increased ventilatory effort; successively, when falling asleep again, the new $PaCO_2$ levels reached will lead to a CSA, also called post-arousal apnea.

As far as pathologic conditions are concerned, ICSD-3 provides eight main CSA syndromes:

- CSA with Cheyne-Stokes breathing (CSB)
- CSA due a medical disorder without CSB
- CSA due to high altitude periodic breathing
- CSA due to a medication or substance
- Primary CSA
- Treatment-emergent central sleep apnea

- CSA of infancy
- CSA of prematurity

The pathogenesis of such conditions varies widely, but the two main mechanisms are represented by i) respiratory instability and ii) depression of the brainstem respiratory centers or chemoreceptors.

i. Respiratory instability occurs when the respiratory control system generates over-responses or under-responses to minimal changes in nocturnal $PaCO_2$ (i.e., high "loop gain"). Loop gain is an engineering term used to describe how a system (e.g., the respiratory control system) responds to disturbances, in this case to respiratory ones. A loop gain includes three components: (1) the controller gain (i.e., the respiratory pontomedullary center that sends ventilatory commands based on $PaCO_2$ and PaO_2 changes); (2) the plant gain (i.e., the lungs and airways ventilatory response); and (3) the mixing gain (i.e., the circulatory time needed for changes in $PaCO_2$ and PaO_2 in pulmonary capillaries to be detected by the chemoreceptors). The higher the loop gain, the higher the overventilation or underventilation responses to variations in $PaCO_2$ and PaO_2.
ii. Central chemoreceptors may be found in the retrotrapezoid nucleus of the ventrolateral medulla and are responsible for the ventilatory output based on $PaCO_2$ and PaO_2 changes. A depression of the brainstem respiratory centers or central chemoreceptors may occur anytime any noxa (e.g., strokes, tumors, opioid use) involves such regions. CSA is meant as a failure of this controller during sleep.

Risk Factors

CSA prevalence appears to be higher among particular populations of subjects. In particular, the risk to develop CSA is higher among males, old adults, people suffering from congestive heart failure (CHF), subjects who develop a stroke, opioid users or patients who undergo CPAP therapy.

- *Sex.* Prevalence of CSA is higher in males than in women. Such difference may be due to the effect of sexual hormones on $PaCo_2$ apneic threshold. In particular, studies show how testosterone may be responsible for an increase of such threshold during NREM sleep.
- *Age.* An observational study of 741 randomly selected adults showed how CSA syndrome (Central AHI >10) prevalence tends to increase with age. Such phenomenon may find an explanation in the elderly higher prevalence of comorbidities (e.g., CHF, stroke, atrial fibrillation) or in the ageing process altering the sleep structure, inducing a higher prevalence of CSA.
- *Congestive heart failure (CHF).* CSA is a frequent finding in people affected by CHF. One of the mechanisms is linked to the augmented circulation time in such patients, but the pathophysiology will be discussed more in detail below.
- *Stroke or structural brainstem lesions.* Strokes may alter brain breathing control system, even if such alteration may occur just during the acute phase. Moreover, since the ventilatory control nuclei are located in the brainstem, any lesion at this level may compromise breathing, particularly during sleep.
- *Opioid use.* Opioid drugs increase the risk of CSA acting on μ receptors, able to produce ventilatory depression.
- *Continuous Positive Airway Pressure - CPAP.* This therapy resolves OSA episodes in most cases, but it is sometimes associated with the development CSAs, especially during the initial period of its use. This phenomenon is known as treatment-emergent CSA.

Clinical Presentation

The clinical presentation of patients with CSA depends on the cause of the apnea. For example, in hypercapnic CSA common findings are: respiratory failure, cor pulmonale, polycythemia, daytime sleepiness and snoring; in nonhypercapnic CSA, instead, we can find: daytime sleepiness, insomnia (i.e., restless sleep), mild and intermittent snoring, awakenings (± choking, or shortness of breath), normal body habitus. Patients with alveolar hypoventilation (i.e., waking hypercapnia), a small percentage of patients with CSA, present with symptoms suggestive of ventilatory failure, including cor pulmonale, peripheral edema, and polycythemia. Restless sleep and daytime sleepiness are also commonly reported in these patients. On the other hand, non-hypoventilating (normocapnic) patients with idiopathic CSA show no symptoms of ventilatory failure; these patients have a constellation of symptoms that may be similar to that of patients with obstructive apnea, although differences do exist. Idiopathic CSA patients complain daytime hypersomnolence less commonly than patients with OSA, and their principal symptoms are constituted by insomnia, restless sleep, or frequent awakenings during the night accompanied by gasping for air or shortness of breath. These patients also tend to have a normal body habitus, contrary to obesity in patient with obstructive apneas.

As expected, arterial oxygen desaturations occur during central apneas. The extent to which the saturation falls during a given apnea is likely to be related to the saturation (or to the PaO_2) at the time ventilation ceases, to the duration of the apnea, and to the lung volume at which the apnea occurs.

Few studies are published about hemodynamic consequences of central apneas: Schroeder and colleagues reported that pulmonary artery pressures increased from 26/16 mmHg during wakefulness to 41/26 mmHg during central apneic episodes and it seems highly probable that any elevation in pulmonary pressure will result from hypoxemia and hypercapnia.

Moreover, as far as sleep is concerned, some studies suggested that the frequent arousals and awakenings generally associated with hypercapnia after an apnea can lead to disruption of the normal distribution of sleep stages.

Diagnosis

The diagnosis of CSA is based on full-night recording of standard polysomnographic variables.

A central apnea is characterized by no inspiratory effort throughout the event. This is most effectively and consistently accomplished with an esophageal balloon catheter recording intrathoracic pressure swings that reflect ventilatory effort. However, this method is not possible in clinical practice, so other strategies have been used. Most evidence suggests that respiratory inductive plethysmography is a valid alternative method. If there is a complete absence of thoracoabdominal motion throughout an apnea, this strongly suggests that the event is central in origin.

In adults, according to the third International Classification of Sleep Disorders (ICSD-3), the polysomnographic criteria defining CSA are: an AHI > 5 events per hour of sleep, with more than 50% of these events being due to central apneas or hypopneas. In central apnea and hypopnea there are specific polysomnographic characteristics like the absence of snoring during the event or positive airway pressure device flow signal compared to baseline breathing. A crescendo-decrescendo shape in the inspiratory flow, limited desaturation following the event, as well as arousal occurring in the middle of the ventilatory upturns, are useful to identify the central cause of a respiratory event.

During the diagnosis is important to differentiate subtypes of CSA depending on wakefulness $PaCO_2$ levels: this information distinguish hypercapnic from eucapnic/hypocapnic CSA. Hypercapnic CSA and hypoventilation are due to functional or anatomical lesions at the level of the respiratory centers as occurs in congenital central alveolar hypoventilation syndrome, idiopathic central alveolar hypoventilation syndrome, stroke, medications use, brain tumors, Chiari's syndrome; neuromuscular disorders like motor neuron disease, poliomyelitis, neuropathies, myopathies and restrictive thoracic disorders cause a non adequate ventilation. In eucapnic/hypocapnic CSA, the main underlying mechanism is the instability in ventilatory control.

TREATMENT

The different therapeutic approaches depend mainly on the specific cause of the central apnea.

For the hypercapnic patient, nocturnal ventilatory assistance is the most appropriate approach. Recent studies demonstrate that nocturnal ventilatory assistance with a nasal mask and a pressure- or volume-cycled ventilator is more effective than invasive ventilation. CPAP alone worsens the number of central apneas and does not improve nocturnal hypoxemia.

For patients with CSA due to opioids, the first approach is to reduce dose since the effect on central apneas is dose dependent. If the dose cannot be decreased, bilevel positive pressure with a fast back-up rate (12 to 16 breaths per minute) or adaptive servoventilation may be useful.

For symptomatic patients with idiopathic CSA and insomnia, restless sleep, daytime hypersomnolence, and mild to moderate nocturnal hypoxemia several pharmacologic approaches can be attempted.

Acetazolamide, a carbonic anhydrase inhibitor, has been used to treat CSA, but several studies have reported the development of obstructive apnea. Theophylline, naloxone and medroxyprogesterone acetate show little efficacy in the treatment of central apnea. Benzodiazepines, on the other hand, can significantly reduce the number of central events. However, theophylline improved CSA in a patient with damaged brainstem. Inhalation of O_2 and CO_2 proved to be an effective therapy for some patients with CSA. Several studies suggest that oxygen may be a useful method of treating CSA dead space in patients with idiopathic CSA.

In patients who both have central apneas and a large component of obstructive events, it is important to treat the obstruction of the airways with beneficial effects on both types of apnea.

The treatment of Cheyne-Stokes respiration requires a special comment because it has been the subject of a large number of studies. First, heart failure (if present) should be treated as aggressively as possible. An innovative treatment for Cheyne-Stokes sees the positioning of a neurostimulation lead either into the right brachiocephalic vein or into the left pericardiophrenic vein to stimulate the phrenic nerve. Early clinical experience is encouraging. Data from large studies are still needed to confirm safety and efficacy.

We will now discuss the principal CSA syndromes and their possible specific management.

CSA with Cheyne-Stokes Breathing (CSB)

Congestive heart failure (CHF) represents the first cause of CSA, even if CSB pattern has been described in other conditions (e.g., strokes or renal failure) too. In the case of CHF, CSA with CSB is meant to be the result of a high loop gain, where the prolonged circulation time due to reduced ejection fraction (<45%) represents the key feature. Nevertheless, prolonged circulation time alone appears to be not sufficient to generate CSA, highlighting how in CHF alterations in the controller gain (increased chemoreceptors sensitivity) and in the plant gain (venous pulmonary congestion and low pulmonary functional residual capacity) are present too. The result of these alterations is a particular ventilatory pattern depending on controller gain overshooting and undershooting during $PaCO_2$ oscillations. When observing PSG, we will notice cycles of 3 consecutive central apneas or hypopneas separated by a crescendo–decrescendo shape tidal volume (Figure 1).

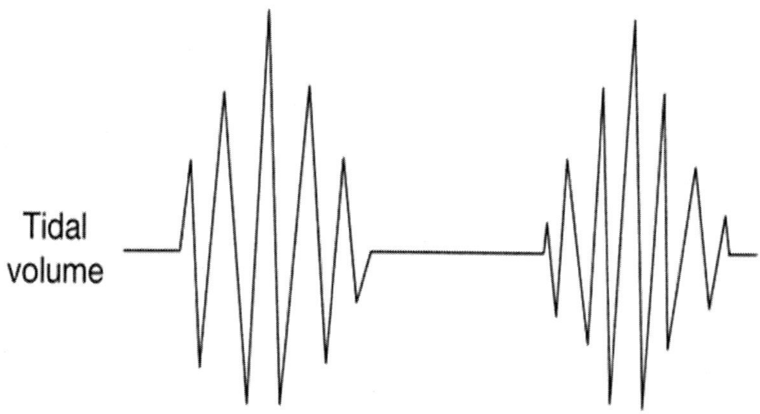

Figure 1. Simplicistic schematization of CSB pattern.

According to ICSD-3, the diagnostic criteria for CSA with CSB are the following:

- the presence of symptoms (A) OR atrial fibrillation/flutter, CHF, or a neurologic disorder (B)
- AND specific PSG characteristics (C)
- AND the disorder results to be not better explained by any other cause (D)

The symptoms criterion (A) includes one or more of the following: daytime sleepiness; difficulty initiating or maintaining sleep, frequent awakenings, or non-restorative sleep; awakening shortness of breath; snoring; witnessed apneas. PSG findings (C) should present ALL of the following: >5 central apneas/central hypopneas per hour of sleep; central events are >50% of all events; the pattern of ventilation meets criteria for CSB.

As already mentioned, CSB may be present after a stroke too, usually appearing in the acute phases. CSB tends to recover in the next weeks or months and it is not known its influence on stroke recovery.

As far as treatment is concerned, the first interventions aim to treat the medical condition underlying such disorder. In the case of the most frequent one, i.e., CHF, treatment options include diuretics, angiotensin- converting enzyme inhibitors (ACE-I) and beta-blockers; such therapeutical approaches seem to improve even AHI and quality of life in patients with CSA and CSB. Other therapeutic approaches applied in advanced CHF, like resynchronizing therapy, may also have a beneficial effect on CSA. However, despite the optimal CHF therapy, the presence of CSA requires specific treatment. The golden standard is application of positive airway pressure during sleep, although other non-positive airway pressure treatment modalities have been tried too.

CSA due to Medical Conditions without CSB

CSA may be a frequent finding in several diseases that may be systemic (e.g., diabetes mellitus, end-stage renal disease - ESRD), localized to the plant gain (e.g., interstitial lung disease, pulmonary hypertension), or to the controller gain (e.g., brainstem strokes, tumors). To note that even acromegaly is a condition which may often present CSA, even if, like the other ones mentioned above, OSA may coexist too. Regarding neurological affections, there are several diseases associated with CSA. Particularly, it can be the first manifestation of multiple system atrophy, can be found multiple sclerosis (i.e., brainstem demyelinating plaques) or Chiari type 1 malformation. Moreover, infectious diseases involving brainstem may trigger CSA too, as in the case of Listeria Monocytogenes rhombencephalitis.

The key for management here is to identify the medical condition that may cause CSAs and apply a specific therapy for it, while ventilatory management does not differ from the one applied to other syndromes. As far as ESRD CSA is concerned, possible strategies that revealed to be effective in reducing AHI and CSAs include supplemental nocturnal oxygen, bicarbonate buffer use during dialysis, and nocturnal dialysis.

CSA due to High Altitude Periodic Breathing

The higher the altitude, the lower the barometric pressure (PB), with a reduction of ambient $P0_2$ while the fraction of inspired oxygen remains constant at 20.93%. Reaching altitudes of 3500m or above, PB and PO_2 reach critical levels able to determine hypoxemia, with consequential hyperventilation. During sleep, such alterations establish a periodic pattern during which hypoxemia triggers hyperventilation, while consequent hypocapnia triggers CSAs. Such findings are frequent in lowlanders climbing at high altitudes, while tend to disappear with time thanks to adaptative mechanisms. Here, central apnea may respond to treatment with supplemental oxygen. Unfortunately, this type of CSA is difficult to treat and is likely to lead to a higher level of untreated OSA among these patients. An alternative treatment modality (with O_2 more effective than CPAP/Bilevel PAP) results in an optimal/good opportunity in patients developing central apnea at high altitude.

CSA due to a Medication or Substance

The medications or substances involved most in respiratory alterations are represented by opioids. Opioids are natural or synthetic agents able to activate some particular classes of G protein-coupled receptors (i.e., δ, k and μ) localized in central and peripheral nervous system and in the respiratory tract. Such receptors are involved in pain processing and other neurologic functions. In particular, the stimulation of μ receptors causes respiratory depression, inducing a dose-dependent reduction in respiratory rate and tidal volume. Moreover, opioids tend to decrease hypoxic and hypercapnic ventilatory responsiveness. All these alterations are responsible for a higher risk of sleep-related breathing disorders (SBD), with a predisposition for central apneas. CSA during opioids therapy may occur with two patterns: cluster breathing and ataxic/Biot's breathing. The former is composed of variable duration CSAs separated by cyclic hyperventilation with constant tidal volume, while the latter is made up of a breath with variable amplitude and rate of tidal volume, with intermittent variable CSAs. As already mentioned above, the first therapeutical approach aims to reduce opioid doses, since the effect on central apneas is dose dependent. If such therapeutical variation is not possible, bilevel positive pressure with a fast back-up rate (12 to 16 breaths per minute) or adaptive servoventilation may be useful for the treatment of such condition.

Primary CSA

This condition is identifiable when no other causative etiology or any pathognomonic respiratory pattern (e.g., CSB) is found, so that we talk about idiopathic CSA (ICSA). Furthermore, PSG diagnostic criteria establish that 5 or more events of central apneas/hypopneas (representing more than 50% of the total number of apneas/hypopneas) need to be identified. The pathophysiology is attributable to a high controller and plant gain, while no increase in effective circulatory time is observed. Here, repetitive episodes of CSA are detectable during N1 and N2 phases of NREM sleep, with periodic breathing cycles of 20-40s length (shorter than CSB). Particularly, the apnea event ends with a large breath, concomitant with an arousal. Moreover, no crescendo-decrescendo ventilatory pattern is observed in the periodic breathing.

ICSA shows an infrequent occurrence, therefore there is limited evidence about specific therapeutic interventions and just few studies may be found. Apart from PAP, a significant reduction in AHI, CSA index and an amelioration of symptoms has been detected administering nocturnal carbon dioxide, using acetazolamide therapy, zolpidem, or triazolam. Since the associated risk of respiratory depression, zolpidem or triazolam therapy should be used as last choice.

Treatment-Emergent Central Sleep Apnea

Previously called Complex CSA, this form of apnea was practically born together with CPAP therapy. The diagnostic criteria see the presence of 5 or more events of obstructive sleep apneas/hypopneas per hour during a diagnostic PSG followed by, successively, the presence of 5 or more events of central sleep apneas/hypopneas per hour (representing > 50% of total apneas/hypopneas) during the CPAP titration. Several authors consider treatment-emergent CSA as the result of sleep fragmentation and sleep stage shift occurring during initial phases of CPAP therapy. Moreover, it seems to be a self-limiting disorder, resolving spontaneously in 50-90% of patients undergoing CPAP therapy. As far as pathogenesis is concerned, treatment-emergent CSA includes both an increased upper airway resistance with elevated critical closing pressure (Pcrit), accompanied by increased ventilatory effort. Once on CPAP, CSA physiology will predominate or emerge with the absence of ventilatory effort during apneas likely due to chemoresponsive ventilatory dysregulation (high loop gain).

The treatment options are to either continue using CPAP assessing whether central apneas naturally resolve (which occurs frequently, as already mentioned) or using positive airway pressure (PAP) to either bilevel mode (BPAP) with a backup rate or adaptive servoventilation (ASV).

CSA of Infancy and of Prematurity

In addition to adult syndromes, it is worth to cite that CSA may occur in the infancy too. The pathophysiologic mechanism starts with an arousal or a desaturation that triggers a brief hyperventilation with a concomitant sudden reduction of $PaCo_2$ levels, reaching the apnea threshold. So, a CSA occurs, determining a rapid desaturation again, since the low functional residual lung capacity (FRC) in infants. Some infants may show an elevated CSA number, configuring a pathologic condition that is more frequent in premature ones, due to an immature respiratory control system.

When therapy is required, the approaches to CSA in infancy include the use of respiratory stimulants (methylxanthines), as well as stabilizers of respiratory control (oxygen with or without ventilatory support). Methylxanthines (caffeine and theophyllines) resulted to be effective for CSA treatment in premature infants. Since hypoxia is a trigger for periodic breathing and central apneas in infants, another therapeutical approach is constituted by nocturnal supplemental oxygen. Evidence revealed how such therapy leads to a reduction in the number of central apneas and to an abolition of periodic breathing. A reduction in central apneas with oxygen treatment has also been reported in infants with Prader–Willi syndrome.

HYPOVENTILATION SYNDROMES

Among sleep breathing disorders (SBDs) associated with a reduced ventilatory effort it is worth to cite hypoventilation syndromes. The main characteristic of such syndromes is a rise in blood $PaCo_2$ during NREM sleep, which may persist even during wakefulness. Pathogenetically, the alveolar hypoventilation may be due to a reduced respiratory rate (RR) or to an increase of the dead space volume (V_d), which is not useful for gas exchange. The cause of the former may reside in ventilatory control abnormalities, while the latter may be due to alterations in pulmonary mechanics.

The ICSD-3 describes six subtypes of hypoventilation disorders in the chapter of SBDs[3]:

- Obesity hypoventilation syndrome (OHS)
- Congenital central alveolar hypoventilation syndrome (CCHS)
- Late-onset central hypoventilation syndrome with hypothalamic dysfunction (LO-CHS/HD)
- Idiopathic central alveolar hypoventilation
- Sleep related hypoventilation due to a medication or substance
- Sleep related hypoventilation due to a medical disorder

We will discuss the main characteristics and management of such syndromes.

Obesity Hypoventilation Syndrome

Obesity hypoventilation syndrome (OHS, also historically described as the Pickwickian syndrome) is defined as BMI > 30 Kg/m^2 combined with sleep disordered breathing and daytime hypercapnia ($PaCo_2$ > 45mmHg), not otherwise explained by any other condition. In the general population prevalence is around 0.15-0.30%, while among OSA patients who refer to a sleep center it may be calculated around 10% and it increases with the increase of BMI.

Pathogenesis sees three main alterations: i) obesity-related changes in the respiratory system (i.e., restrictive syndrome due to fat deposit limiting diaphragm and rib cage movements, with an increased effort required for breathing that needs to be compensated by an augmented drive from the respiratory centers); ii) alterations in respiratory drive (firstly REM sleep hypoventilations occur, maybe due to a leptin resistance leading to reduced central drive, secondly the hypoventilation perpetuates even during wakefulness); and iii) breathing abnormalities during sleep (i.e., obstructive sleep apneas).

Clinically, OHS patients tend to be severely obese (BMI ⩾40 kg/m^2), to show OSAs (AHI ⩾ 30) and they are typically hypersomnolent. Moreover, patients with OHS are more likely to report dyspnea and to manifest pulmonary hypertension compared to patients with eucapnic OSA and similar BMI.

OHS is typically diagnosed either when an affected patient reaches a state of acuity, in the form of acute-on-chronic hypercapnic respiratory failure, or, alternatively, when performing ambulatory visits by pulmonary or sleep specialists. Blood gas analysis and PSG are central diagnostic tools able to demonstrate hypercapnia (even during wakefulness) and sleep disordered breathing, respectively.

As far as therapeutic interventions are concerned, the principal one is constituted by positive airway pressure (PAP) treatment. Both CPAP and NIV are effective, even if the former will be better for OHS patients presenting several OSAs, while the latter will be better for patients showing severe alterations in respiratory mechanics, severe hypercapnia and typical REM sleep hypoventilation. In addition to classic ventilatory interventions, it is even necessary a multimodal therapeutic approach combining strategies aimed at weight loss and increased physical activity. In the case of an acute-on-chronic hypercapnic respiratory failure, NIV should administered within one hour since the presentation to the emergency department and should be used as much as tolerated for the first 24 hours.

Congenital Central Alveolar Hypoventilation Syndrome (CCHS)

Also known as Ondine's curse, is a rare disease due to a mutation in the PHOX2B gene of chromosome 4p12. The spectrum of hypoventilation is varied, most cases are found in newborns, even if mild cases may be identified in adults too. During perinatal sleep, particularly NREM sleep, it is possible to note nocturnal shallow breathing or central apneas with cyanosis. The pathogenesis is not completely understood, but authors hypothesized that the alteration may lay in brain areas assigned to the integration of afferent chemoreceptor signals for ventilation. During wakefulness such alterations may not be present, thanks conscious behaviors. Unfortunately, the mortality rate is around 38% at about 3 months of life. Moreover, CCHS may be associated with other pathological conditions, such as Hirschsprung disease (aganglionic megacolon), neural crest tumors (e.g., neuroblastomas), and ocular abnormalities (e.g., strabismus).

Diagnosis sees PSG as first approach, showing hypoventilation (hypercapnia and hypoxemia), typically more severe during NREM sleep than REM one or wakefulness. The typical pattern is a reduction in RR and of airflow and tidal volume; low or absent ventilatory responses to hypercapnia or hypoxia may be present too. When in presence of the above-mentioned PSG findings, diagnosis may be confirmed by PHOX2B genetic testing.

As far as respiratory management is concerned, cyclic respiratory assessments are needed during lifetime, at least annually. Regarding therapeutic interventions, the only available options are constituted by ventilatory support: i) Positive pressure ventilation via tracheostomy, ii) Positive pressure ventilation via mask, iii) Phrenic nerve pacing, iv) and Negative pressure ventilation. The choice of intervention and the change from one to another are influenced by a several factors, such as patient's age, disease onset age, duration of ventilator dependency, and the patient's and families' wishes. The decision should be individualized, taking into account risks and benefits of each therapy. Finally, therapeutic interventions may include CCHS associated conditions too (e.g., gastroenteric or cardiologic support).

Late-Onset Central Hypoventilation Syndrome with Hypothalamic Dysfunction

Late-onset central hypoventilation syndrome with hypothalamic dysfunction (LO-CHS/HD) usually presents with sleep related hypoventilation episodes after the first year of life. Moreover, patients present with obesity, endocrine abnormalities referrable to hypothalamic dysfunction, tumors of neural crest origin and mood disorders or abnormal behaviors (at least two out of these four findings are required). As additional criteria, mutations of the PHOX2B-gene and other disorders explaining hypoventilation have to be excluded. Diagnosis is based on the recognition of central sleep hypoventilation at PSG, together with at least two of the up mentioned clinical characteristics (imaging, blood samples and cognitive evaluation are requested).

Ventilatory support does not substantially differ from the other syndromes, while here a multimodal approach is needed with hormonal correction (hypothalamus-hypophysis axis dysfunction) and child psychiatric support.

Idiopathic Central Alveolar Hypoventilation

Idiopathic central alveolar hypoventilation is a diagnosis of exclusion, that can be suspected if any alteration of lung parenchyma, airways, rib cage or neuromuscular diseases (NMD), drug treatment, obesity or congenital hypoventilation is ruled out. The pathophysiology is not clear yet, though it could possibly involve an impairment of the hypercapnic and hypoxic chemoresponsiveness and respiratory drive. The management of this disorder does not differ from CCHS one.

Sleep Related Hypoventilation due to a Medication or Substance

Certain drugs, which act depressing ventilatory drive or impairing muscle function, may sometimes be the cause of sleep related hypoventilations (SRHs). The drugs associated most with this phenomenon are constituted by opiates and benzodiazepine receptor agonists (BRAs), and their effect is more frequent in populations with risk factors for hypoventilation (e.g., obesity, respiratory or neuromuscular disease, preexisting OSA). As far as opiates are concerned, the mechanism may be due to a reduction of upper airway muscle tone or to a reduction of respiratory rate and irregular breathing (ataxic breathing). As per BRAs, they reduce muscle tone in the upper airway, as well as reduce the chemoreceptor response to hypoxia.

To manage drug-induced hypoventilation during sleep, a dose reduction or a complete termination of the drug treatment must first be considered, monitoring the effects of such dose reduction on respiratory function. If the treatment with the specific medication needs to be continued, a specific treatment for SRH must be initiated and noninvasive ventilation (e.g., bilevel) is recommended.

Sleep Related Hypoventilation due to a Medical Disorder

This condition may be found when hypoventilation is present in a patient with alterations of lung parenchyma, airways (e.g., chronic obstructive lung disease, advanced restrictive syndromes). Here ventilatory drive is preserved, but gas exchange is limited by airway resistance or parenchymal damage. Furthermore, other etiologies may involve neuromuscular diseases (e.g., spinal muscular atrophy, myotonic dystrophy), chest wall abnormalities (e.g., kyphoscoliosis) or neurologic alterations (e.g., cervical spinal cord injury or brainstem pathologic involvement). Apart from PSG, that shows sleep related hypoventilation episodes, diagnostics may include lung function tests, imaging (i.e., thoracic CT scan, brain and/or spinal cord MRI) or a specialist consult. As far as therapy is concerned, it should be focused on resolving the main causal condition of hypoventilation.

References

Alattar MA, Scharf SM. Opioid-associated central sleep apnea: a case series. *Sleep Breath* 2009; 13(2):201-206.

Alexiev F, Brill AK, Ott SR, Duss S, Schmidt M, Bassetti CL. Sleep-disordered breathing and stroke: chicken or egg? *J Thorac Dis.* 2018; 10 (Suppl 34): S4244-S4252. doi: 10.21037/jtd.2018.12.66.

American Academy of Sleep Medicine. *International Classification of Sleep Disorders*, 3rd ed. Darien, IL: American Academy of Sleep Medicine, 2014.

Amiel J, Laudier B, Attié-Bitach T, et al. Polyalanine expansion and frameshift mutations of the paired like homeobox gene PHOX2B in congenital central hypoventilation syndrome. *Nat Genet* 2003; 33:459-61.

Antic NA, Malow BA, Lange N, McEvoy RD, Olson AL, Turkington P, Windisch W, Samuels M, Stevens CA, Berry-Kravis EM, Weese-Mayer DE. PHOX2B mutation-confirmed congenital central hypoventilation syndrome: presentation in adulthood. *Am J Respir Crit Care Med.* 2006 Oct 15; 174(8):923-7. doi: 10.1164/rccm. 200605-607CR. Epub 2006 Jul 27. PMID: 16873766.

Aurora, R. Nisha, Susmita Chowdhuri, Kannan Ramar, Sabin R. Bista, Kenneth R. Casey, Carin I. Lamm, David A. Kristo, Jorge M. Mallea, James A. Rowley, Rochelle S. Zak, Sharon L. Tracy, The Treatment of Central Sleep Apnea Syndromes in Adults: Practice Parameters with an Evidence-Based Literature Review and Meta-Analyses, *Sleep,* Volume 35, Issue 1, 1 January 2012, Pages 17–40, https://doi.org/10.5665/sleep.1580.

Balachandran JS, Masa JF, Mokhlesi B. Obesity Hypoventilation Syndrome Epidemiology and Diagnosis. *Sleep Med Clin.* 2014; 9(3):341-347. doi: 10.1016/j.jsmc.2014.05.007.

Bassetti C, Aldrich MS. Sleep apnea in acute cerebrovascular diseases: final report on 128 patients. *Sleep.* 1999 Mar 15;22(2):217-23. doi: 10.1093/sleep/22.2.217. PMID: 10201066.

Berry RB, et al. (2012) Rules for scoring respiratory events in sleep: update of the 2007 AASM Manual for the Scoring of Sleep and Associated Events. Deliberations of the Sleep Apnea Definitions Task Force of the American Academy of Sleep Medicine. *J Clin Sleep Med* 8(5):597–619.

Bixler EO, Vgontzas AN, Lin HM, Ten Have T, Rein J, Vela-Bueno A, Kales A. Prevalence of sleep-disordered breathing in women: effects of gender. *Am J Respir Crit Care Med.* 2001 Mar;163 (3 Pt 1):608-13. doi: 10.1164/ajrccm.163.3.9911064. PMID: 11254512.

Bixler EO, Vgontzas AN, Ten Have T, Tyson K, Kales A. Effects of age on sleep apnea in men: I. Prevalence and severity. *Am J Respir Crit Care Med.* 1998 Jan; 157(1):144-8. doi: 10.1164/ajrccm.157. 1.9706079. PMID: 9445292.

Böing S, Randerath WJ. Chronic hypoventilation syndromes and sleep-related hypoventilation. *J Thorac Dis.* 2015; 7(8):1273-1285. doi: 10.3978/j.issn.2072-1439.2015.06.10.

Bonnet M, Dexter J, Arand D. The effect of triazolam on arousal and respiration in central sleep apnea patients. *Sleep* 1990; 13:31-41.

Bradley TD, Floras JS. Sleep apnea and heart failure: Part II: central sleep apnea. *Circulation.* 2003 Apr 8;107(13):1822-6. doi: 10.1161/01.CIR.0000061758.05044.64. PMID: 12682029.

Bradley TD, McNicholas WT, Rutherford R, et al. Clinical and physiologic heterogeneity of the central sleep apnea syndrome. *Am Rev Respir Dis* 1986; 134:217-221.

Braley TJ, Boudreau EA. Sleep disorders in multiple sclerosis. *Curr Neurol Neurosci Rep.* 2016; 16:50.

Braley TJ, Segal BM, Chervin RD. Sleep-disordered breathing in multiple sclerosis. *Neurology.* 2012; 79:929–936.

Cassel W et al. (2011) A prospective polysomnographic study on the evolution of complex sleep apnoea. *Eur Respir J* 38(2): 329–337.

Cutrufello NJ, Ianus VN, Rowley JA. Opioids and sleep. *Curr Opin Pulm Med.* 2020 Nov; 26(6):634-641. doi: 10.1097/MCP.0000000000000733. PMID: 32925368.

De Backer W, Verbraecken J, Willemen M, Wittesaele W, De Cock W, Van de Heyning P. Central apnea index decreases after prolonged treatment with acetazolamide. *Am J Respir Crit Care Med* 1995; 151:87-91.

De Pontual L, Trochet D, Caillat-Zucman S, Abou Shenab OA, Bougneres P, Crow Y, Cunningham S, Esteva B, Heberle LC, Leger J, Pinto G, Polak M, Shafik MH, Straus C, Trang H, Munnich A, Lyonnet S, Desguerre I, Amiel J. Delineation of late onset hypoventilation associated with hypothalamic dysfunction syndrome. *Pediatr Res.* 2008 Dec; 64(6):689-94. doi: 10.1203/PDR.0b013e318187dd0e. PMID: 18670370.

De Stefano, A., Di Giovanni, P., Kulamarva, G., Gennachi, S., Di Fonzo, F., Sallustio, V., Patrocinio, D., Candido, S., Lamarca, G., Dispenza, F. Oropharyngeal dysphagia in elderly population suffering from mild cognitive impairment and mild dementia: Understanding the link (2020) *American Journal of Otolaryngology - Head and Neck Medicine and Surgery,* 41 (4), art. no. 102501.

De Stefano, A., Dispenza, F., Kulamarva, G., Lamarca, G., Faita, A., Merico, A., Sardanelli, G., Gabellone, S., Antonaci, A. Predictive factors of severity and persistence of oropharyngeal dysphagia in sub-acute stroke (2020) *European Archives of Oto-Rhino-Laryngology,* doi: 10.1007/s00405-020-06429-2.

Donovan LM, Kapur VK. Prevalence and Characteristics of Central Compared to Obstructive Sleep Apnea: Analyses from the Sleep Heart Health Study Cohort. *Sleep.* 2016 Jul 1; 39(7):1353-9. doi: 10.5665/sleep.5962.

Eckert DJ, Jordan AS, Merchia P, Malhotra A. Central sleep apnea: pathophysiology and treatment. *Chest.* 2007; 131(2):595–607.

Edwards BA, Malhotra A, Sands SA. Adapting our approach to treatment-emergent central sleep apnea. *Sleep.* 2013; 36(8):1121-1122. Published 2013 Aug 1. doi: 10.5665/sleep.2862.

Fahey PJ, Hyde RW. "Won't breathe" vs "can't breathe." Detection of depressed ventilatory drive in patients with obstructive pulmonary disease. *Chest* 1983; 84:19-25.

Ferini-Strambi L, Marelli S. Sleep dysfunction in multiple system atrophy. *Curr Treat Options Neurol.* 2012; 14:464–473.

Ferre A, Poca MA, de la Calzada MD, et al. Sleep-related breathing disorders in Chiari malformation type 1: a prospective study of 90 patients. *Sleep.* 2017;40.

Findley LJ, Ries AL, Tisi GM, et al. Hypoxemia during apnea in normal subjects: mechanisms and impact of lung volume. *J Appl Physiol* 1983; 55:1777-1783.

Glenn W, Phelps M, Gersten L, Diaphragm pacing in the management of central alveolar hypoventilation. In: Guilleminault C, Dement W, editors. *Sleep apnea syndromes,* New York: Alan R Liss; 1978. p. 333-345.

Grote L. Drug-Induced Sleep-Disordered Breathing and Ventilatory Impairment. *Sleep Med Clin.* 2018 Jun;13(2):161-168. doi: 10.1016/j.jsmc.2018.03.003. PMID: 29759267.

Guilleminault C, Stoohs R, Schneider H, et al. Central alveolar hypoventilation and sleep. Treatment by intermittent positivepressure ventilation through nasal mask in an adult. *Chest* 1989; 96:1210-1212.

Guilleminault C, van den Hoed J, Mitler MM. Clinical overview of the sleep apnea syndromes. In: Guilleminault C, Dement W, editors. *Sleep apnea syndromes.* New York: Alan R Liss; 1978. p.1-12.

Hanly P, Pierratos A. Improvement of sleep apnea in patients with chronic renal failure who undergo nocturnal hemodialysis. *N Engl J Med* 2001; 344:102-7.

Henderson-Smart DJ, De Paoli AG. Methylxanthine treatment for apnoea in preterm infants. *Cochrane Database Syst Rev* 2010; 12: CD000140.

Hernandez AB, Patil SP. Pathophysiology of central sleep apneas. *Sleep Breath.* 2016; 20:467–482.

Javaheri S, Malik A, Smith J, et al. Adaptive pressure support servoventilation: a novel treatment for sleep apnea associated with use of opioids. *J Clin Sleep Med* 2008; 4:305-310.

Javaheri S, Parker TJ, Liming JD, Corbett WS, Nishiyama H, Wexler L, Roselle GA. Sleep apnea in 81 ambulatory male patients with stable heart failure. Types and their prevalences, consequences, and presentations. *Circulation.* 1998 Jun 2; 97(21):2154-9. doi: 10. 1161/01.cir.97.21.2154. PMID: 9626176.

Javaheri S, Smith J, Chung E (2009). The prevalence and natural history of complex sleep apnea. *J Clin Sleep Med* 5(3):205–211 163.

Javaheri S.: "Sleep disorders in systolic heart failure: a prospective study of 100 male patients. The final report." *Int J Cardiol* 2006; 106: 21.

Jean G, Piperno D, Francois B, Charra B. Sleep apnea incidence in maintenance hemodialysis patients: influence of dialysate buffer. *Nephron* 1995; 71:138-42.

Johnson PL, Edwards N, Burgess KR, Sullivan CE. Sleep architecture changes during a trek from 1400 to 5000 m in the Nepal Himalaya. *J Sleep Res.* 2010 Mar; 19(1 Pt 2):148-56. doi: 10.1111/j.1365-2869.2009.00745.x. Epub 2009 Aug 3. PMID: 19663929.

Kumagai T, Ishibashi Y, Kawarazaki H, et al. Effects of nocturnal oxygen therapy on sleep apnea syndrome in peritoneal dialysis patients. *Clin Nephrol* 2008; 70:332-9.

Kuzniar TJ et al. (2008) Natural course of complex sleep apnea – a retrospective study. *Sleep Breath* 12(2):135–139.

Lamba J, Simpson CS, Redfearn DP, Michael KA, Fitzpatrick M, Baranchuk A (2011) Cardiac resynchronization therapy for the treatment of sleep apnoea: a meta-analysis. *Europace* 13(8):1174–1179.

Launois SH, Siyanko N, Joyeux-Faure M, et al. Acquired c entral hypoventilation following Listeria monocytogenes rhombencephalitis. *Thorax.* 2017; 72:763–765.

Lee WY, Mokhlesi B. Diagnosis and management of obesity hypoventilation syndrome in the ICU. *Crit Care Clin* 2008; 24: 533-549.

Lorusso, F., Martines, F., Mistretta, A., ...Dispenza, F., Gallina, S.Effects of adenotonsillectomy on neurocognitive and behavioural function in pediatric obstructive sleep apnea syndrome. *B-ENT* 2018; 14:113-118.

Malhotra A, Bertisch S, Wellman A (2008). Complex sleep apnea: it isn't really a disease. *J Clin Sleep Med* 4(5):406–408.

Manning DJ, Stothers JK. Sleep stage, hypoxia and periodic breathing in the neonate. *Acta Paediatr Scand* 1991; 80: 763–769.

Martin RJ, Sanders MH, Gray BA, et al. Acute and long-term ventilatory effects of hyperoxia in the adult sleep apnea syndrome. *Am Rev Respir Dis* 1982; 125:175-180.

Martins RT, Eckert DJ. Central sleep apnea due to other medical disorders. *Sleep Med Clin.* 2014; 9:57–67.

Masa JF, Corral J, Alonso ML, et al. Efficacy of different treatment alternatives for obesity hypoventilation syndrome. Pickwick Study. *Am J Respir Crit Care Med* 2015; 192: 86-95.

Masa JF, Corral J, Caballero C, et al. Non-invasive ventilation in obesity hypoventilation syndrome without severe obstructive sleep apnoea. *Thorax* 2016; 71: 899-906.

Masa JF, Pépin JL, Borel JC, et al. Obesity hypoventilation syndrome. *Eur Respir Rev* 2019; 28: 180097.

Mellins RB, Balfour HH Jr, Turino GM, Winters RW. Failure of automatic control of ventilation (Ondine's curse). Report of an infant born with this syndrome and review of the literature. *Medicine* (Baltimore). 1970; 49(6):487–504.

Mokhlesi B, Kryger MH, Grunstein RR. Assessment and management of patients with obesity hypoventilation syndrome. *Proc Am Thorac Soc.* 2008; 5(2): 218-25. https://doi.org/10.1513/pats.200708-122MG.

Mokhlesi B. Obesity hypoventilation syndrome: a state-of-the-art review. *Respir Care* 2010; 55: 1347-1362.

Orr JE, Malhotra A, Sands SA. Pathogenesis of central and complex sleep apnoea. *Respirology.* 2017 Jan; 22(1):43-52. doi: 10.1111/ resp.12927. Epub 2016 Oct 31. PMID: 27797160; PMCID: PMC5161664.

Pagel, J F et al. "The effects of altitude associated central apnea on the diagnosis and treatment of obstructive sleep apnea: comparative data from three different altitude locations in the mountain west." Journal of clinical sleep medicine: *JCSM: official publication of the American Academy of Sleep Medicine* vol. 7,6 (2011): 610-5A. doi: 10.5664/jcsm.1462.

Piper AJ. Obesity hypoventilation syndrome - the big and the breathless. *Sleep Med Rev.* 2011; 15(2):79-89. https://doi.org/10. 1016/j.smrv.2010.04.002.

Quadri S, Drake C, Hudgel DW. Improvement of idiopathic central sleep apnea with zolpidem. *J Clin Sleep Med* 2009; 5:122-9.

Raetzo MA, Junod AF, Kryger MH. Effect of aminophylline and relief from hypoxia on central sleep apnea due to medullary damage. *Bull Eur Physiopathol Respir* 1987; 23:171-175.

Randerath W, Verbraecken J, Andreas S, Arzt M, Bloch KE, Brack T, Buyse B, De Backer W, Eckert DJ, Grote L, Hagmeyer L, Hedner J, Jennum P, La Rovere MT, Miltz C, McNicholas WT, Montserrat J, Naughton M, Pepin JL, Pevernagie D, Sanner B, Testelmans D, Tonia T, Vrijsen B, Wijkstra P, Levy P. Definition, discrimination, diagnosis and treatment of central breathing disturbances during sleep. *Eur Respir J.* 2017 Jan 18; 49(1):1600959. doi: 10.1183/ 13993003.00959-2016. PMID: 27920092.

Randerath WJ, Treml M, Priegnitz C, et al. Evaluation of a noninvasive algorithm for differentiation of obstructive and central hypopneas. *Sleep.* 2013; 36:363–368.

Ratz D, Wiitala W, Badr MS, Burns J, Chowdhuri S. Correlates and consequences of central sleep apnea in a national sample of US veterans. *Sleep.* 2018; 41(9): zsy058. doi: 10.1093/sleep/zsy058.

Rigatto H, Brady JP. Periodic breathing and apnea in preterm infants. II. Hypoxia as a primary event. *Pediatrics* 1972; 50: 219–228.

Roehrs T, Conway W, Wittig R, et al. Sleep–wake complaints in patients with sleep-related respiratory disturbances. *Am Rev Respir Dis* 1985; 132:520-523.

Schroeder JS, Motta J, Guilleminault C. Hemodynamic studies in sleep apnea. In: Guilleminault C, Dement W, editors. *Sleep apnea syndromes,* New York: Alan R Liss; 1978. p. 177-196.

Simakajornboon N, Beckerman RC, Mack C, et al. Effect of supplemental oxygen on sleep architecture and cardiorespiratory events in preterm infants. *Pediatrics* 2002; 110: 884–888.

Sleep disorders medicine basic science, technical considerations and clinical aspects, BJ Selim et al., S. Chokroverty (ed.), *Sleep Disorders Medicine*, chapter 33 - Central Sleep Apnea, Hypoventilation Syndrome, and Sleep in High Altitude. Springer Science+Business Media New York 2017. doi: 10.1007/978-1-4939-6578-6_33.

Tamura A, Kawano Y, Naono S, Kotoku M, Kadota J (2007) Relationship between beta-blocker treatment and the severity of central sleep apnea in chronic heart failure. *Chest* 131(1):130–135.

Terziyski K, Draganova A. Central Sleep Apnea with Cheyne-Stokes Breathing in Heart Failure - From Research to Clinical Practice and Beyond. *Adv Exp Med Biol.* 2018; 1067:327-351. doi: 10.1007/5584_2018_146. PMID: 29411336.

Trang H et al. (2005) The French congenital central hypoventilation syndrome registry: General data, phenotype, and genotype. *Chest* 127(1):72–79.

Trang H, Samuels M, Ceccherini I, et al. Guidelines for diagnosis and management of congenital central hypoventilation syndrome. *Orphanet J Rare Dis.* 2020; 15(1):252. Published 2020 Sep 21. doi: 10.1186/s13023-020-01460-2.

Urquhart DS, Gulliver T, Williams G, et al. Central sleep-disordered breathing and the effects of oxygen therapy in infants with Prader-Willi syndrome. *Arch Dis Child;* 2013; 98: 592–595.

Urquhart DS, Tan HL. Sleep disordered breathing at the extremes of age: infancy. *Breathe (Sheff).* 2016; 12(1): e1-e11. doi: 10.1183/20734735.001016.

Walsh JT, Andrews R, Starling R, Cowley AJ, Johnston ID, Kinnear WJ (1995). Effects of captopril and oxygen on sleep apnoea in patients with mild to moderate congestive cardiac failure. *Br Heart J* 73(3): 237–241.

Xie A et al. (1994) Interaction of hyperventilation and arousal in the pathogenesis of idiopathic central sleep apnea. *Am J Respir Crit Care Med* 150(2):489–495.

Xie A et al. (1995) Hypocapnia and increased ventilatory responsiveness in patients with idiopathic central sleep apnea. *Am J Respir Crit Care Med* 152(6 Pt 1):1950–1955.

Xie A, Rankin F, Rutherford R, et al. Effects of inhaled CO2 and added dead space on idiopathic central sleep apnea. *J Appl Physiol* 1997; 82:918-926.

Xie A, Skatrud JB, Puleo DS, Rahko PS, Dempsey JA. Apnea-hypopnea threshold for CO2 in patients with congestive heart failure. *Am J Respir Crit Care Med.* 2002; 165:1245–50. [PubMed: 11991873].

Zhou XS, Rowley JA, Demirovic F, Diamond MP, Badr MS. Effect of testosterone on the apneic threshold in women during NREM sleep. *J Appl Physiol* (1985). 2003 Jan; 94(1):101-7. doi: 10.1152/jappl physiol.00264.2002. Epub 2002 Sep 13. PMID: 12391093.

Zutler M, Holty JE. Opioids, sleep, and sleep-disordered breathing. *Curr Pharm Des.* 2011;17(15):1443-9. doi: 10.2174/138161211796 197070. PMID: 21476955.

In: Advances in Sleep Apnea
Editors: F. Lorusso et al.
ISBN: 978-1-53619-758-7

Chapter 6

ADVANCES IN MANAGEMENT OF PEDIATRIC SLEEP APNEA

Antonella Mistretta, Alessia Ceraso, Rosalia Gargano, Salvatore Gallina and Francesco Lorusso*
Department of Otolaryngology, Head and Neck Surgery,
Policlinico Paolo Giaccone University of Palermo, Palermo, Italy

ABSTRACT

Numerous studies document that OSA in children shows peculiarities compared to adults, in particular from the clinical and prognostic pathophysiological aspect. Child is not a small adult and the pediatric OSAS has clinical characteristics that are completely different from those of the adult, so much so that while presenting some similarities with that of the adult, it is very different so as to make the definitions and criteria used for the diagnosis of OSA in the adult, not applicable to the pediatric age. Sleep disturbances in children includes snoring, upper airway resistance syndrome, nocturnal hypoventilation and OSAS in order of severity. The incidence of Obstructive sleep apnea syndrome

* Corresponding Author's Email: dott.francescolorusso@gmail.com.

(OSAS) in the pediatric population is about 2%. The diagnosis is based on the employment of questionnaires, but they are unable to differentiate OSAS from primary snoring. Instrumental differential diagnostic criteria between different conditions such as simple snoring, obstructive hypoventilation and OSAS are not yet well standardized and polysomnography (PSG) that is the gold standard also among children.

INTRODUCTION

Some epidemiological data: the age most involved is that between 2 and 6 years. Simple snoring is more common in children between the ages of 3 and 6. As for OSAS, the peak is found around 2.5 years in males and 4 years in females. There is no significant gender prevalence. Compared to adults, respiratory sleep disorders in pediatric age have some peculiarities that affect the risk of underestimation.

First of all, a higher frequency of obstructive hypoventilation is observed in children rather than periodic and distinct apnoic events. Furthermore, there is a poor correlation between the clinical data, daytime symptoms and OSAS severity.

Finally, the instrumental differential diagnostic criteria between different conditions such as simple snoring, obstructive hypoventilation and OSAS are not yet well standardized.

In particular, it is important to remember that in children OSAS is diagnosed even in the presence of an apnea-hypopnea index greater than 1 and that the syndrome is defined as severe when this index is greater than 10 events per hour.

Even mild-moderate forms can be responsible for neurobehavioral disorders with repercussions on psycho-physical development, and for reduced growth.

In severe forms, there may be important disorders affecting the cardiovascular system, therefore, it is necessary to arrive at an early and accurate diagnosis to prevent possible complications. It was also highlighted an increased energy consumption during sleep due to the high respiratory effort. Making an accurate diagnosis has important implications for treatment planning. It is in fact fundamental to formulate a balance of severity of the problem and consequently predict the degree of peri and post operative morbidity. Young patients affected by OSAS have an increased risk of developing peri and post-operative complications, especially in the presence of comorbidities and severe OSAS.

The management of these patients must involve different specialists (pediatrician, ENT and orthodontist) and must necessarily include a sleep study. From an anamnestic point of view in adults there are essential diagnostic elements such as daytime sleepiness associated with snoring and respiratory pauses.

In the child, however, the clinical picture is more nuanced and for this reason the simple clinical evaluation is often misleading. In fact, apneas occur mainly in the rem phase and therefore in the terminal phases of sleep when the parents are asleep. In addition, many ailments in the child are characterized by periods of sub-obstruction and hypoventilation without apnea. Another limitation of taking anamnesis is that many parents tend to overestimate their child's problem.

In the child, it is based on the parental anamnesis performed through the administration of questionnaires that have an high sensitivity and specificity, but in the various studies in the literature no reference is ever made to the AHI. As already mentioned, OSAS in pediatric patients has a multifactorial genesis.

The adeno-tonsillar hypertrophy, along with obesity, is one of the most frequent causes. More rarely, OSAS can be caused by craniofacial malformations and neuromuscular diseases. Pediatric OSA occurs mostly in infants and children below 6 years of age. Not all children with marked tonsillar hypertrophy are affected by OSA so there is an individual variability regarding the muscle tone of the VAS. In particular in obese children, tonsillar hypertrophy does not play a decisive role in the genesis of OSA. The presence of "dento-facial" anomalies is a frequent contributing cause of OSAS. For this reason, it is also important to involve the orthodontist in the clinical management of these young patients.

MAIN CHARACTERISTICS OF OSAHS IN CHILDREN

OSAHS (Obstructive sleep apnea/hypopnea syndrome) represents the most severe expression of sleep disordered breathing (SBD) in children. OSAHS is "is a disorder of breathing during sleep, characterised by prolonged partial upper airway obstruction and/or intermittent complete obstruction (obstructive apnoea), which disrupts normal ventilation during sleep and normal sleep patterns."

Several studies confirm how, despite the similar incidence between the two ages (2-4% vs 1-3%), pediatric OSAHS shows different clinical and prognostic pathophysiological peculiarities than in adult.

As confirmed by the ERS guidelines, the main risk factors for pediatric OSAHS are:

- adenotonsillar hypertrophy.
- Obesity.
- Allergic rhinitis (AR).
- Craniofacial dysmorphism.
- Neuromuscular pathologies.

Adenotonsillar hypertrophy is the main predisposing factor for the development of OSAHS in pediatric age, not by chance the peak incidence of both between 2 and 6 years coincides.

Obesity is the second most frequent risk factor for pediatric OSAHS. Each increase in BMI above the 50th percentile is associated with about 10% increased risk of OSAHS.

The coexistence of adenotonsillar hypertrophy and obesity leads to a higher risk of persistence of the pathology after adeno-tonsillectomy, as demonstrated by numerous studies.

Many studies have been conducted on the effectiveness of weight loss in adults with OSAHS, few in children; adequate long-term dietotherapy can provide great benefits and even healing from OSAHS in children who do not present other risk factors and comorbidity, as Andersen demonstrated in his recent study, confirming that in such cases first-line therapy is weight loss.

Allergic rhinitis can affect night rest in several ways; nasal congestion due to inflammation of the mucous membranes, causes an increase in resistances of the upper airways resulting in oral breathing and sleep disturbances.

With regard to dysmorphism and craniofacial paramorphisms, the ones that predispose to OSAHS are: retrognatics, micrognathia, mandibular or jaw hypoplasia, vertical craniofacial growth and a class II of malocclusion. We have alto to consider craniofacial dysmorphisms in the context of syndromic pathologies (such as Down syndromes, Crouzon, Apert, Prader-Willy) mandibular hypoplasia in syndromic contexts (such as Pierre Robin syndrome, Treacher-Collins, Goldenhar) with retrognathia or micrognathia, atresia or stenosis of the coanes, and partial or complete labio-palatoschisis.

Pediatric OSAHS differs from adult's one about etiopathogenetic, clinical and prognostic point of view. The question is whether these are different pathological processes or an identical pathology with different age-related manifestations. In current opinion, the first hypothesis seems to be correct; a patient suffering from OSAHS in childhood and, later, as an adult, is not affected by recurrence but by a new kind of pathology.

Obvious differences between adults and children already emerge from the polysomnographic study. Polysomnographic alterations of mild or medium severity in the adult correspond to a considerable severity in children, probably because oxygen desaturation may occur during short apnea, due to reduced lung functional capacity and more frequent respiratory rhythm that characterize this age; different classification of severity stages between adults and children has to be referred also to the important consequences that OSAHS has during development during growth.

Comparing electroencephalographic parameters in children and adults affected by OSAHS the first ones show a less fragmented sleep architecture; the result is a considerable limitation of daytime hypersomnia which is instead one of the most frequent clinical manifestations of OSAHS in adults. The negative consequence of this aspect is that less awakenings induce long and uninterrupted periods of obstructive hypoventilation.

In children a sleep that is insufficient or disturbed in its full performance and in the correct alternation of the phases that compose it, is the basis of the pathogenesis of neurocognitive and neurobehavioral disorders as well as reduced height-weight growth. Most of the data on this evidence was collected in children with SDB; in these patients the pathogenic mechanism is mainly related to two factors:

- hypoxia, due to obstructive apnea/hypopnea
- altered architecture of sleep.

As regards the symptoms of OSAHS from two years of age, we can divide them according to their day or night presentation.

Nocturnal Symptomatology

During the night, children suffering from OSAHS may show: *habitual snoring*, which is certainly one of the most frequent symptoms, but also difficult, noisy, and almost exclusive *oral breathing* in all cases of adenoid hypertrophy, in which the nasal airflow is obstructed, presence of *apneas* and *hypopneas, restlessness in sleep, profuse sweats, awakenings during night, nocturnal enuresis*. The re-proposal of nocturnal enuresis (at least three times a week for two weeks) after a period of absence of at least six months, in a child over 5 years of age if female, 6 if male, leads of course to the exclusion of pathologies such as diabetes mellitus, insipid diabetes, epilepsy and OSAHS.

Daytime Symptomatology

In children main daytime symptoms are hyperactivity, low concentration capacity, attention deficit, reduced learning skills, resulting in poor school performance. It is thought that nocturnal hypoxia and altered sleep architecture can cause such neurobehavioral and neurocognitive disorders.

In our Institute we carried out a study which analyzed the consequences of OSAHS on cognitive and neuro-behavioral profile of children; we assessed the benefits obtained by adeno-tonsillectomy on these subjects using two questionnaires:

- questionnaire for the evaluation of sleep disorders (SDSC-*Sleep Disturbance Scale for Children*, Bruni 1996),
- questionnaire for the evaluation of cognitive and behavioral disorders in wakefulness*(Conners scale,* Conners 1998, mod.).
- We compared the scores of the pre- and post-operative questionnaires, showing statistically significant results:
- Alteration of daytime cognitive and behavioral functions in patients with OSAHS.
- Resolution of the pathology after adeno-tonsillectomy in almost all cases.
- Drastic post-operative improvement of sleep quality and cognitive and behavioral disorders.

There are conflicting views in the literature on this symptomatic aspect of the OSAHS.

The randomized CHAT study pointed out that in patients affected by OSAHS who underwent AT, intellectual performance remains worse than healthy controls (perhaps related to persistent neurological hypoxic damage).

Growth Failure and OSAHS

While childhood obesity is a very important risk factor for OSAHS, growth failure in children can be a severe consequence of the disease. The causes seem to include low caloric intake associated with adenotonsillar hypertrophy, excessive caloric expenditure secondary to increased respiratory work, and an abnormal release of growth hormone, secondary to non-REM deep sleep loss.

Several studies show that the impaired quality of sleep in subjects with OSAHS, results in impaired functioning of GH production and, to a greater extent, of IGF-1, which is the main effector in growing mechanism.

In 2018, in our Institute we carried out a study on children with OSAHS (degree from mild to severe) between 3 and 7 years, in whom the main cause of pathology was adenotonsillar hypertrophy without comorbidity (obesity, craniofacial malformations, allergic rhinitis, etc.); these patients had reduced blood values of IGF-1 (normal GH values) and a reduced growth rate compared to healthy controls, evaluated using BMI values (% correct for sex and age), weight growth rate and height. After AT, the blood values of IGF-1 increased (statistically significantly) 3 months after surgery and control 12 months later. Similarly, the values of the auxological parameters returned to normal 12 months after AT (referring to the Italian growth curves of Cacciari).

According to ERS guidelines [5] the stepwise treatment approach to OSAHS has to be implemented until complete resolution of the disease.

The steps are the following:

1. Weight loss if child is overweight or obese.
2. Nasal corticosteroids and/or montelukast p.o.
3. Adenotonsillectomy.
4. Rapid maxillary expansion or orthodontic appliances.
5. CPAP or NPPV (for nocturnal hypoventilation).
6. Craniofacial surgery.
7. Tracheostomy.

Is nowadays confirmed the decisive role of adeno-tonsillectomy in the resolution of OSAHS when the main cause of pathology il adenotonsillar hypertrophy (AT leads in the various cases to an improvement and healing in 78-85% of cases).

ORAL EFFECT OF OBSTRUCTIVE SLEEP APNEA

The incorrect action of the buccinators, which can even be four times higher than normal, is the one we can see earlier, from the change in the inclination of the teeth of the lateral sectors (lingualization of the arches).

Normally the teeth should have an alignment that brings the forces to converge at the level of the crista galli lamina, point of discharge of the activation forces of cranial motility. In the presence of buccinator imbalances, on the other hand, we see a tendency to convergence of the teeth, the palate is ogival but also in cases where the palate remains more or less wide, however the size of the dental arch is reduced. When the palate is too narrow, orthodontic intervention is required very early because a language cannot be taught to swallow properly if the palate is too narrow.

One of the effects of the narrowing of the palate due to the action of the buccinators is the difficulty of eruption of the canines, a problem that occurs quite frequently, because the restriction of the palate occurs mainly at the level of the intercanine diameter. This is related to the fact that the fibers of the buccinator on one side pass under the orbicular and intersect with those of the buccinator on the opposite side.

Another consequence is represented by dental crowding, and the difficulty of exchange. But the palate that narrows is a palate that makes the mandible unstable, because by creating a disproportion between the lower arch and the narrow upper arch, it will no longer be possible to have consistent dental contacts, i.e., there will no longer be contact between a cusp and a fossa but often contacts will be created between the cusp and the cusp and therefore the lower arch will tend to move to the right or left to seek these coherent contacts, and at this point the position of the mandible will be decided by the muscle tone and the inclination of a cusp with respect to to the other, giving rise to the cruciate bite with the displacement of the midline. In fact, to obtain the maximum closure during swallowing, necessary to promote trigeminal stimulation, the strongest muscle will drag the jaw from that side, giving rise in many cases to the creation of a cross bite, which in cascade will drag a whole series of postural problems.

If we see that the mouth is centered in opening, but it moves in closing, we will know that it is not the jaw that is twisted but that it is deflected by the muscles during the occlusion.

Tongue-Mediated Actions

Several situations of imbalance can arise; the growing patient may present:

a situation in which the action of m. of the lips, of the orbicularis, with a tongue that pushes slightly forward, this will lead to teeth that tend to verticalize. The verticalization of the teeth always means mandibular retrusion with the mandible that work more posteriorly and the occlusion muscles that work no longer as an agonist - antagonist but in co-contraction. This is the most expensive mechanism that is used to operate the muscles and also the one that does the most damage to the joints.

We can have the lips and tongue more or less in balance, in this case the damage will initially be inapparent at the oral level, with a localization in other district.

Thrust of the tongue greater than the resistance capacity of the lips, in this case we will have a fanning of the teeth or diastemas will be created, it will be the easiest case to diagnose.

Due to its position and movement, the tongue can behave as a motive force or an inhibiting force or at the same time inhibiting and motive.

The tongue acts as an impeding force when it is interposed between the two dental arches and by interposing it inhibits their extrusion by preventing mutual contact: anterior or lateral open bite. The tongue acts as a driving force when it pushes on the teeth, especially the anterior ones, creating: diastemas, cross bites, or malocclusions such as the 2nd and 3rd dental classes.

Tongue as a driving force can also give paradontosis. In this pathology much importance has always been given to bacterial etiology, but it has been seen that the dysfunction often causes periodontal disease, and this is highlighted with the Payne technique which highlights the stress of the tongue right on the teeth where periodontosis is located.

A pathognomonic sign of dysfunctional swallowing is tartar on the vestibular surface of the teeth which is an expression of the thrust of the tongue on the teeth and therefore of the thrust of saliva through them.

The narrowing of the palate and its simultaneous elevation in the nasal cavities will lead as a further consequence to their narrowing, up to a possible deviation of the nasal septum. At this point we are witnessing a change in the respiratory dynamics that passes from nasal to oral breathing.

Facial Effects of Oral Breathing

Oral breathing continues even after an adenotonsillectomy and only after myofunctional therapy can we observe a return to nasal breathing. The pressure changes that are created in dysfunctional swallowing give rise to various pathologies of the ear: due to the positive pressure that occurs in the rear part of the pharynx during dysfunctional swallowing, there will no drainage of the secretions from the Eustachian tube into the pharynx, an action that normally takes place during every swallowing act, but there will be a stagnation or even an inversion of the flow of secretions inside the tubes that will tend to be pushed towards the ear causing a decrease in the vibratility of the tympanic membrane with possible catarrhal or purulent otitis and consequent transmission type hearing loss.

Craniofacial malformations such as orofacial cleft, craniostosis and mandibular dysostosis or craniofacial macroscopies are the most common at birth and are very often due to the use of teratogens such as drugs, high-dose ionizing radiation, viruses and maternal diseases For example, phenylketonuria or diabetes during gestation, can give craniofacial anomalies. For this reason, the correct medical history can help to understand any disorders in the child.The upper airways are like a collapsible tube and their flexibility increases during the rest, therefore extrinsic factors such as atypical craniofacial features can increase the risk of collapse of the airways.

Damages of the Extrinsic Musculature of the Upper Airways

Let's try to clarify the fetal and newborn development of the face and oral cavity: the first face shape appears around the fourth week of fetal development and by the twelfth week the first areas of ossification appear and the bone replaces. At the same time, postnatal development is rapid too: the head, which accounts for nearly a quarter of the child's length at birth, is about 12 percent of what it will be in adulthood. Sixty percent of the adult-sized face develops around six years of age. During infancy and early childhood, the skull base increases in length through endochondral ossification which occurs at important growth sites called synchondrosis, two of these growth centers: intermaxillary synchondrosis and the dental alveolus ligament, are active until at puberty. Skull base growth is the essential engine of facial growth through ossification. The maxillary bone and mandible are pulled down and forward by the muscles to which they are attached.

The development of the oral cavity and tongue: begins around the second month of pregnancy, when the cells of the neural crest migrate. The movement of the fetal tongue between the sixth and tenth gestational week allows the closure of the primitive mouth of the fetus (the stomodeo).

Importance of physiological nasal breathing: there are studies that show how the limitation of nasal airflow, posteriorly up to the nasopharynx, influences the correct development of both the jaw and the sinus paranasal, since bone resorption of the periosteum is not favored. From these studies it appears that if the nasal cavity is narrowed to one side, there will be a palatal asymmetry with hypoplasia of the side of the palate corresponding to the nasal cavity hypoplasia and decreases in size.

The turbinates then usually decrease in size rapidly, but at birth they participate in the high nasal resistance. The usual rapid reduction in the size of the turbinates will not occur if there is inflammation of the nasal mucosa. Nasal breathing is not the only function with a very important role in orofacial development. Coordination between nasal breathing and sucking must also develop very early in life. An increased resistance to nasal breathing leads to an abnormal orofacial development of the mandible and therefore according to these studies, by maintaining adequate lumen of the upper airways, the onset of OSA can be prevented.

Correlation between prematurity and AHI: from various studies it appears that in full term babies, the average palatal length (hard palate) is 24 mm, in pre-term babies it seems to be 16 mm. AHI in preterm births on polysomnography is 0.3, pre-term babies appear to be much more. Therefore, there is a correlation between premature and elevated AHI and a shorter palatal length. In preterm births, the type of breathing is more oral than in term births, associated with hypotonia of the muscles.

During the first two years of life, the skull grows very quickly and triples its volume, to adapt to the expansion of the brain mass, until it reaches 95% of its development around 10 years.

The facial mass, on the other hand, at the same age, only completed 75% of its growth, and then became more active with the development of the upper jaw and mandible, as well as with the completion of the permanent dentition.

More specifically, the response of the maxilla stops 18/24 months before the mandible and the latter ends its growth about 2 years after the end of the statural growth.

Patients in this phase have various associated problems including dental crowding and non-definitive deciduous teeth, a growt of the skull that is not perfectly concluded, a reduced compliance in assessing the right consistencies of foods. In addition, an ENT that evaluates the problematic swallowing/adenoid hypertrophy and tonsillar hypertrophy under various aspects, must also evaluate the various objective parameters of the polygraphic examination, the AHI (Apnea Hypopnea Index), the patient's clinic, at the same time direct the patient for evaluation dentistry and speech therapy and review the patient in light of all these investigations.

A separate chapter is represented by children with craniofacial malformations. Typically, 60% of these patients require airway surgery, in most cases within the first month of life. The type of intervention varies and is modulated according to the degree and level of obstruction.

Also, in the context of children with craniofacial malformations, in mild to moderate forms, positional therapy or the use of a nasopharyngeal brace or CPAP may be sufficient. In severe forms, if mandibular hypoplasia is present, primary osteodistraction is indicated. In some cases, tracheostomy may also be indicated.

References

Akre H, Overland B, Asten P, et al. Obstructive sleep apnea in Treacher Collins syndrome. *Eur Arch Otorhinolaryngol* 2012; 269: 331–337.

American Academy of Pediatrics. Clinical practice guideline: diagnosis and management of childhood obstructive sleep apnea syndrome. *Pediatrics.* 2002 Apr; 109(4):704-12.

American Thoracic Society. Standards and indications for cardiopulmonary sleep studies in children. *Am J Respir Crit Care Med.* 1996; 153:866–878.

Andersen, IG, Holmb, JC, Homøea, P. Impact of weight-loss management on children and adolescents with obesity and obstructive sleep apnea. *Int. J. Pediatr. Otorhinolaryngol.* 2019, 123, 57–62.

Bruni, Oliviero, et al. "The Sleep Disturbance Scale for Children (SDSC) Construct ion and validation of an instrument to evaluate sleep disturbances in childhood and adolescence." *Journal of sleep research* 5.4 (1996): 251-261.

Bruno A, Di Sano C, Lorusso F, Dino P, Russo D, Ballacchino A, Gallina S, Modica DM, Chiappara G, Simon HU, Pace E. Notch-1 decreased expression contributes to leptin receptor downregulation in nasal epithelium from allergic turbinates. *Biochim Biophys Acta Mol Basis Dis.* 2019 Jun 1;1865(6):1642-1650.

Burton MJ, Glasziou PP. Tonsillectomy or adeno-tonsillectomy versus nonsurgical treatment for chronic/recurrent acute tonsillitis. *Cochrane Database Syst Rev.* 2009;(1):CD001802.

Cassano, M., et al. "Modification of growth, immunologic and feeding parameters in children with OSAS after adenotonsillectomy." *Acta Otorhinolaryngologica Italica* 38.2 (2018): 124.

Cassano P, Cassano M. *Roncopatia in età pediatrica* [*Snoring in the pediatric age*]. Clinica ORL, facoltà di medicina, Università degli studi di Foggia. Congresso nazionale SIO (Società italiana di Otorinolaringologia e Chirurgia Cervico-facciale) 2004.

Choi JH, Kim EJ, Choi J, Kwon SY, Kim TH, Lee SH, Lee HM, Shin C, Lee SH. Obstructive sleep apnea syndrome: a child is not just a small adult. *Ann Otol Rhinol Laryngol.* 2010 Oct; 119(10):656-61. doi: 10.1177/000348941011901002. PMID: 21049849.

Conners, C. Keith, et al. "The revised Conners' Parent Rating Scale (CPRS-R): factor structure, reliability, and criterion validity." *Journal of abnormal child psychology* 26.4 (1998): 257-268.

De Jong T, Bannink N, Bredero-Boelhouwer HH, et al. Long-term functional outcome in 167 patients with syndromic craniosynostosis; defining a syndrome-specific risk profile. *J Plast Reconstr Aesthet Surg* 2010; 63: 1635–1641.

De Stefano, A., Di Giovanni, P., Kulamarva, G., Gennachi, S., Di Fonzo, F., Sallustio, V., Patrocinio, D., Candido, S., Lamarca, G., Dispenza, F. Oropharyngeal dysphagia in elderly population suffering from mild cognitive impairment and mild dementia: Understanding the link (2020) *American Journal of Otolaryngology - Head and Neck Medicine and Surgery,* 41 (4), art. no. 102501

De Stefano, A., Dispenza, F., Kulamarva, G., Lamarca, G., Faita, A., Merico, A., Sardanelli, G., Gabellone, S., Antonaci, A. Predictive factors of severity and persistence of oropharyngeal dysphagia in sub-acute stroke (2020) *European Archives of Oto-Rhino-Laryngology,* doi: 10.1007/s00405-020-06429-2.

Eliot S. Katz, Renee H. Moore, Carol L. Rosen, Ron B. Mitchell, Raouf Amin, Raanan Arens, Hiren Muzumdar, Ronald D. Chervin, Carole L. Marcus, Shalini Paruthi, Paul Willging and Susan Redline. Growth After Adenotonsillectomy for Obstructive Sleep Apnea: An RCT. *Pediatrics* 2014; 134; 282; originally published online July 28, 2014. doi: 10.1542/peds.2014-0591.

Flores-Mir C, Korayem M, Heo G, et al. Craniofacial morphological characteristics in children with obstructive sleep apnea syndrome: a systematic review and meta-analysis. *J Am Dent Assoc* 2013; 144: 269–277.

Garliner D. *Myofunctional Therapy.* W. B. Saunders Co., 1981.

Gozal D, Serpero LD, Kheirandish-Gozal L, Capdevila OS, Khalyfa A, Tauman R. Sleep measures and morning plasma TNF-α levels in children with sleepdisordered breathing. *Sleep.* 2010; 33(3):319-325.

Gozal D. Sleep disordered breathing in school aged children: impact on school performance. *Pediatrics* 1998; 102:616-20.

Guilleminault C, Stoohs R. Chronic snoring and obstructive sleep apnea syndrome in children. *Lung,* 1990;168:912-919.

Hannon, TS, Rofey, DL, Ryan, CM, Clapper, DA, Chakravorty, S, Arslanian, SA. Relationships among obstructive sleep apnea, anthropometric measures, and neurocognitive functioning in adolescents with severe obesity. *J. Pediatr.* 2012, 160, 732–735.

Huang YS, Guilleminault C. Pediatric Obstructive Sleep Apnea: Where Do We Stand? *Adv Otorhinolaryngol.* 2017; 80:136-144. doi: 10. 1159/000470885. Epub 2017 Jul 17. PMID: 28738322.

Jennum P, et al. *Thorax* 2013; 68:949–954. doi: 10.1136/thoraxjnl-2012-202561.

Kaditis, AG, Alonso Alvarez, ML, Boudewyns, A, Alexopoulos, EI, Ersu, R, Joosten, K, Larramona, H, Miano, S, Narang, I, Trang, H. et al. Obstructive sleep disordered breathing in 2- to 18-year-old children: Diagnosis and management. *Eur. Respir. J.* 2016, 47, 69–94.

Kimple, A, Ishman, S, Allergy and sleep-disordered breathing. *Curr. Opin. Otolaryngol. Head Neck Surg.* 2013, 21, 277–281.

Kiris M, Muderris T, Celebi S, Cankaya H, Bercin S. Changes in serum IGF-1 and IGFBP-3 levels and growth in children following adenoidectomy, tonsillectomy or adenotonsillectomy. *Int J Pediatr Otorhinolaryngol.* 2010; 74(5):528-531.

Lo Bue A, Salvaggio A, Insalaco G. Obstructive sleep apnea in developmental age. A narrative review. *Eur J Pediatr.* 2020 Mar; 179(3):357-365. doi: 10.1007/s00431-019-03557-8. Epub 2020 Jan 15. PMID: 31940071.

Lorusso F, Dispenza F, Modica DM, Gallina S. The Role of Modified Expansion Sphincter Pharyngoplasty in Multilevel Obstructive Sleep Apnea Syndrome Surgery. *Int Arch Otorhinolaryngol.* 2018 Oct; 22(4):432-436.

Lorusso F, Dispenza F, Saraniti C, Sireci F, Modica DM, Gallina S. Sleep disordered breathing: evaluation of dynamic patterns of the upper airways in obese subjects. *Otorinolaringologia* 2014; 64:57–64.

Lorusso F, Gallina S, Modica DM, Di Salvo N, Riggio F. Bipolar Quantum Molecular Resonance versus *Blunt Dissection tonsillectomy. B-ENT* 2015; 11(02):101–108.

Lorusso, F, Dispenza, F, Martinciglio, G, ...Battaglia, A, Gallina, S. Postural changes in patients undergoing hyoid surgery for OSAS. *Euro Mediterranean Biomedical Journal,* 2017; 12(29):140-143.

Lorusso, F, Martines, F, Mistretta, A, ...Dispenza, F, Gallina, S. Effects of adenotonsillectomy on neurocognitive and behavioural function in pediatric obstructive sleep apnea syndrome. *B-ENT* 2018; 14:113-118.

Maclean JE, Waters K, Fitzsimons D, et al. Screening for obstructive sleep apnea in preschool children with cleft palate. *Cleft Palate Craniofac J* 2009; 46: 117–123.

Magliulo, G, Iannella, G, Ciofalo, A, Polimeni, A, de Vincentiis, M, Pasquariello, B, Montevecchi, F, Vicini, C. Nasal pathologies in patients with obstructive sleep apnoea. *Acta Otorhinolaryngol. Ital.* 2019.

Marcus CL, Moore RH, Rosen CL, et al. A randomized trial of adenotonsillectomy for childhood sleep apnea. *N Engl J Med.* 2013; 368(25):2366–2376. doi: 10.1056/NEJMoa1215881.

Marcus CL. Sleep-disordered breathing in children. *Am J Respir Crit Care Med.* 2001;164:16–30.

Marcus, CL, Brooks, LJ, Draper, KA, Gozal, D, Halbower, AC, Jones, J, Schechter, MS, Ward, SD, Sheldon, SH, Shiman, RN, et al. Diagnosis and Management of Childhood Obstructive Sleep Apnea Syndrome. *Pediatrics* 2012, 130, 576–584.

McNamara F, Issa FG, Sullivan CE. Arousal pattern following central and obstructive breathing abnormalities in infant and children. *J appl Physiol* 1996; 81:2651-2657.

Mitchell RB. Adenotonsillectomy for obstructive sleep apnea in children: outcome evaluated by pre- and postoperative polysomnography. *Laryngoscope.* 2007; 117(10):1844-1854.

Mitchell, RB, Kelly, J. Outcome of adenotonsillectomy for obstructive sleep apnea in obese and normal-weight children. *Otolaryngol. Head Neck Surg.* 2007, 137, 43–48.

Modica DM, Lorusso F, Presti G, Fasola S, Gallina S. Our Assessment Using Palate Postoperative Problems Score (PPOPS): Tool for the Evaluation of Results in Palatal Surgery Techniques. *Indian J Otolaryngol Head Neck Surg.* 2019 Oct; 71(Suppl 1):766-770.

Modica DM, Marchese D, Lorusso F, Speciale R, Saraniti C, Gallina S. Functional Nasal Surgery and Use of CPAP in OSAS Patients: Our Experience. *Indian J Otolaryngol Head Neck Surg.* 2018 Dec; 70(4):559-565.

Nieminen P, Löppönen T, Tolonen U, Lanning P, Knip M, Löppönen H. Growth and biochemical markers of growth in children with snoring and obstructive sleep apnea. *Pediatrics.* 2002; 109(4):55.

O'Brien, IM, Sitha, S, Baur, LA, Waters, KA. Obesity increases the risk for persisting obstructive sleep apnea after treatment in children. *Int. J. Pediatr. Otorhinolaryngol.* 2006, 70, 1555–1560.

Profitt WR, McGlone RE, Barrett MJ. Lip and tongue pressures related to dental arch and oral cavity size in Australian Aborigenes. *Jour. Dent. Res.* 1975.54:1161-1172.

Schlaud M, Urschitz MS, Urschitz-Duprat PM, Poets CF. The German study on sleep-disordered breathing in primary school children: epidemiological approach, representativeness of study sample, and preliminary screening results. *Paediatr Perinat Epidemiol* 2004; 18:431-40.

Shintani T, Asakura K, Kataura A. The effect of adenotonsillectomy in children with OSA. *Int J Pediatr Otorhinolaryngol* 998; 44:51–58.

Straub WJ. The etiology of the perverted swallowing habit. *Am. J. Orthod.* 951; 1:603-612.

Tahara, Shinsaku, Hirotaka Hara, and Hiroshi Yamashita. "Evaluation of body growth in prepubertal Japanese children with obstructive sleep apnea after adenotonsillectomy over a long postoperative period." *International journal of pediatric otorhinolaryngology* 79.11 (2015): 1806-1809.

Tahara, Shinsaku, Hirotaka Hara, and Hiroshi Yamashita. "Evaluation of body growth in prepubertal Japanese children with obstructive sleep apnea after adenotonsillectomy over a long postoperative period." *International journal of pediatric otorhinolaryngology* 79.11 (2015): 1806-1809.

Ye J, Liu H, Zhang GH, et al. Outcome of adenotonsillectomy for obstructive sleep apnea syndrome in children. *Ann Otol Rhinol Laryngol.* 2010; 119(8):506-513.

Young T, Palta M, Dempsey J, Skatrud J, Weber S, Badr S. The occurrence of sleep disorders among middle–age adults. *Engl J Med* 1993; 328:1230-1235.

In: Advances in Sleep Apnea
Editors: F. Lorusso et al.
ISBN: 978-1-53619-758-7

Chapter 7

OBSTRUCTIVE SLEEP APNEA AND CARDIOVASCULAR DISEASE

Ludovico Rossetto*[*], *Enrico Bonnì* and *Giuseppina Novo
Department PROMISE, University of Palermo, Italy

ABSTRACT

Obstructive Sleep Apnea (OSAS) is related to different types of cardiovascular disease (CVD): arterial hypertension, coronary artery disease, heart failure (HF), atrial fibrillation (AF), strokes and pulmonary hypertension. OSAS is associated with increased risk of mortality or major cardiovascular events and its prevalence in patients with CVD is estimated between 40% to 60%. Pathophysiological link between OSAS and CVD is represented by intermittent hypoxiemia (IH) that induces oxidative stress, endothelial dysfunction with systemic and vascular inflammation and the increase of sympathetic activation and blood pressure (BP) elevation. Continuous Positive Airway Pressure (CPAP) is the gold standard therapy for OSAS patients. CPAP decreasing Apnea–Hypopnea Index (AHI) may improve patients' quality life

* Corresponding Author's Email: ludovico.rossetto1@gmail.com.

but its role on reduction of cardiovascular outcomes remains unclear.

Prevalence of OSAS in hypertensive patients is over 30% and around 80% in patients with drug resistant hypertension. Randomized controlled trials (RCTs) and meta-analysis have demonstrated a modest efficacy of CPAP on reduction of blood pressure. Patients with resistant hypertension, with poor adherence to CPAP had an increased risk of cerebrovascular events and hypertensive crises. IH induced by OSAS may promote arterial plaque development and growing, accelerating atherogenesis. Studies suggest that OSAS is associated with the presence of unstable plaque characteristics in patients with coronary artery disease. It's currently unclear if CPAP could positively affect CV outcome, however therapeutic adherence seems to play a fundamental role in order to ameliorate clinical status of patients and with the proposal of reduce CV events. The prevalence of atrial fibrillation (AF) in OSAS patients is about 5%, while 30-50% of AF patients are diagnosed with OSAS. The mechanisms promoting AF in OSAS patients include: intermittent nocturnal hypoxemia/hypercapnia, sympathovagal imbalance and neurohumoral activation, intrathoracic pressure shifts, oxidative stress, inflammation and atrial remodelling. OSAS has been shown to reduce the efficacy of antiarrhythmic drugs (AADs) and the success rate of both electrical cardioversion and catheter ablation in AF. CPAP treatment may reduce AF recurrences and ameliorate rhythm control.

Considering the wide spectrum of organs and neuroendocrine system involved by OSAS, a multidisciplinary approach must underlie the diagnostic and the therapeutic process. As for all therapeutics solutions, the adherence to CPAP therapy seems to play a key role in order to impact to cardiovascular outcomes. CPAP may have different impact in various phenotype of OSAS. In this perspective, a personalized medicine approach should be the new goal in diagnostic and therapeutic management.

Introduction

In the last decades, medical literature has widely demonstrated the close relationship existing between Obstructive Sleep Apnea (OSAS) and Cardiovascular Disease (CVD).

OSAS is associated with increased risk of mortality or major cardiovascular events and its prevalence in patients with CVD is estimated between 40% to 60%.

OSAS is related to different types of CVD: arterial hypertension, coronary artery disease, heart failure (HF), atrial fibrillation (AF), strokes and pulmonary hypertension.

Obstructive Apnea is characterized by repeated episodes of narrowing or collapse of the pharyngeal airway during sleep which causes partial (hypopnea) or complete (apnea) airflow cessation despite thoracoabdominal effort. The apneic events lead to recurrent cycles of intermittent hypoxemia (IH), reductions in intrathoracic pressure and arousals. Pathophysiological link between OSAS and CVD is represented by IH that induces oxidative stress, endothelial dysfunction with systemic and vascular inflammation and the increase of sympathetic activation and blood pressure (BP) elevation. Furthermore repetitive variations of intrathoracic pressure results in changing stroke volume and cardiac output.

In consideration of close connection between OSAS and CVD, a careful cardiological evaluation should be offered to OSAS patients to attempt a strict control of cardiovascular risk factors and an adequate specialized treatment.

Continuous Positive Airway Pressure (CPAP), which deliver air flow to maintain patents upper airway, is considered the gold standard therapy for OSAS patients; nevertheless CPAP improves quality life, reduces Apnea–Hypopnea Index (AHI) and may contribute to ameliorate some clinical and subclinical cardiovascular surrogate endpoint, its role in the reduction of cardiovascular outcomes remains unclear.

OSAS AND HYPERTENSION

The relationship between OSAS and hypertension has been clearly shown in the literature. Among patients with OSAS, the prevalence of hypertension is estimated between 30% to 70%. Prevalence of OSAS in hypertensive patients is over 30% and around 80% in patients with drug resistant hypertension.

Hypertension has a multifactorial pathogenesis in OSAS for different reasons: hyperactivation of the sympathetic tone, peripheral vasoconstriction, endothelial dysfunction, altered baroceptor reflex and increased activation of renin-angiotensin-aldosterone system. Typically OSAS patients present nocturnal catecholamine surges which determines an increase in heart rate and in peripheral vascular resistance. This abnormal response, during time, may contribute to the loss of nocturnal physiological fall of blood pressure values (non dipping pattern) exposing the patients to an additional increase of cardiovascular risk.

Osas and Hypertension are linked by a dose response relationship that is independent of common confounding risk factor. A recent meta-analysis showed that the risk of essential hypertension increased by 17% for every 10 events/h increase in the AHI (OR = 1.17, 95% CI (1.07, 1.27), $p = 0.001$).

Randomized controlled trials (RCTs) and meta-analysis have demonstrated a modest efficacy of CPAP on reduction of blood pressure. A meta-analysis of studies that have examined the effect of CPAP on BP in patients with resistant hypertension showed a favourable impact of CPAP with a reduction of - 6.74 mmHg [95% CI: -9.98 to -3.49; $P < 0.001$; I^2 61%] for systolic BP and - 5.94 mmHg (95% CI: - 9.40 to - 2.47; $P = 0.001$; I^2 76%) for diastolic BP. In a most recent meta-analysis, including 68 RCTs, it has been shown that CPAP is associated with an average BP reduction of -2.09 (-2.78, -1.40) mmHg [mean (95% CI)] for the systolic and of -1.92 (-2.40, -1.43) mmHg [mean (95% CI)] for the diastolic BP. Younger age, uncontrolled blood pressure and severe OSA-related oxygen desaturations, have been recognized as positive predictors of a favourable response to OSA treatment. Nevertheless a modest reduction of BP values, it should be remembered that also small variations confer a reduced cardiovascular risk.

In addition to conventional medical therapy, the use of CPAP, in patients with resistant hypertension, seems to offer a noticeable contribute. Indeed it was observed that patients with resistant hypertension, with poor adherence to CPAP have an increased risk of cerebrovascular events and hypertensive crises. Probably OSAS could play a key role in the pathogenesis of resistant hypertension, interfering in pathophysiological mechanisms that are poorly affected by conventional antihypertensive drug.

In consideration of these data, it appears reasonable to investigate for OSAS in patients with resistant arterial hypertension, regardless of evident signs or symptoms related to sleep disorders.

OSAS AND CORONARY ARTERY DISEASE

The main pathogenic mechanism of CAD in OSAS patients, in common with other CVD, was previously described, adjunctive mechanisms include: hypoxia, oxidative stress, hyperactivation of procoagulant state, insulin resistance and metabolic dysregulation. IH plays the main role in the negative complex response lead to atherosclerosis. Indeed, as well established, atherogenesis mainly consists of chronic inflammatory disease and IH, via activation of the transcription factor NF-κB, promotes systemic inflammation. Data derived from animal studies shown that inflammation induced by IH is a key factor in generation of pre-atherosclerotic lesions. IH may also promote maladaptive metabolic responses leading to adipocytes dysfunction and increased risk of type 2 diabetes. These pathological processes, accelerating atherogenesis, promote arterial plaque development and growing. However, the role of IH is not only negative, indeed some studies suggest positive cardiac effect through ischaemic preconditioning and the development of coronary collateral circles.

Zhang et al. have shown that Gensini score (an angiographic scoring system for determination of severity of coronary artery disease) was higher in moderate to severe OSAS patients with CAD. A retrospective analysis, made using intracoronary optical frequency-domain imaging (instrumental modality for evaluation of the characteristics of atherosclerotic plaque), in OSAS and non OSAS patients with CAD undergoing percutaneous coronary intervention (PCI), showed that in the OSAS group there was higher prevalence of thinned cap fibroatheroma (67% vs. 35%, $P = 0.014$) and microchannels (86% vs. 55%, $P = 0.014$); these results suggest that OSAS could be associated with the presence of unstable plaque characteristics in CAD patients. Reducing apneic events, CPAP should theoretically have a positive effects on underlying pathogenetic factors induced by OSAS. Several observational studies, in patients with CAD and OSAS, found a significative reduction of cardiovascular outcomes, in patients treated with CPAP. Neverthless, The Save Study, a randomised controlled trial designed to determine OSAS treatment efficacy with CPAP in reducing the risk of cardiovascular events in patients with established CVD, failed to demonstrate a significative reduction of primary outcome (a composite of cardiovascular death, myocardial infarction, stroke, hospitalization for unstable angina, heart failure (HF), or transient ischemic attack). However in this trial, mean utilization of CPAP, in OSAS group, was 3.3 hours per night. A meta-analysis of randomized controlled trials (including also The Save Study) comparing CPAP with medical therapy alone, in OSAS patients, who reported cardiovascular outcomes, confirmed that CPAP therapy was not associated with reduction of MACE, nevertheless an improvement of cardiac outcomes was observed in the subgroup that wore CPAP > 4 hours per night.

It's currently unclear if CPAP could positively affect CV outcome, however therapeutic adherence seems to play a fundamental role in order to ameliorate clinical status of patients and with the proposal of reduce CV events.

In light of these data, and in the hypothesis that CPAP utilisation may have different impact in various OSAS phenotype, further studies are needed.

OSAS, Atrial Fibrillation and Other Arrhytmias

AF is common in the general population and its prevalence is about 2%. The prevalence of AF in OSAS patients is about 5%, while 30-50% of AF patients are diagnosed with OSAS and an independent association between the two disorders have been demonstrated even if many confounding conditions exist, such as systemic hypertension, obesity, and HF. Furthermore, it is well established that the association between OSAS and AF increases risk of mortality or major cardiovascular events.

The mechanisms promoting AF in OSAS patients include: intermittent nocturnal hypoxemia/hypercapnia, sympathovagal imbalance and neurohumoral activation, intrathoracic pressure shifts, oxidative stress, inflammation and atrial remodelling.

During an apneic episode, vagal tone is stimulated causing transient bradycardia, atrial effective refractory period shortening and consequently increasing in susceptibility to excitatory stimuli; moreover, hypoxemia increases sympathetic and activation of the renin–angiotensin system, determining AF threshold reducing.

Exaggerated intrathoracic pressure shifts are seen during apneic events and they cause acute atrial dilation and increased frequency of premature beats. Chronic repetitive apneic events are associated with progressive left atrial dilation and fibrosis as well as left ventricular hypertrophy and diastolic dysfunction.

OSAS has been shown to reduce the efficacy of antiarrhythmic drugs (AADs) and the success rate of both electrical cardioversion and catheter ablation in AF. In the ORBIT-AF (Outcomes Registry for Better Informed Treatment of Atrial Fibrillation), which included >10 000 AF patients, those with coexisting OSAS had significantly worse AF symptoms, an increased risk of AF relapses and worse outcomes after catheter ablation. Importantly, there is evidence that CPAP treatment may reduce AF recurrences and ameliorate rhythm control in AF patients. In the ORBIT-AF, CPAP treatment significantly reduced the progression to permanent AF. Moreover, a meta-analysis have demonstrated that the risk of AF recurrence after catheter ablation in OSAS patients treated with CPAP was not significantly different from a control population without OSA and this risk was significantly reduced of about 57% compared to OSAS patients not treated with CPAP ($P < 0.001$). Furthermore, recent studies have shown that an aggressive risk-factor reduction programme focusing on weight, hyperlipidaemia, OSAS, hypertension, diabetes, smoking cessation, and alcohol-intake reduction significantly reduced AF burden after AF catheter ablation.

For these reasons Heart Rhythm Society Expert Consensus Statement on catheter and surgical ablation of AF (2017) suggests diagnostic testing with either Home Sleep Apnea Testing (HSAT) or polysomnography in patients with suspected sleep apnea when catheter ablation is planned. AF is not the only arrhythmia linked to

OSAS. Brady-tachy syndrome (condition characterized by alternating episodes of bradycardia or pauses and supraventricular tachycardia or atrial fibrillation) and even ventricular arrhythmias have been shown in OSAS patients, in particular: ventricular ectopy, nonsustained ventricular tachycardia and, importantly, an increased risk of sudden cardiac death has been reported in patients with severe OSAS, particularly among those observed to have nocturnal oxygen desaturation to <78%.

The efficacy of CPAP treatment on reducing rhythm disturbances in patients with OSA is not clear and additional study are needed.

OSAS and Heart Failure

Sleep-disordered breathing (SDB) is common in HF patients. The most common types are: central sleep apnoea (CSA, similar to Cheyne Stokes respiration), OSAS and a mixed pattern of the two. Other causes of sleep disturbance include anxiety, depression, decubitus or paroxysmal pulmonary congestion (orthopnoea and paroxysmal nocturnal dyspnoea) and diuretic therapy causing nocturnal diuresis. SDB occurs in more than two-third of patients with HF and its prevalence is even higher in acute HF. In particular, CSA accounts for approximately two thirds of the sleep apnea, while OSAS comprises a significant minority.

It has been demonstrated that SDB increases the risk of adverse outcomes, including mortality, in patients with HF.

As explained above, OSAS produces sympathetic nervous system hyperactivation, preload and afterload increase consequent to intrathoracic pressure shifts while attempting to inspire against occluded airways, systemic hypertension, high burden of atrial and ventricular arrhythmias and an elevated risk of coronary events. All of these conditions are important to understand the connection between OSAS and HF.

The pathogenesis of CSA is uncertain, but one of the hypothesis is based on the observation that patients who have HF and CSA tend to have lower arterial carbon dioxide tensions ($PaCO2$) than patients who have heart failure without CSA. For this reason apnea starts when

PaCO2 level is below the apneic threshold. After the apneic phase, hypercapnia stimulates hyperpnea, which yields marked hypocapnia and allows the cycle of events to repeat.

Since HSAT have not been validated to diagnose CSA, current guidelines recommend polysomnography as the preferred diagnostic modality for patients with HF.

CPAP treatment benefits seen in AF are not clear for HF. The CANPAP (Canadian Continuous Positive Airway Pressure for Patients with Central Sleep Apnea and Heart Failure) trial did not found any benefit in HF patients with CSA treated with CPAP although a post hoc analysis suggested a reduction in mortality among patients for whom CPAP therapy resulted in a significant improvement in AHI (to <15 events/h). Furthermore, reductions in pro-arrhythmic state, risk of AF relapsing and sympathetic nervous system stimulation have been observed in patients with both OSAS and CSA treated with CPAP. Finally, CPAP results in favourable hemodynamic effects, including improved left ventricular systolic function in OSA patients with high wedge pressures. For these reasons current guidelines suggest CPAP in class IIB.

Adaptive servoventilation (ASV) has been tried in patients with HF and CSA. This is a bi-level positive airway pressure (Bi-PAP) therapy in which the degree of pressure support varies between respiratory cycles in order to maintain stable minute ventilation and a backup rate is programmed to trigger breaths during periods of central apnea.

The SAVIOR-C (Study of the Effects of Adaptive Servo-ventilation Therapy on Cardiac Function and Remodeling in Patients with Chronic Heart Failure) trial failed to show an improvement in ejection fraction or brain natriuretic peptide (BNP) level and the SERVE-HF (Treatment of Sleep-Disordered Breathing with Predominant Central Sleep Apnea by Adaptive Servo Ventilation in Patients with Heart Failure) trial led to an increase in both all-cause and cardiovascular mortality, although both trials revealed improvements in quality of life and clinical status. It has been supposed that the failure is due to the reduction of cardiac output related to the higher levels of PAP delivered in ASV mode. The ongoing ADVENT-HF (Effect of Adaptive Servo Ventilation on Survival and Hospital Admissions in Heart Failure) trial is investigating the effect of ASV therapy on mortality and morbidity in HF patients (left ventricular ejection fraction ≤45%) with SDB using an updated algorithm. At the present time, treatment of ASV is contraindicated in patients with HF and CSA.

Implantable phrenic nerve stimulation is an alternative approach to treat CSA in HF patients. Costanzo MR et al. studied this treatment in 96 HF patients with CSA and found that it reduces CSA severity and was associated with benefits on HF quality of life.

OSAS and Pulmonary Hypertension

Osas and Pulmonary hypertension (PH), despite theirs clinical and prognostic impact, are currently two underdiagnosed disorder. The prevalence of pulmonary hypertension in OSA ranges from 17% to 53%. Hypercapnia and nocturnal episodes of hypoxia cause pulmonary arteriolar constriction leading to acute elevation in pulmonary artery pressures. Different factors are implicated in hypoxic vasoconstriction in PH: nitric oxide, endothelin, angiopoietin-1, serotonin, and NADPH-oxidase. Furthermore, chronic hypoxia, stimulating additional inflammatory pathways, lead to pulmonary vascular remodelling and irreversible increasing in pulmonary vascular resistance.

Vascular remodelling and pulmonary vascular resistance increasing lead to rise of right ventricle after-load, moreover negative inspiratory intrathoracic pressure, generated during apneic episode, causes an increase in venous return augmenting right ventricular pre-load.

In addition, adrenergic hyperactivity, the rise of peripheral vascular resistance induced by OSAS during time, lead to diastolic dysfunction and left HF.

The mechanism described above produce a mixed pattern of PH: pre-capillary and post-capillary. Importantly the presence of PH in OSAS may aggravate the patient clinical status and the prognosis. The literature suggests that treatment with CPAP may improve pulmonary artery systolic pressure but further randomized controlled trial are needed.

In the light of high prevalence of nocturnal hypoxaemia and OSAS in PH, in agreement with 2015 ESC/ERS Guidelines for the Diagnosis and Treatment of Pulmonary Hypertension, overnight oximetry or polysomnography should be performed in case of suspicious of OSAS or hypoventilation.

Conclusion

Considering the wide spectrum of organs and neuroendocrine system involved by OSAS, a multidisciplinary approach must underlie the diagnostic and the therapeutic process. In cardiac patients, risk factors control, medical therapy, interventional and surgical approach, as indicated in the international guidelines, are the cornerstone of therapeutic management. However, in light of frequently overlapping between OSAS and CVD, adequate therapeutic solution for reduces apneic events, could ameliorate patients' quality life, the control of cardiovascular risk factor and surrogate endpoint. In this view cardiologists should investigate for OSAS in their patients, especially in presence of typical signs and symptoms.

As for all therapeutics solutions, the adherence to CPAP therapy seems to play a key role in order to impact to cardiovascular outcomes. Despite OSAS is a multifactorial and complex disorder its severity is currently stratified only by AHI. A wide heterogeneity exist in OSAS patients in term of: pathogenic causes, symptoms, disease impact on quality of life and prognostic outcome. Furthermore the studies suggest that CPAP may have different impact in various phenotype of OSAS. In this perspective, a personalized medicine approach should be the new goal in diagnostic and therapeutic management of these patients.

Our OSAS perception remain just the tip of the iceberg, hence a stronger diagnostic and therapeutic effort is required in order to provide best management suited.

References

Abuzaid, AS; Al Ashry, HS; Elbadawi, A; et al. Meta-analysis of cardiovascular outcomes with continuous positive airway pressure therapy in patients with obstructive sleep apnea. *Am J Cardiol.*, 2017, 120(4), 693-699.

Ahmad, M; Makati, D; Akbar, S. Review of and Updates on Hypertension in Obstructive Sleep Apnea. *Int J Hypertens.*, 2017, 2017, 1848375. doi: 10.1155/2017/1848375.

Albuquerque, FN; Calvin, AD; Sert Kuniyoshi, FH; Konecny, T; Lopez-Jimenez, F; et al. Sleep-disordered breathing and excessive daytime sleepiness in patients with atrial fibrillation. *Chest.*, 2012, 141, 967–973.

Aronson, D; Lavie, L; Lavie, P. Does OSA Upregulate Cardioprotective Pathways to an Ischemic Insult? *Chest*, 2018, 153, 295-7. 10.1016/j.chest.2017.07.036.

Atul Malhotra, James C Fang, Safwan Badr, M; April F Eichler. Sleep-disordered breathing in heart failure. In: *UpToDate*, Post TW (Ed), UpToDate, Waltham, MA. (Accessed on Novembre 06, 2020).

Bisogni, V; Pengo, MF; Maiolino, G; Rossi, GP. The sympathetic nervous system and catecholamines metabolism in obstructive sleep apnoea. *J Thorac Dis.*, 2016, 8(2), 243-254. doi: 10.3978/j.issn.2072-1439.2015.11.14.

Bradley, TD; Hall, MJ; Ando, S; Floras, JS. Hemodynamic effects of simulated obstructive apneas in humans with and without heart failure. *Chest.*, 2001, 119, 1827–1835.

Bradley, TD; Logan, AG; Kimoff, RJ; Sériès, F; Morrison, D; et al. CANPAP Investigators. Continuous positive airway pressure for central sleep apnea and heart failure. *N Engl J Med.*, 2005, 353, 2025–2033.

Calkins, H; Hindricks, G; Cappato, R; Kim, YH; Saad, EB; et al. 2017 HRS/EHRA/ECAS/APHRS/SOLAECE expert consensus statement on catheter and surgical ablation of atrial fibrillation: executive summary. *J Arrhythm.*, 2017, 33, 369–409.

Cioffi, G; Russo, TE; Stefenelli, C; Selmi, A; Furlanello, F; et al. Severe obstructive sleep apnea elicits concentric left ventricular geometry. *J Hypertens.*, 2010, 28, 1074–1082.

Costanzo, MR; Ponikowski, P; Coats, A; Javaheri, S; Augostini, R; et al. Phrenic nerve stimulation to treat patients with central sleep apnoea and heart failure. *Eur J Heart Fail.*, 2018 Dec, 20(12), 1746-1754. doi: 10.1002/ejhf.1312. Epub 2018 Oct 10.

Deacon, NL; Jen, R; Li, Y; Malhotra, A. Treatment of Obstructive Sleep Apnea. Prospects for Personalized Combined Modality Therapy. *Ann Am Thorac Soc.*, 2016, 13(1), 101-108. doi: 10.1513/AnnalsATS.201508-537FR.

Dewan, NA; Nieto, FJ; Somers, VK. Intermittent hypoxemia and OSA: implications for comorbidities. *Chest.*, 2015, 147(1), 266-274. doi: 10.1378/chest.14-0500.

Drager, LF; Bortolotto, LA; Pedrosa, RP; Krieger, EM; Lorenzi-Filho, G. Left atrial diameter is independently associated with arterial stiffness in patients with obstructive sleep apnea: potential implications for atrial fibrillation. *Int J Cardiol.*, 2010, 144, 257–259.

Elmasry, A; Lindberg, E; Hedner, J; Janson, C; Boman, G. Obstructive sleep apnoea and urine catecholamines in hypertensive males: a population-based study. *Eur Respir J.*, 2002, 19(3), 511-517. doi: 10.1183/09031936.02.00106402.

Galiè, N; Humbert, M; Vachiery, JL; Gibbs, S; Lang, I; Torbicki, A; Simonneau, G; Peacock, A; Vonk Noordegraaf, A; Beghetti, M; Ghofrani, A; Gomez Sanchez, MA; Hansmann, G; Klepetko, W; Lancellotti, P; Matucci, M; McDonagh, T; Pierard, LA; Trindade, PT; Zompatori, M; Hoeper, M. 2015 ESC/ERS guidelines for the diagnosis and treatment of pulmonary hypertension. *Eur Heart J.*, 2016, 69, 177.

Gami, AS; Olson, EJ; Shen, WK; Wright, RS; Ballman, KV; et al. Obstructive sleep apnea and the risk of sudden cardiac death: a longitudinal study of 10,701 adults. *J Am Coll Cardiol.*, 2013, 62, 610–616.

Hindricks, G; Potpara, T; Dagres, N; et al. 2020 ESC Guidelines for the diagnosis and management of atrial fibrillation developed in collaboration with the European Association of Cardio-Thoracic Surgery (EACTS) [published online ahead of print, 2020 Aug 29]. *Eur Heart J.*, 2020, ehaa612. doi: 10.1093/eurheartj/ehaa612.

Holmqvist, F; Guan, N; Zhu, Z; Kowey, PR; Allen, LA; et al. Impact of obstructive sleep apnea and continuous positive airway pressure therapy on outcomes in patients with atrial fibrillation—results from the Outcomes Registry for Better Informed Treatment of Atrial Fibrillation (ORBIT-AF). *Am Heart J.*, 2015, 169, 647–654.e642.

Hou, H; Zhao, Y; Yu, W; et al. Association of obstructive sleep apnea with hypertension: A systematic review and meta-analysis. *J Glob Health.*, 2018, 8(1), 010405. doi: 10.7189/jogh.08.010405.

Iftikhar, IH; Valentine, CW; Bittencourt, LR; et al. Effects of continuous positive airway pressure on blood pressure in patients with resistant hypertension and obstructive sleep apnea: a meta-analysis. *J Hypertens.*, 2014, 32(12), 2341-2350. doi: 10.1097/HJH. 0000000000000372.

Javaheri, S. Effects of continuous positive airway pressure on sleep apnea and ventricular irritability in patients with heart failure. *Circulation.*, 2000, 101, 392–397.

Johnson, KG; Johnson, DC. Frequency of sleep apnea in stroke and TIA patients: a meta-analysis. *J Clin Sleep Med.*, 2010, 6, 131–137.

Kaneko, Y; Floras, JS; Usui, K; Plante, J; Tkacova, R; et al. Cardiovascular effects of continuous positive airway pressure in patients with heart failure and obstructive sleep apnea. *N Engl J Med.*, 2003, 348, 1233–1241.] and diastolic function Arias MA, García-Río F, Alonso-Fernández A, Mediano O, Martínez, I, Villamor J, Obstructive sleep apnea syndrome affects left ventricular diastolic function: effects of nasal continuous positive airway pressure in men. *Circulation.*, 2005, 112, 375–383.

Kapur, VK; Auckley, DH; Chowdhuri, S; Kuhlmann, DC; Mehra, R; et al. Clinical practice guideline for diagnostic testing for adult obstructive sleep apnea: an American Academy of Sleep Medicine clinical practice guideline. *J Clin Sleep Med.*, 2017, 13, 479–504.

Kasai, T. Sleep apnea and heart failure. *J Cardiol.*, 2012 Aug, 60(2), 78-85. doi: 10.1016/j.jjcc.2012.05.013. Epub 2012 Jul 21. PMID: 22824295.

Kent, BD; McNicholas, WT; Ryan, S. Insulin resistance, glucose intolerance and diabetes mellitus in obstructive sleep apnoea. *J Thorac Dis*, 2015, 7, 1343-57.

Kholdani, C; Fares, WH; Mohsenin, V. Pulmonary hypertension in obstructive sleep apnea: is it clinically significant? A critical analysis of the association and pathophysiology. *Pulm Circ.*, 2015, 5, 220–227

Konishi, T; Kashiwagi, Y; Funayama, N; et al. Obstructive sleep apnea is associated with increased coronary plaque instability: an optical frequency domain imaging study. *Heart Vessels*, 34. 1266–1279, (2019). https://doi.org/10.1007/s00380-019-01363-8.

Lavie, L; Lavie, P. Molecular mechanisms of cardiovascular disease in OSAHS: the oxidative stress link. *Eur Respir J.*, 2009, 33(6), 1467-1484. doi: 10.1183/09031936.00086608.

Lévy, P; Ryan, S; Oldenburg, O; et al. Sleep apnoea and the heart. *Eur Respir Rev*, 2013, 22, 333-52. 10.1183/09059180.00004513.

Li, L; Wang, ZW; Li, J; Ge, X; Guo, LZ; et al. Efficacy of catheter ablation of atrial fibrillation in patients with obstructive sleep apnoea with and without continuous positive airway pressure treatment: a meta-analysis of observational studies. *Europace.*, 2014, 16, 1309–1314.

Linz, D; Hohl, M; Khoshkish, S; Mahfoud, F; Ukena, C; et al. Low-level but not high-level baroreceptor stimulation inhibits atrial fibrillation in a pig model of sleep apnea. *J Cardiovasc Electrophysiol.*, 2016, 27, 1086–1092.

Logan, AG; Perlikowski, SM; Mente, A; et al. High prevalence of unrecognized sleep apnoea in drug-resistant hypertension. *Journal of Hypertension.*, 2001 Dec, 19(12), 2271-2277. doi: 10.1097/00004872-200112000-00022.

Logan, AG; Tkacova, R; Perlikowski, SM; Leung, RS; Tisler, A; et al. Refractory hypertension and sleep apnoea: effect of CPAP on blood pressure and baroreflex. *Eur Respir J.*, 2003, 21, 241–247.

Lyons, OD; Floras, JS; Logan, AG; Beanlands, R; Cantolla, JD; et al. ADVENT-HF Investigators. Design of the effect of adaptive servo-ventilation on survival and cardiovascular hospital admissions in patients with heart failure and sleep apnoea: the ADVENT-HF trial. *Eur J Heart Fail.*, 2017, 19, 579–587.

Mandal, S; Kent, BD. Obstructive sleep apnoea and coronary artery disease. *J Thorac Dis.*, 2018 Dec, 10(Suppl 34), S4212-S4220. doi: 10.21037/jtd.2018.12.75. PMID: 30687537, PMCID: PMC6321892.

Marrone, O; Bonsignore, MR. Pulmonary haemodynamics in obstructive sleep apnoea. *Sleep Med Rev.*, 2002, 6(3), 175-193. doi: 10.1053/smrv.2001.0185.

McEvoy, RD; Antic, NA; Heeley, E; Luo, Y; Ou, Q; Zhang, X; Mediano, O; Chen, R; Drager, LF; Liu, Z; Chen, G; Du, B; McArdle, N; Tripathi, M; Billot, L; Li, Q; Lorenzi-Filho, G; Barbe, F; Redline, S;

Wang, J; Arima, H; Neal, B; White, DP; Grunstein, RR; Zhong, N; Anderson, CS. CPAP for prevention of cardiovascular events in obstructive sleep apnea. *N Engl J Med.*, 2016, 375, 919–931.

Mehra, R; Benjamin, EJ; Shahar, E; Gottlieb, DJ; Nawabit, R; et al. Association of nocturnal arrhythmias with sleep-disordered breathing: the Sleep Heart Health Study. *Am J Respir Crit Care Med.*, 2006, 173, 910–916.

Momomura, S; Seino, Y; Kihara, Y; Adachi, H; Yasumura, Y; et al. SAVIOR-C Investigators . Adaptive servo-ventilation therapy for patients with chronic heart failure in a confirmatory, multicenter, randomized, controlled study. *Circ J.*, 2015, 79, 981–990.

Navarro-Soriano, C; Martínez-García, MA; Torres, G; Barbé, F; Sánchez-de-la-Torre, M; Caballero-Eraso, C; Lloberes, P; Cambriles, TD; Somoza, M; Masa, JF; González, M; Mañas, E; de la Peña, M; García-Río, F; Montserrat, JM; Muriel A; Oscullo, G; García-Ortega, A; Posadas, T; Campos-Rodríguez, F, on behalf the Spanish Sleep Network. Long-term Effect of CPAP Treatment on Cardiovascular Events in Patients With Resistant Hypertension and Sleep Apnea. Data From the HIPARCO-2 Study. *Arch Bronconeumol.*, 2020 Feb 3, S0300-2896(19)30612-X. English, Spanish. doi: 10.1016/j.arbres.2019.12.006. Epub ahead of print. PMID: 32029279.

Oldenburg, O; Lamp, B; Faber, L; Teschler, H; Horstkotte, D; Töpfer, V. Sleep-disordered breathing in patients with symptomatic heart failure: a contemporary study of prevalence in and characteristics of 700 patients. *Eur J Heart Fail.*, 2007, 9, 251–257.

Oldenburg, O; Wellmann, B; Buchholz, A; Bitter, T; Fox, H; et al. Nocturnal hypoxaemia is associated with increased mortality in stable heart failure patients. *Eur Heart J.*, 2016, 37, 1695–1703.

Patel, N; Donahue, C; Shenoy, A; Patel, A; El-Sherif, N. Obstructive sleep apnea and arrhythmia: a systemic review. *Int J Cardiol.*, 2017, 228, 967–970.

Pathak, RK; Middeldorp, ME; Lau, DH; Mehta, AB; Mahajan, R; et al. Aggressive risk factor reduction study for atrial fibrillation and implications for the outcome of ablation: the ARREST-AF cohort study. *J Am Coll Cardiol*, 2014, 6 4, 22222231.

Pathak, RK; Middeldorp, ME; Meredith, M; Mehta, AB; Mahajan, R; et al. Longterm effect of goal-directed weight management in an atrial fibrillation cohort: a long-term follow-up study (LEGACY). *J Am Coll Cardiol*, 2015, 65, 21592169.

Peker, Y; Carlson, J; Hedner, J. Increased incidence of coronary artery disease in sleep apnoea: a long-term follow-up. *Eur Respir J.*, 2006, 28, 596–602.

Pengo, MF; Soranna, D; Giontella, A; Perger, E; Mattaliano, P; Schwarz, EI; Fava, C. Obstructive sleep apnoea treatment and blood pressure: which phenotypes predict a response? A systematic review and meta-analysis. *European Respiratory Journal*, (2020), 1901945. doi: 10.1183/13993003.01945-2019.

Ponikowski, P; Voors, AA; Anker, SD; Bueno, H; Cleland, JGF; et al. 2016 ESC Guidelines for the diagnosis and treatment of acute and chronic heart failure: The Task Force for the diagnosis and treatment of acute and chronic heart failure of the European Society of Cardiology (ESC) Developed with the special contribution of the Heart Failure Association (HFA) of the ESC. *Eur Heart J.*, 2016, Jul 14, 37(27), 2129-2200. doi: 10.1093/eurheartj/ehw128.

Sajkov, D; Wang, T; Saunders, NA; Bune, AJ; Mcevoy, RD. Continuous positive airway pressure treatment improves pulmonary hemodynamics in patients with obstructive sleep apnea. *Am J Respir Crit Care Med.*, 2002, 165, 152–158.

Sharma, BK; Bakker, JP; McSharry, DG; Desai, AS; Javaheri, S; Malhotra, A. Adaptive servoventilation for treatment of sleep-disordered breathing in heart failure: a systematic review and meta-analysis. *Chest.*, 2012, 142, 1211–1221.

Simantirakis, EN; Schiza, SI; Marketou, ME; Chrysostomakis, SI; Chlouverakis, GI; et al. Severe bradyarrhythmias in patients with sleep apnoea: the effect of continuous positive airway pressure treatment: a long-term evaluation using an insertable loop recorder. *Eur Heart J.*, 2004, 25, 1070–1076.

Tietjens, JR; Claman, D; Kezirian, EJ; et al. Obstructive Sleep Apnea in Cardiovascular Disease: A Review of the Literature and Proposed Multidisciplinary Clinical Management Strategy. *J Am Heart Assoc.*, 2019, 8(1), e010440. doi: 10.1161/JAHA.118.010440.

Usui, K; Bradley, TD; Spaak, J; Ryan, CM; Kubo, T; et al. Inhibition of awake sympathetic nerve activity of heart failure patients with obstructive sleep apnea by nocturnal continuous positive airway pressure. *J Am Coll Cardiol.*, 2005, 45, 2008–2011.

Weitzenblum, E. Chronic cor pulmonale. *Heart.*, 2003, 89, 225–230.

Wong, HS; Williams, AJ; Mok, Y. The relationship between pulmonary hypertension and obstructive sleep apnea. *Curr Opin Pulm Med.*, 2017 Nov, 23(6), 517-521. doi: 10.1097/MCP.0000000000000421. PMID: 28786883.

Xia, W; Huang, Y; Peng, B; et al. Relationship between obstructive sleep apnoea syndrome and essential hypertension: a dose-response meta-analysis. *Sleep Med.*, 2018, 47, 11-18. doi: 10.1016/j.sleep.2018.03.016.

Zhang, J; Song, Y; Ji, Y; et al. Correlation between coronary artery disease and obstructive sleep apnea syndrome and analysis of risk factors. *Exp Ther Med.*, 2018, 15(6), 4771-4776. doi: 10.3892/etm.2018.6070.

In: Advances in Sleep Apnea
Editors: F. Lorusso et al.
ISBN: 978-1-53619-758-7

Chapter 8

ADVANCES IN OBSTRUCTIVE SLEEP APNEA SYNDROME AND DYSMETABOLIC PATHOLOGY

Alessandro Mattina[1,*] and Elisa Calzolari[2]
[1]Diabetes and Islet Transplantation Unit,
Department of Diagnostic and Therapeutic Services,
IRCCS ISMETT (Istituto Mediterraneo per i Trapianti e Terapie ad Alta Specializzazione), UPMC Italy, Palermo, Italy
[2]Allergy and Respiratory Diseases, IRCCS Policlinico San Martino,
University of Genoa, Department of Internal Medicine (DIMI),
Genoa, Italy

ABSTRACT

The relationship between obstructive sleep apnea (OSA) syndrome and metabolic diseases is bidirectional. Sleep fragmentation and intermittent hypoxemia present in OSA, can affect insulin resistance, systemic inflammatory state and, consequently, the related metabolic pathologies. On the other hand, obesity, metabolic syndrome, glucose intolerance, diabetes

* Corresponding Author's Email: alessandromattina@gmail.com.

and other diseases associated with insulin resistance such as the non-alcoholic fatty liver disease (NAFLD), may be implicated in the development and worsening of OSA. Moreover, patients with OSA are already at high cardiovascular risk, and the association with metabolic diseases significantly increases their risk.

The pathophysiological pathways linking OSA to metabolic diseases have not been fully explained. Intermittent hypoxia and sleep fragmentation may play a key role as main triggers in the etiopathogenetic chain of progression of OSA to metabolic alterations and cardiovascular damage. Intermittent hypoxia causes an altered production of reactive oxygen species with consequent oxidative stress. This is related to a state of general inflammation and to functional alterations of the hypothalamus-pituitary-adrenal axis. The continual micro arousals are also associated with an inappropriate activation of the sympathetic system, which determines an altered release of adipokine and proinflammatory cytokines. All these factors are closely linked to one another, resulting in the onset or worsening of insulin resistance and increased metabolic risk.

The treatment of OSA may stabilize some metabolic alterations and is strongly recommended to reduce cardiovascular risk and improve quality of life. Though the direct beneficial effect of cPAP on metabolism has not been unequivocally confirmed, weight loss and lifestyle intervention have been shown to affect the common therapeutic outcomes of OSA and metabolic diseases.

A multidisciplinary approach is the most effective pathway for the therapeutic management of these patients. Furthermore, given the increasing prevalence of both OSA and metabolic pathologies, international guidelines converge on the need for accurate screening programs.

INTRODUCTION

The link between arterial hypertension, insulin resistance, dyslipidemia, central obesity, and obstructive sleep apnea (OSA) had already been studied in 1998, by Ian Wilcox, who coined the term "Syndrome Z" to indicate a condition characterized by the simultaneous presence of OSA and metabolic syndrome. It was known that understanding the common mechanisms underlying these pathologies could help to assess the cardiovascular risk associated with them. In fact, patients with OSA are already at high cardiovascular risk, and the association with metabolic diseases significantly increases their risk.

OSA syndrome is related to dysmetabolic pathology with a bidirectional relationship based on some common pathophysiological aspects. It is closely related to the presence of obesity, diabetes, dyslipidemia, insulin resistance, and other metabolic diseases such as non-alcoholic fatty liver disease (NAFLD).

Obesity

The high prevalence of OSA worldwide in recent years is strongly intertwined with obesity.

According to data provided by the World Health Organization (WHO), the number of obese people in the world has doubled since 1980: in 2016, over 1.9 billion adults were overweight, including over 650 million obese.

The link between OSA and obesity is constant, though not always present, both due to the mechanical obstructions caused by the excessive accumulation of fat in the respiratory area, and to more complex dysfunction of the adipose tissue as endocrine organ. Therefore, age-adjusted rates of OSA are 4- to 10-fold higher with obesity, especially with central obesity. Central obesity is typical of the metabolic syndrome and appears to be more closely correlated with OSA than obesity in general. Obese patients with OSA have a higher proportion of visceral fat than obese controls with similar BMI[5]. Also high apnea-hypopnea index (AHI), the most common parameter used to measure the degree of OSA, is significantly associated with a larger visceral adipose tissue area.

Diabetes and Insulin Resistance

The prevalence of OSA worldwide is also strongly associated with the recent diabetes epidemic crisis. Though obese patients with OSA have an increased risk of developing type 2 diabetes (T2D), other evidence has shown that OSA itself represents a risk of developing a glucose alteration regardless of obesity.

In 2019, the International Diabetes Federation announced that approximately 460 million people are living with T2D, and this number is expected to increase to 700 million in 2045.

In the T2D population the prevalence of OSA is very high and can reach 23%[8]. When associated with obesity, OSA exceeded 80%.

This common ground is partly represented by insulin resistance, a condition in which normal insulin concentration produces a lower-than-normal biological response. The presence of sleep-disordered breathing in the general population has been shown to be independently associated with insulin resistance.

This could explain the occurrence of OSA in a phase of pre-diabetes in which a state of insulin resistance is already present. Pre-diabetes is a condition characterized by increased insulin resistance and impaired glucose tolerance, with blood glucose values not falling within the diagnostic criteria for T2D. One in 13 adults (374 million people) have impaired glucose tolerance worldwide. This disease is often recognized with a diagnostic delay, and with repercussions on other risk factors and also on the possible diagnosis of OSA.

In type 1 diabetes (T1D), a high prevalence of OSA has been found compared to the general population. T1D is much less common than T2D, and accounts for approximately 5-10% of diabetes globally. It is caused by the autoimmune response against pancreatic β cells. So, the pathogenesis of T1D is very different from that of T2D, as are the underlying mechanisms in common with OSA. There are only hypotheses confirmed by a few studies that explain the relationship with OSA. The increased susceptibility to OSA in T1D patients may be secondary to the desensitization of the carotid body caused by a state of chronic hyperglycemia or by mechanisms related to diabetes complications, neuropathy in particular. In fact, patients with T1D and OSA have an increased prevalence of autonomic and peripheral neuropathy compared to T1D patients not suffering from OSA.

Indeed, not only in T1D neuropathy is associated with the severity of OSA. In general, the vascular complications of diabetes can be affected by the presence and severity of OSA. Sleep-disordered breathing have been associated with a higher risk of diabetic nephropathy and its severity. OSA was also related to diabetic retinopathy and its progression.

Finally, the relationship between diabetes and OSA during REM sleep is of particular interest. In general, obstructive events that occur during REM sleep are more harmful than those that occur during non-REM sleep. Glycated hemoglobin and mean glucose values are independently associated with the severity of OSA during REM sleep. Furthermore, REM sleep apneas and hypopneas are independently associated with an increased insulin resistance.

Lipids and NAFLD

OSA is often associated with an atherogenic type of dyslipidemia characterized by an increase in triglyceride levels, a reduction in high-density lipoprotein (HDL) levels and the presence of small and dense low-density lipoprotein (LDL). Furthermore, AHI has been shown to independently correlate with low HDL cholesterol values.

The accumulation of lipids in the liver with a mechanism not attributable to excessive alcohol consumption is the characteristic of another emerging metabolic disease, the non-alcoholic fatty liver disease (NAFLD). Also for the development of NAFLD the mechanism of action is generally linked to a state of insulin resistance. About 25% of the general population suffer from NAFLD. Among these patients, about 15% have a more severe form characterized by inflammation and fibrosis, non-alcoholic steatohepatitis (NASH), which can progress to cirrhosis and hepatocellular carcinoma. Patients with OSA show a far higher than 50% incidence of NAFLD; polysomnographic parameters such as AHI and oxygen desaturation index (ODI) are also significantly higher in patients with NAFLD. These data confirm the need for careful monitoring of the development and progression of NAFLD/NASH in patients with severe nocturnal hypoxia.

Pathophysiological and Causal Pathways

The intermediate mechanisms that link OSA to metabolic diseases have not been fully explained. It is generally accepted that intermittent hypoxia and sleep fragmentation play a key role as main triggers in the etiopathogenetic chain of progression of OSA to the metabolic alterations and cardiovascular damage.

Obesity-related upper airway anatomy alterations could explain the strong link between OSA and obesity from a purely mechanical point of view. The accumulation of fat along the circumference of the neck, at the level of the soft palate and submental area, leads to an extrinsic narrowing of the collapsible area of the pharynx. This structural alteration causes a mechanical obstruction to the air flow, thus leading to the greatest risk of OSA in obese patients.

However, central obesity, typical of the metabolic syndrome, may be more closely correlated with OSA than obesity in general. In fact, patients with OSA have a higher proportion of visceral fat than obese controls with a similar BMI.

The hyperactivation of the sympathetic system is probably the most important factor involved in the origin and development of metabolic alterations in OSA. It plays a role in the regulation of glucose metabolism and adipose tissue, through an increase in catecholamine secretion. The sympathetic (autonomic) nervous activity does not return to basal levels after each apnea, but progressively increases in the succession of apneic events, and can persist in the subsequent daytime phases. This sympathoexcitation leads to increased insulin and glucagon secretion, increased hepatic gluconeogenesis and attenuation of the response of incretin hormones to blood glucose.

The fragmentation of sleep may also cause a stress-related increase of hypothalamus-pituitary-adrenal (HPA) axis activity, with consequent elevation of growth hormone (GH) and cortisol circulating levels. Glucose impairment and insulin resistance are the main effects of GH and cortisol on glucose metabolism. Their contribution to the risk of developing T2D is well known.

The recurrence of apneic events can lead to an increased production and accumulation of redox species, with activation of oxidative stress and a systemic inflammatory state. In particular, the production of superoxide anions from neutrophils and monocytes, and the alteration of circulating cytokines, can direct the progression of OSA towards insulin resistance and various degrees of β cell dysfunction due to intermittent hypoxia. Sympathoexcitation itself, with the increased production of catecholamines, can exert pro-inflammatory effects through β1-adrenoceptor – triggered pathways.

The dyslipidemia present in OSA may be secondary to the other associated metabolic pathologies, but may also be a consequence of the increased production of catecholamines and reactive oxygen species (ROS). Intermittent episodes of hypoxia can affect the activation of regulatory genes of liver lipogenesis and the phenomena of lipid peroxidation.

These mechanisms are also the basis of endothelial dysfunction, the increased risk of hypertension, and the progression of atherosclerotic disease in patients with OSA, confirming the strong relationship between cardiovascular, and metabolic and sleep breathing disorders. Furthermore, endothelial dysfunction, identified through cellular, intercellular, and vascular adhesion molecules, is in turn associated with metabolic dysfunction, and considered predictive of T2D.

In addition, the plasma adipokines associated with OSA, released by adipocytes and stimulated by acute sleep deprivation, are able to exert complex actions on lipid metabolism and leptin secretion.

Leptin is one of the principal hormones produced by adipose tissue. The greater activity in the sense of satiety is mediated by specific receptors at the hypothalamic level, where leptin can inhibit the expression of the neuropeptide Y (NPY), which is a powerful stimulator of appetite. The downregulation of NPY is associated with increased sympathetic autonomic activity and energy metabolism. Since leptin levels are higher in obese patients, it has been hypothesized that the presence of a state of leptin resistance is associated with obesity. The relationship between OSA and hyperleptinemia is less clear, and studies have at times offered contradictory opinions. However, patients with OSA have much higher circulating leptin levels than non-OSA subjects of the same age, sex and BMI, suggesting the presence of a state of leptin resistance also in this condition. Furthermore, the possibility of identifying different OSA phenotypes by circulating leptin levels has recently been suggested.

The underlying mechanism between OSA and NAFLD is a complex of oxidative stress, insulin resistance, lipid profile, and the inflammatory state. In general, the relationship can be partially explained by the activation of hypoxia-inducible factors (HIF) and to endoplasmic reticulum stress in conditions of chronic hypoxemia.

The described mechanisms of sympathetic activation, HPA axis alterations, oxidative stress, activation of inflammatory pathways, and changes in adipokine profile lead to inexorable vicious circles characterized by insulin resistance, increase in systemic inflammatory state, and worsening of OSA.

The link to OSA is likely to have a different basis in T1D patients. The hypoxia threshold could be altered by hyperglycemia itself, since its chronic exposure can cause chemoreceptors degeneration of the carotid body and its discharge rate. This mechanism may partly explain the predisposition to OSA in T1D. Moreover, both autonomic and peripheral neuropathy may play a role in neuromuscular dysfunction of the upper airway dilator muscle, as well as in the alteration of central and peripheral chemoreceptors.

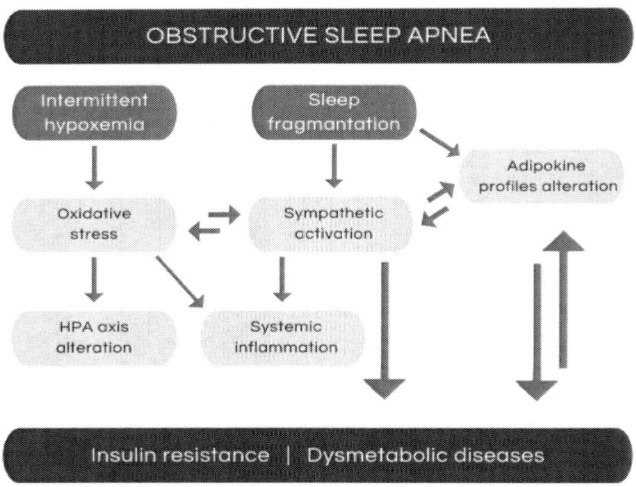

Figure 1. Obstructive sleep apneas and hypopneas are characterized by intermittent hypoxemia and sleep fragmentation. Intermittent hypoxemia causes an altered production of reactive oxygen species with consequent oxidative stress. This is related to a state of general inflammation and to functional alterations of the hypothalamus-pituitary-adrenal (HPA) axis. The continual micro arousals are also associated with an inappropriate activation of the sympathetic system, which determines an altered release of adipokine and proinflammatory cytokines. All these factors are closely linked to one another, resulting in the onset or worsening of insulin resistance and increased risk of metabolic disorders such as obesity and type 2 diabetes.

Treatment

While the treatment for OSA, such as lifestyle modification, continuous positive airway pressure (cPAP), oral appliances, and surgery have shown a reduction of cardiovascular risk factors and improvement on quality of life, the evidence for a beneficial effect on insulin resistance and glucose metabolism are conflicting.

The first line treatment in OSA is the use of nighttime cPAP. The delivery of a continuous positive pressure is able to mechanically maintain the upper airway patency, and reduce the apneic component during sleep. Even if the patient's compliance is one of the most important challenges for the physician, the treatment is usually well tolerated.

As previously mentioned, REM sleep apneas are associated with insulin resistance, and their effect is much more detrimental. In OSA, using cPAP for at least 4 hours per night results in only 25-40% coverage of REM sleep, which generally occurs in the second half of the night. Using cPAP ventilation for at least 7 hours per night, REM sleep will cover approximately 87%, resulting in better control of potentially damaging obstructive events.

The cPAP not only prevents the events of desaturation and hypoxemia, but also reduces nocturnal micro-arousals associated with an increase in adrenergic tone and, consequently, with alterations in blood pressure and metabolic control.

Numerous studies have explored the effects of treatment for OSA regarding metabolic outcomes on populations of normoglycemic, pre-diabetic and diabetic patients.

One of the main studies on non-diabetic patients is by Chirinos et al.. They highlight how only the combined treatment of cPAP and weight loss of about 7 kg can be associated with an improvement in insulin sensitivity measured by intravenous glucose tolerance test. CPAP alone did not demonstrate significant modifications in glucose metabolism in this subtype of patients.

The results of the studies on patients affected with pre-diabetes are those with the greatest discrepancy: different glycemic levels and different degrees of adherence to cPAP therapy are considered, such as presence of additional lifestyle interventions (i.e., weight loss and physical activity).

A randomized controlled trial by Pamidi et al., compared a group of patients with OSA, an AHI greater than 5, and on cPAP therapy for at least 8 hours per night with a group treated only with oral placebo. Correct use of nighttime ventilation for about two weeks demonstrated superiority over placebo in improving oral glucose tolerance and increasing insulin sensitivity. Furthermore, the use of cPAP has shown a reduction in circulating noradrenaline levels, and an improvement in systolic-diastolic blood pressure values. These results prove that cPAP therapy may lead to a reduction in cardio-metabolic risk factors in a potentially reversible condition such as pre-diabetes.

The effect of cPAP in patients with T2D is equally controversial. There are various randomized trials that evaluate the potential benefits of OSA therapy on T2D patients using different level of adherence to therapy, different follow-up times, and different markers of glucose metabolism.

A study by Mokhlesi et al., which involved better adherence to nocturnal ventilotherapy (more than 7 hours per night) resulted in an improvement in plasma glucose and insulin levels.

Another study demonstrating a benefit of cPAP therapy featured patients with OSA and moderately controlled T2D on oral hypoglycemic and/or insulin therapy; in these patients following a treatment of about 6 months, a reduction of HbA1c of 0.4% was found. This value, albeit limited, may result in a clear reduction in the risk of microvascular complications. However, cPAP showed no benefit on diabetic macular edema and visual acuity in patients with T2D and severe OSA after 12 months of therapy.

Other studies have not been able to demonstrate clear metabolic benefits related to treatment with cPAP. Shaw et al., found no improvement in HbA1c and fast blood glucose in patients on cPAP therapy for 6 months for at least 4 hours per night.

Treatment of OSA with cPAP for 6 months also appears to be associated with a reduction in circulating leptin levels, with a mechanism that is not fully known. Some plausible explanations have included body composition modification, with a reduction in the accumulation of visceral fat, a reduction in the sympathoexcitation, in stress markers levels, and in insulin resistance. Increase in lean mass can better explain the improvement in insulin sensitivity, especially when associated with cPAP treatment.

Adherence to ventilation therapy with cPAP is one of the key points for a good quality treatment. The benefits in terms of improved quality of life due to the reduction of daytime sleepiness and greater control of blood pressure values are widely attested to. Further randomized studies are needed to evaluate the real connotative effects of noninvasive ventilation, with adequate therapeutic compliance on OSA-related dysmetabolic pathology.

However, in the literature, opinion is unanimous on the beneficial effects in these patients of interdisciplinary programs with association of cPAP therapy, weight loss, and lifestyle improvement.

Weight loss, whether achieved through medical nutrition, pharmacological therapy or bariatric surgery, has a dual effect on the reduction of obstructive events and improvement of the metabolic profile. Combined treatment of cPAP and weight loss or weight loss alone are associated with a reduction in insulin resistance and serum triglyceride levels.

The AHEAD study, published in 2009, showed in T2D patients how an intensive lifestyle intervention based on weight loss and physical activity programs, compared to an educational support mainly focused on the diabetes management, can lead to a better improvement in the severity of OSA. In 1 year, authors found a reduction in AHI of about 9.7 events per hour in patients with a weight loss of 10 kg or more. Same patients were re-evaluated after 4 and 10 years to verify long-term effect of lifestyle modifications. After 4 years, intensive lifestyle modifications aimed at weight reduction were more effective in reducing AHI, despite 50% of the weight being regained. A study done 10 years after confirmed that lifestyle modification and, therefore, weight reduction is more effective than diabetes education support in improving OSA.

Two antidiabetic drug classes, widely used in T2D, have recently demonstrated cardiovascular protection, weight reduction, and other extra-glycemic effects: glucagon-like peptide 1 receptor agonists (GLP-1RA) and sodium-glucose co-transporter-2 inhibitors (SGLT2i). GLP-1RA are used in the treatment of obesity as a secondary indication. In the "SCALE Sleep Apnea" study, carried out in 2016, on non-diabetic patients with obesity and OSA, it was shown that the use of Liraglutide 3 mg/day for about 8 months was associated with a net weight loss, reduction of HbA1c levels and AHI (about 6 events/h).

The most recent ROMANCE study, designed to compare treatment with liraglutide alone, cPAP alone or the combined treatment for 26 weeks, in a group of patients with T2D, obesity and OSA have no results published at this time.

SGLT2i was found to improve moderate to severe OSA in a few studies with small size samples. Nevertheless, the reduction of AHI seemed not to be linked only to weight loss, perhaps due to the effect of SGLT2i on diuresis and body composition.

Conclusion

The relationship between OSA and metabolic diseases is bidirectional. On the one hand, sleep fragmentation and intermittent hypoxemia present in OSA, through sympathetic activation, HPA axis alterations, oxidative stress, activation of inflammatory pathways, and changes in adipokine profiles, influence insulin sensitivity and, consequently, all the metabolic pathologies related to it.

At the same time, obesity, metabolic syndrome, glucose intolerance, and T2D may be implicated in the development and worsening of OSA.

Furthermore, patients with OSA are already at high cardiovascular risk, and the association with metabolic diseases, diabetes foremost, significantly increases their risk.

Given their high prevalence in the general population, the screening for metabolic diseases in patients with OSA and for sleep-disordered breathing in patients with metabolic disorders is of pivotal importance. Many patients with OSA are diagnosed with incident metabolic diseases, particularly T2D, and vice versa.

International guidelines agree on the need to pay attention to any symptoms suggestive of OSA, such as heavy snoring, witnessed apneas, and excessive daytime sleepiness in patients with prediabetes, T2D, NAFLD or other metabolic diseases. The American Diabetes

Association recommends evaluation with a sleep specialist and a polysomnogram, if indicated.

On the other hand, patients with OSA should be screened for the presence and severity of metabolic disease, T2D, and NAFLD for the possible implementation of appropriate treatment strategies.

Though the direct beneficial effect on metabolism has not been unequivocally confirmed, the treatment of OSA is strongly recommended for evidence on the reduction of cardiovascular risk factors and the improvement in quality of life. However, cPAP can stabilize some metabolic alterations, and other therapeutic indications for OSA often overlap with those for obesity or diabetes. Apart from cPAP and dental appliances, the International Diabetes Federation recommends glucose control, weight reduction, and reduction in alcohol intake for the treatment of OSA associated with diabetes.

The most effective pathway for the therapeutic management of these patients should be a collaboration between various professional figures specialized in sleep and metabolism disorders, such as diabetologists, endocrinologists, dieticians, pulmonologists, and otolaryngologists acting in an integrated way. A multidisciplinary approach to therapy would allow a highly personalized treatment to achieve the best health and quality of life outcomes.

References

"*IDF Atlas 9th edition and other resources.*"

Adderley N. J. et al., "Obstructive sleep apnea, a risk factor for cardiovascular and microvascular disease in patients with type 2 diabetes: Findings from a population-based cohort study," *Diabetes Care*, vol. 43, no. 8, pp. 1868–1877, 2020, doi: 10.2337/dc19-2116.

Adedayo A. M. et al., "Obstructive sleep apnea and dyslipidemia: Evidence and underlying mechanism," *Sleep and Breathing*, vol. 18, no. 1. Springer Verlag, pp. 13-18, 2014, doi: 10.1007/s11325-012-0760-9.

Altaf Q. A. et al., "Obstructive sleep apnea and retinopathy in patients with type 2 diabetes: A longitudinal study," *Am. J. Respir. Crit. Care*

Med., Vol. 196, no. 7, pp. 892-900, Oct. 2017, doi: 10.1164/rccm.201701-0175OC.

Alvarez-Buylla R. and E. R. de Alvarez-Buylla, "Carotid sinus receptors participate in glucose homeostasis," *Respir. Physiol.,* Vol. 72, no. 3, pp. 347–359, Jun. 1988, doi: 10.1016/0034-5687(88)90093-X.

Alzoubaidi M. and B. Mokhlesi, "Obstructive sleep apnea during rapid eye movement sleep: Clinical relevance and therapeutic implications," *Current Opinion in Pulmonary Medicine*, vol. 22, no. 6. Lippincott Williams and Wilkins, pp. 545–554, Oct. 2016, doi: 10.1097/MCP.0000000000000319.

American Diabetes Association, "Standards of Medical Care in Diabetes - 2020," *Diabetes Care*, vol. 43, no. SUPPL. 1. American Diabetes Association Inc., Jan. 2020, doi: 10.2337/diacare.27.2007.s15.

Andrews R. C. and B. R. WALKER, "Glucocorticoids and insulin resistance: old hormones, new targets," *Clin. Sci.,* Vol. 96, no. 5, pp. 513-523, May 1999, doi: 10.1042/cs0960513.

Baiceanu A., P. Mesdom, M. Lagouge, and F. Foufelle, "Endoplasmic reticulum proteostasis in hepatic steatosis," *Nature Reviews Endocrinology*, vol. 12, no. 12. Nature Publishing Group, pp. 710–722, Dec. 2016, doi: 10.1038/nrendo.2016.124.

Balks H. J., J. J. Holst, A. von zur Mühlen, and G. Brabant, "Rapid Oscillations in Plasma Glucagon-Like Peptide-1 (GLP-1) in Humans: Cholinergic Control of GLP-1 Secretion via Muscarinic Receptors1," *J. Clin. Endocrinol. Metab.*, Vol. 82, no. 3, pp. 786–790, Mar. 1997, doi: 10.1210 / jcem.82.3.3816.

Banghoej A. M. et al., "Obstructive sleep apnoea is frequent in patients with type 1 diabetes," *J. Diabetes Complications*, vol. 31, no. 1, pp. 156–161, Jan. 2017, doi: 10.1016/j.jdiacomp.2016.10.006.

Bibbins-Domingo K. et al., "Screening for obstructive sleep apnea in adults us preventive services task force recommendation statement," *JAMA - Journal of the American Medical Association*, vol. 317, no. 4. American Medical Association, pp. 407–414, Jan. 2017, doi: 10.1001/jama.2016.20325.

Blackman A. et al., "Effect of liraglutide 3.0 mg in individuals with obesity and moderate or severe obstructive sleep apnea: The scale sleep apnea randomized clinical trial," *Int. J. Obes.*, Vol. 40, no. 8, pp. 1310–1319, Aug. 2016, doi: 10.1038/ijo.2016.52.

Bloom S. R., A. V. Edwards, and R. N. Hardy, "The role of the autonomic nervous system in the control of glucagon, insulin and pancreatic polypeptide release from the pancreas.," *J. Physiol.*, Vol. 280, no. 1, pp. 9–23, Jul. 1978, doi: 10.1113/jphysiol.1978. sp012369.

Bolinder J. et al., "Effects of dapagliflozin on body weight, total fat mass, and regional adipose tissue distribution in patients with type 2 diabetes mellitus with inadequate glycemic control on metformin," *J. Clin. Endocrinol. Metab.*, Vol. 97, no. 3, pp. 1020-1031, Mar. 2012, doi: 10.1210/jc.2011-2260.

Bonsignore M. R., W. T. McNicholas, J. M. Montserrat, and J. Eckel, "Adipose tissue in obesity and obstructive sleep apnoea," *European Respiratory Journal*, vol. 39, no. 3. European Respiratory Society, pp. 746–767, Mar. 2012, doi: 10.1183 / 09031936.00047010.

Börgel J. et al., "Obstructive sleep apnoea and its therapy influence high-density lipoprotein cholesterol serum levels," *Eur. Respir. J.*, vol. 27, no. 1, pp. 121–127, Jan. 2006, doi: 10.1183/09031936.06. 00131304.

Bottini P., S. Redolfi, M. L. Dottorini, and C. Tantucci, "Autonomic neuropathy increases the risk of obstructive sleep apnea in obese diabetics," *Respiration*, vol. 75, no. 3, pp. 265-271, Mar. 2008, doi: 10.1159/000100556.

Bozkurt N. C., S. Beysel, B. Karbek, I. O. Unsal, E. Cakir, and T. Delibasi, "Visceral obesity mediates the association between metabolic syndrome and obstructive sleep apnea syndrome," *Metab. Syndr. Relat. Disord.*, Vol. 14, no. 4, pp. 217–221, May 2016, doi: 10.1089/met. 2015.0086.

Bruno A., Di Sano C., Lorusso F., Dino P., Russo D., Ballacchino A., Gallina S, Modica DM, Chiappara G, Simon HU, Pace E. Notch-1 decreased expression contributes to leptin receptor downregulation in nasal epithelium from allergic turbinates. *Biochim Biophys Acta Mol Basis Dis.* 2019 Jun 1; 1865(6):1642-1650.

Cakmak E. et al., "Association between the severity of nocturnal hypoxia in obstructive sleep apnea and non-alcoholic fatty liver damage," *Hepat. Mon.*, vol. 15, no. 11, Nov. 2015, doi: 10.5812/ hepatmon.32655.

Caro J. F., M. K. Sinha, J. W. Kolaczynski, P. L. Zhang, and R. V. Considine, "Leptin: The tale of an obesity gene," *Diabetes*, vol. 45, no. 11. American Diabetes Association Inc., pp. 1455–1462, Jan. 1996, doi: 10.2337 / diab.45.11.1455.

Chami H. A., D. J. Gottlieb, S. Redline, and N. M. Punjabi, "Association between glucose metabolism and sleep-disordered breathing during REM sleep," Am. *J. Respir. Crit. Care Med.*, Vol. 192, no. 9, pp. 1118-1126, Nov. 2015, doi: 10.1164 / rccm.201501-0046OC.

Chin K. et al., "Changes in intra-abdominal visceral fat and serum leptin levels in patients with obstructive sleep apnea syndrome following nasal continuous positive airway pressure therapy," *Circulation*, vol. 100, no. 7, pp. 706-712, Aug. 1999, doi: 10.1161 / 01.CIR.100.7. 706.

Chirinos J. A. et al., "CPAP, Weight Loss, or Both for Obstructive Sleep Apnea," *N. Engl. J. Med.*, Vol. 370, no. 24, pp. 2265–2275, Jun. 2014, doi: 10.1056 / nejmoa1306187.

Fendri S., D. Rose, S. Myambu, S. Jeanne, and J. D. Lalau, "Nocturnal hyperglycaemia in type 2 diabetes with sleep apnoea syndrome," *Diabetes Res. Clin. Pract.*, Vol. 91, no. 1, Jan. 2011, doi: 10.1016 / j.diabres.2010.09.029.

Flier J. S. and E. Maratos-Flier, "Obesity and the hypothalamus: Novel peptides for new pathways," *Cell*, vol. 92, no. 4. Cell Press, pp. 437-440, Feb. 1998, doi: 10.1016/S0092-8674(00)80937-X.

Foster G. D. et al., "A randomized study on the effect of weight loss on obstructive sleep apnea among obese patients with type 2 diabetes: The sleep AHEAD study," *Arch. Intern. Med.*, Vol. 169, no. 17, pp. 1619–1626, 2009, doi: 10.1001/archinternmed.2009. 266.

Foster G. D. et al., "Obstructive sleep apnea among obese patients with type 2 diabetes," *Diabetes Care*, vol. 32, no. 6, pp. 1017-1019, Jun. 2009, doi: 10.2337/dc08-1776.

Fujihara K. et al., "The Relationship between Diabetic Neuropathy and Sleep Apnea Syndrome: A Meta-Analysis," *Sleep Disord.*, Vol. 2013, pp. 1–7, 2013, doi: 10.1155/2013/150371.

Furukawa S. et al., "The effectiveness of dapagliflozin for sleep-disordered breathing among Japanese patients with obesity and type 2 diabetes mellitus," *Endocr. J.,* vol. 65, no. 9, pp. 953–961, 2018, doi: 10.1507/endocrj.EJ17-0545.

Gage J. R., G. Fonarow, M. Hamilton, M. Widawski, O. Martínez-Maza, and DL Vredevoe, "Beta Blocker and Angiotensin-Converting Enzyme Inhibitor Therapy Is Associated with Decreased Th1 / Th2 Cytokine Ratios and Inflammatory Cytokine Production in Patients with Chronic Heart Failure," *Neuroimmunomodulation*, vol. 11, pp. 173-180, 2004, doi: 10.1159/000076766.

Goldberger J. J. et al., "American Heart Association/American College of Cardiology Foundation/Heart Rhythm Society scientific statement on noninvasive risk stratification techniques for identifying patients at risk for sudden cardiac death: A scientific statement from the American Heart Association Council on Clinical Cardiology Committee on Electrocardiography and Arrhythmias and Council on Epidemiology and Prevention, "Circulation, vol. 118, no. 14. *Circulation*, pp. 1497–1518, Sep. 2008, doi: 10.1161/CIRCULATIONAHA.107.189375.

Gordon P. and M. H. Sanders, "Sleep 7: Positive airway pressure therapy for obstructive sleep apnoea/hypopnoea syndrome," *Thorax*, vol. 60, no. 1. BMJ Publishing Group, pp. 68–75, Jan. 2005, doi: 10.1136/thx.2003.007195.

Grimaldi D., G. Beccuti, C. Touma, E. Van Cauter, and B. Mokhlesi, "Association of obstructive sleep apnea in rapid eye movement sleep with reduced glycemic control in type 2 diabetes: Therapeutic implications," *Diabetes Care*, vol . 37, no. 2, pp. 355–363, Feb. 2014, doi: 10.2337/dc13-0933.

Heinzer R. et al., "Prevalence of sleep-disordered breathing in the general population: THE HypnoLaus study," *Lancet Respir. Med.*, Vol. 3, no. 4, pp. 310-318, Apr. 2015, doi: 10.1016/S2213-2600 (15) 00043-0.

Iftikhar I. H., C. M. Hoyos, C. L. Phillips, and U. J. Magalang, "Meta-analyzes of the Association of Sleep Apnea with Insulin Resistance, and the Effects of CPAP on HOMA-IR, Adiponectin, and Visceral Adipose Fat," *J. Clin. Sleep Med.*, Vol. 11, no. 04, pp. 475–485, Apr. 2015, doi: 10.5664/jcsm.4610.

International Diabetes Federation, "*The IDF Consensus Statement on Sleep Apnoea and Type 2 Diabetes*," pp. 1–24, 2008.

Ip M. S. M., B. Lam, M. M. T. Ng, W. K. Lam, K. W. T. Tsang, and K. S. L. Lam, "Obstructive sleep apnea is independently associated with insulin resistance," *Am. J. Respir. Crit. Care Med.*, Vol. 165, no. 5, pp. 670–676, Mar. 2002, doi: 10.1164/ajrccm.165.5.2103001.

Kakkar R. K. and R. B. Berry, "Positive airway pressure treatment for obstructive sleep apnea," *Chest*, vol. 132, no. 3. American College of Chest Physicians, pp. 1057-1072, 2007, doi: 10.1378/chest.06-2432.

Kendzerska T., A. S. Gershon, G. Hawker, G. Tomlinson, and R. S. Leung, "Obstructive sleep apnea and incident diabetes a historical cohort study," *Am. J. Respir. Crit. Care Med.*, Vol. 190, no. 2, pp. 218-225, Jul. 2014, doi: 10.1164/rccm.201312-2209OC.

Kline D. D., Y. J. Peng, D. J. Manalo, G. L. Semenza, and N. R. Prabhakar, "Defective carotid body function and impaired ventilatory responses to chronic hypoxia in mice partially deficient for hypoxia-inducible factor 1α," *Proc. Natl. Acad. Sci. U. S. A.*, vol. 99, no. 2, pp. 821–826, Jan. 2002, doi: 10.1073/pnas.022634199.

Kozu Y. et al., "Cluster analysis identifies a pathophysiologically distinct subpopulation with increased serum leptin levels and severe obstructive sleep apnea," *Sleep Breath.*, 2020, doi: 10.1007/s11325-020-02160-8.

Kritikou I. et al., "Sleep apnoea, sleepiness, inflammation and insulin resistance in middle-aged males and females," *European Respiratory Journal*, vol. 43, no. 1. European Respiratory Society, pp. 145–155, Jan. 2014, doi: 10.1183/09031936.00126712.

Kuna S. T. et al., "Effects of Weight Loss on Obstructive Sleep Apnea Severity: 10-year Results of the Sleep AHEAD Study," *Am. J. Respir. Crit. Care Med.*, Jul. 2020, doi: 10.1164/rccm.201912-2511oc.

Kuna S. T. et al., "Long-term effect of weight loss on obstructive sleep apnea severity in obese patients with type 2 diabetes," *Sleep*, vol. 36, no. 5, pp. 641–649, May 2013, doi: 10.5665/sleep.2618.

Lam J. C. M. et al., "A randomized controlled trial of nasal continuous positive airway pressure on insulin sensitivity in obstructive sleep apnoea," *Eur. Respir. J.*, vol. 35, no. 1, pp. 138–145, Jan. 2010, doi: 10.1183/09031936.00047709.

Lavie L., "Obstructive sleep apnoea syndrome - An oxidative stress disorder," *Sleep Medicine Reviews*, vol. 7, no. 1. W. B. Saunders Ltd, pp. 35–51, 2003, doi: 10.1053/smrv.2002.0261.

Lefere S., C. Van Steenkiste, X. Verhelst, H. Van Vlierberghe, L. Devisscher, and A. Geerts, "Hypoxia-regulated mechanisms in the pathogenesis of obesity and non-alcoholic fatty liver disease," *Cellular and Molecular Life Sciences*, vol. 73, no. 18. Birkhauser Verlag AG, pp. 3419–3431, Sep. 2016, doi: 10.1007/s00018-016-2222-1.

Leong, W. B., F. Jadhakhan, S. Taheri, G. N. Thomas, and P. Adab, "The Association between obstructive sleep apnea on diabetic kidney disease: A systematic review and meta-analysis," *Sleep*, vol. 39, no. 2, pp. 301–308, Feb. 2016, doi: 10.5665/sleep.5432.

Leong, W. B., F. Jadhakhan, S. Taheri, Y. F. Chen, P. Adab, and G. N. Thomas, "Effect of obstructive sleep apnoea on diabetic retinopathy and maculopathy: A systematic review and meta-analysis," *Diabet. Med.*, Vol. 33, no. 2, pp. 158–168, Feb. 2016, doi: 10.1111/dme.12817.

Lévy P. et al., "Obstructive sleep apnoea syndrome," *Nat. Rev. Dis. Prim.*, Vol. 1, Jun. 2015, doi: 10.1038/nrdp.2015.15.

Li C., ES Ford, G. Zhao, JB Croft, LS Balluz, and AH Mokdad, "Prevalence of self-reported clinically diagnosed sleep apnea according to obesity status in men and women: National Health and Nutrition Examination Survey, 2005-2006," *Prev. Med.* (Baltim)., Vol. 51, no. 1, pp. 18–23, Jul. 2010, doi: 10.1016/j.ypmed.2010.03.016.

Li J., V. Savransky, A. Nanayakkara, P. L. Smith, C. P. O'Donnell, and V. Y. Polotsky, "Hyperlipidemia and lipid peroxidation are dependent on the severity of chronic intermittent hypoxia," *J. Appl. Physiol.*, Vol. 102, no. 2, pp. 557-563, Feb. 2007, doi: 10.1152/japplphysiol.01081.2006.

Li M., X. Li, and Y. Lu, "Obstructive sleep apnea syndrome and metabolic diseases," *Endocrinology*, vol. 159, no. 7, pp. 2670-2675, 2018, doi: 10.1210/en.2018-00248.

Lorusso F, Dispenza F, Modica DM, Gallina S. The Role of Modified Expansion Sphincter Pharyngoplasty in Multilevel Obstructive Sleep Apnea Syndrome Surgery. *Int Arch Otorhinolaryngol.* 2018 Oct; 22(4):432-436.

Lorusso F, Dispenza F, Saraniti C, Sireci F, Modica DM, Gallina S. Sleep disordered breathing: evaluation of dynamic patterns of the upper airways in obese subjects. *Otorinolaringologia* 2014; 64:57–64.

Lorusso F, Gallina S, Modica DM, Di Salvo N, Riggio F. Bipolar Quantum Molecular Resonance versus Blunt Dissection tonsillectomy. *B-ENT* 2015; 11(02):101–108.

Lorusso, F., Dispenza, F., Martinciglio, G., ...Battaglia, A., Gallina, S. Postural changes in patients undergoing hyoid surgery for OSAS. *EuroMediterranean Biomedical Journal*, 2017; 12(29):140-143.

Lorusso, F., Martines, F., Mistretta, A., ...Dispenza, F., Gallina, S. *Effects of adenotonsillectomy on neurocognitive and behavioural function in pediatric obstructive sleep apnea syndrome. B-ENT* 2018; 14:113-118.

Marshall N. S., K. K. H. Wong, C. L. Phillips, P. Y. Liu, M. W. Knuiman, and R. R. Grunstein, "Is sleep apnea an independent risk factor for prevalent and incident diabetes in the Busselton health study ?," *J. Clin. Sleep Med.*, Vol. 5, no. 1, pp. 15-20, Feb. 2009, doi: 10.5664/jcsm.27387.

Martinez-Ceron E. et al., "Effect of continuous positive airway pressure on glycemic control in patients with obstructive sleep apnea and type 2 diabetes a randomized clinical trial," *Am. J. Respir. Crit. Care Med.*, Vol. 194, no. 4, pp. 476–485, Aug. 2016, doi: 10.1164/rccm.201510-1942OC.

Meigs J. B., F. B. Hu, N. Rifai, and J. A. E. Manson, "Biomarkers of thelial Dysfunction and Risk of Type 2 Diabetes Mellitus," *J. Am. Med. Assoc.,* Vol. 291, no. 16, pp. 1978–1986, Apr. 2004, doi: 10.1001/jama.291.16.1978.

Mishra A. and Z. M. Younossi, "Epidemiology and Natural History of Non-alcoholic Fatty Liver Disease," *J. Clin. Exp. Hepatol.*, Vol. 2, no. 2, pp. 135–144, 2012, doi: 10.1016/S0973-6883(12)60102-9.

Modica DM, Lorusso F, Presti G, Fasola S, Gallina S. Our Assessment Using Palate Postoperative Problems Score (PPOPS): Tool for the

Evaluation of Results in Palatal Surgery Techniques. *Indian J Otolaryngol Head Neck Surg.* 2019 Oct; 71(Suppl 1):766-770.

Modica DM, Marchese D, Lorusso F, Speciale R, Saraniti C, Gallina S. Functional Nasal Surgery and Use of CPAP in OSAS Patients: Our Experience. *Indian J Otolaryngol Head Neck Surg.* 2018 Dec; 70(4): 559-565.

Mokhlesi B. et al., "Effect of one week of 8-hour nightly continuous positive airway pressure treatment of obstructive sleep apnea on glycemic control in type 2 diabetes: A proof-of-concept study," *American Journal of Respiratory and Critical Care Medicine*, vol. 194, no. 4. American Thoracic Society, pp. 516-519, Aug. 2016, doi: 10.1164/rccm.201602-0396LE.

Musso G., M. Cassader, C. Olivetti, F. Rosina, G. Carbone, and R. Gambino, "Association of obstructive sleep apnoea with the presence and severity of non-alcoholic fatty liver disease. A systematic review and meta-analysis, "Obesity Reviews, vol. 14, no. 5. *Obes Rev*, pp. 417-431, May 2013, doi: 10.1111/obr.12020.

Narkiewicz K., M. Kato, B. G. Phillips, C. A. Pesek, D. E. Davison, and V. K. Somers, "Nocturnal continuous positive airway pressure decreases daytime sympathetic traffic in obstructive sleep apnea," *Circulation*, vol. 100, no. 23, pp. 2332–2335, Dec. 1999, doi: 10. 1161/01.CIR.100.23.2332.

Nathan D. M. et al., "Impaired fasting glucose and impaired glucose tolerance: Implications for care," in *Diabetes Care*, Mar. 2007, vol. 30, no. 3, pp. 753–759, doi: 10.2337 / dc07-9920.

Newhouse L. P. et al., "Three hours of intermittent hypoxia increases circulating glucose levels in healthy adults," *Physiol. Rep.,* Vol. 5, no. 1, Jan. 2017, doi: 10.14814/phy2.13106.

Nonogaki K., "New insights into sympathetic regulation of glucose and fat metabolism," Diabetologia, vol. 43, no. 5. *Diabetology*, pp. 533-549, 2000, doi: 10.1007/s001250051341.

Pamidi S. et al., "Eight hours of nightly continuous positive airway pressure treatment of obstructive sleep apnea improves glucose metabolism in patients with prediabetes: A randomized controlled trial," *Am. J. Respir. Crit. Care Med.*, Vol. 192, no. 1, pp. 96-105, Jul. 2015, doi: 10.1164/rccm.201408-1564OC.

Paschetta E. et al., "OSAS-Related inflammatory mechanisms of liver injury in nonalcoholic fatty liver disease," *Mediators of Inflammation*, vol. 2015. Hindawi Limited, 2015, doi: 10.1155/2015/815721.

Pereira K., J. Salsamendi, and J. Casillas, "The Global Nonalcoholic Fatty Liver Disease Epidemic: What a Radiologist Needs to Know," *J. Clin. Imaging Sci.*, Vol. 5, no. 1, Jan. 2015, doi: 10.4103/2156-7514.157860.

Pi-Sunyer X. et al., "A Randomized, Controlled Trial of 3.0 mg of Liraglutide in Weight Management," *N. Engl. J. Med.*, Vol. 373, no. 1, pp. 11–22, Jul. 2015, doi: 10.1056/nejmoa1411892.

Punjabi N. M., J. D. Sorkin, L. I. Katzel, A. P. Goldberg, A. R. Schwartz, and P. L. Smith, "Sleep-disordered breathing and insulin resistance in middle-aged and overweight men," *Am. J. Respir. Crit. Care Med.*, Vol. 165, no. 5, pp. 677–682, Mar. 2002, doi: 10.1164/ajrccm.165.5.2104087.

Reutrakul S. and B. Mokhlesi, "Obstructive Sleep Apnea and Diabetes: A State of the Art Review," *Chest*, vol. 152, no. 5, pp. 1070-1086, 2017, doi: 10.1016/j.chest.2017.05.009.

Reutrakul S. and E. Van Cauter, "Interactions between sleep, circadian function, and glucose metabolism: Implications for risk and severity of diabetes," *Ann. N. Y. Acad. Sci.*, Vol. 1311, no. 1, pp. 151–173, 2014, doi: 10.1111/nyas.12355.

Reutrakul S. et al., "Sleep characteristics in type 1 diabetes and associations with glycemic control: systematic review and meta-analysis," *Sleep Med.*, Vol. 23, pp. 26–45, Jul. 2016, doi: 10.1016/j.sleep.2016.03.019.

Romero-Corral A., S. M. Caples, F. Lopez-Jimenez, and V. K. Somers, "Interactions between obesity and obstructive sleep apnea: Implications for treatment," *Chest*, vol. 137, no. 3, pp. 711–719, Mar. 2010, doi: 10.1378/chest.09-0360.

Ronald Kahn C., "Insulin resistance, insulin insensitivity, and insulin unresponsiveness: A necessary distinction," *Metabolism.*, Vol. 27, no. 12, pp. 1893–1902, 1978, doi: 10.1016/S0026-0495 (78) 80007-9.

Sawada K. et al., "Effect of sodium glucose cotransporter 2 inhibitors on obstructive sleep apnea in patients with type 2 diabetes,"

Endocr. J., vol. 65, no. 4, pp. 461–467, 2018, doi: 10.1507/endocrj.EJ17-0440.

Schwartz M. W. and R. J. Seeley, "Neuroendocrine Responses to Starvation and Weight Loss," *N. Engl. J. Med.*, Vol. 336, no. 25, pp. 1802–1811, Jun. 1997, doi: 10.1056/nejm199706193362507.

Seicean S. et al., "Sleep-disordered breathing and impaired glucose metabolism in normal-weight and overweight / obese individuals," *Diabetes Care*, vol. 31, no. 5, pp. 1001-1006, May 2008, doi: 10. 2337/dc07-2003.

Shamsuzzaman A. S. M., B. J. Gersh, and V. K. Somers, "Obstructive Sleep Apnea: Implications for Cardiac and Vascular Disease," *Journal of the American Medical Association*, vol. 290, no. 14. American Medical Association, pp. 1906–1914, Oct. 2003, doi: 10. 1001/jama.290.14.1906.

Shaw J. E. et al., "The effect of treatment of obstructive sleep apnea on glycemic control in type 2 diabetes," *Am. J. Respir. Crit. Care Med.*, Vol. 194, no. 4, pp. 486–492, Aug. 2016, doi: 10.1164/rccm. 201511-2260OC.

Shaw J. E., N. M. Punjabi, J. P. Wilding, K. G. M. M. Alberti, and P. Z. Zimmet, "Sleep-disordered breathing and type 2 diabetes. A report from the International Diabetes Federation Taskforce on Epidemiology and Prevention," *Diabetes Res. Clin. Pract.*, Vol. 81, no. 1, pp. 2-12, Jul. 2008, doi: 10.1016/j.diabres.2008.04.025.

Somers, V. K., M. E. Dyken, M. P. Clary, and F. M. Abboud, "Sympathetic neural mechanisms in obstructive sleep apnea," *J. Clin. Invest.*, Vol. 96, no. 4, pp. 1897–1904, 1995, doi: 10.1172/JCI118235.

Song S. O., K. He, R. R. Narla, H. G. Kang, H. U. Ryu, and E. J. Boyko, "Metabolic consequences of obstructive sleep apnea especially pertaining to diabetes mellitus and insulin sensitivity," *Diabetes Metab. J.,* vol. 43, no. 2, pp. 144–155, 2019, doi: 10.4093/dmj.2018.0256.

Sprung V. S. et al., "Randomized, cOntrolled Multicentre trial of 26 weeks subcutaneous liraglutide (a glucagon-like peptide-1 receptor Agonist), with or without contiNuous positive airway pressure (CPAP), in patients with type 2 diabetes mellitus (T2DM) and obstructive sleep apnoEa (OSA) (ROMANCE): Study protocol assessing the effects of weight loss on the apnea-hypnoea index (AHI)," *BMJ Open*, vol. 10, no. 7, Jul. 2020, doi: 10.1136/bmjopen-2020-038856.

Streba L. A. M., C. C. Vere, I. Rogoveanu, and C. T. Streba, "Nonalcoholic fatty liver disease, metabolic risk factors, and hepatocellular carcinoma: An open question," *World Journal of Gastroenterology*, vol. 21, no. 14. WJG Press, pp. 4103–4110, Apr. 14, 2015, doi: 10.3748/wjg.v21.i14.4103.

Tahrani A. A. et al., "Obstructive sleep apnea and diabetic neuropathy: A novel association in patients with type 2 diabetes," *Am. J. Respir. Crit. Care Med.*, Vol. 186, no. 5, pp. 434–441, Sep. 2012, doi: 10. 1164/rccm.201112-2135OC.

Tang, Y., Q. Sun, X. Y. Bai, Y. F. Zhou, Q. L. Zhou, and M. Zhang, "Effect of dapagliflozin on obstructive sleep apnea in patients with type 2 diabetes: a preliminary study," *Nutr. Diabetes*, vol. 9, no. 1, Dec. 2019, doi: 10.1038/s41387-019-0098-5.

Vgontzas A. N. et al., "Sleep apnea and daytime sleepiness and fatigue: Relation to visceral obesity, insulin resistance, and hypercytokinemia," *J. Clin. Endocrinol. Metab.*, Vol. 85, no. 3, pp. 1151-1158, 2000, doi: 10.1210/jcem.85.3.6484.

Vilgrain V., et al., "Hepatic steatosis: A major trap in liver imaging," *Diagnostic and Interventional Imaging*, vol. 94, no. 7-8. Elsevier Masson SAS, pp. 713-727, 2013, doi: 10.1016/j.diii.2013.03.010.

West S. D. et al., "Continuous positive airway pressure effect on visual acuity in patients with type 2 diabetes and obstructive sleep apnoea: A multicentre randomized controlled trial," *Eur. Respir. J.*, vol. 52, no. 4, p. 1801177, Oct. 2018, doi: 10.1183/13993003. 01177-2018.

West S. D., D. J. Nicoll, and J. R. Stradling, "Prevalence of obstructive sleep apnoea in men with type 2 diabetes," *Thorax*, vol. 61, no. 11, pp. 945–950, Nov. 2006, doi: 10.1136/thx.2005.057745.

Wilcox I., "'Syndrome Z': The interaction of sleep apnoea, vascular risk factors and heart disease," in *Thorax*, 1998, vol. 53, no. SUPPL. 3, p. S25, doi: 10.1136/thx.53.2008.S25.

Xu J., Y. S. Long, D. Gozal, and P. N. Epstein, "β-cell death and proliferation after intermittent hypoxia: Role of oxidative stress,"

Free Radic. Biol. Med., Vol. 46, no. 6, pp. 783–790, Mar. 2009, doi: 10.1016/j.freeradbiomed. 2008.11.026.

Yokoe T., et al., "Intermittent hypoxia reverses the diurnal glucose rhythm and causes pancreatic β-cell replication in mice," *J. Physiol.*, Vol. 586, no. 3, pp. 899-911, Feb. 2008, doi: 10.1113/ jphysiol. 2007.143586.

Zhang R., P. Zhang, F. Zhao, X. Han, and L. Ji, "Association of Diabetic Microvascular Complications and Parameters of Obstructive Sleep Apnea in Patients with Type 2 Diabetes," *Diabetes Technol. Ther.*, Vol. 18, no. 7, pp. 415-420, Jul. 2016, doi: 10.1089/dia.2015.0433.

In: Advances in Sleep Apnea
Editors: F. Lorusso et al.
ISBN: 978-1-53619-758-7

Chapter 9

ADVANCES IN VENTILATORY TREATMENT FOR OSAS

Maria R. Bonsignore*

PROMISE Department, University of Palermo, Palermo, Italy
Institute for Biomedical Research and Innovation (IRIB),
National Research Council (CNR), Palermo, Italy

ABSTRACT

Continuous positive airway pressure (CPAP) is the most widely used treatment for obstructive sleep apnea (OSA), and was established four decades ago. An alternative option is to use bilevel ventilation, in order to improve compliance to treatment especially in patients who need a high therapeutic pressure to prevent nocturnal respiratory events. Automatic CPAP or bilevel ventilation are also established among OSA therapeutic choices, and are generally indicated in cases of highly variable therapeutic pressure. The major advances in the field regard OSAS in the context of uncomplicated obesity hypoventilation syndrome (OHS), in which either CPAP or bilevel ventilation yield comparable results, and the increasingly popular use of telemedicine in OSA management. The COVID-19 pandemic has been a major

---

* Corresponding Author's Email: mariarosaria.bonsignore@unipa.it.

determinant of the shift from traditional clinic-based management to using telemedicine whenever possible. In addition, availability of CPAP data recorded in millions of patients has allowed big-data studies on adherence to CPAP or bilevel ventilation over prolonged periods of time. It can be foreseen that e-Health programs will soon be used for most of the clinical activities in the OSA field.

INTRODUCTION

Obstructive sleep apnea is mostly treated with the application of nasal continuous positive airway pressure (CPAP) since the original studies by Sullivan and coworkers (Sullivan et al., 1981). Properly titrated CPAP abolishes obstructive apneas and hypopneas by splinting the upper airway open. CPAP prevents hypoxemia, respiratory efforts, hypertensive peaks, and OSA-related sleep fragmentation since the first nights of use (Sullivan et al., 1981).

CPAP is applied through a nose or a face mask, and prevention of leaks is essential for optimal treatment. Many models of masks exist, and the best mask fit should always be pursued, since it improves patient's comfort and effectiveness of treatment (Cistulli & Sullivan, 2019).

In patients in whom CPAP treatment requires a very high therapeutic pressure, use of bilevel ventilation has been proposed to decrease mean airway pressure, since the expiratory pressure is maintained relatively low, and the highest pressure is reached only during the inspiratory phase. Alternatively, a minority of patients with associated comorbidities, such as chronic obstructive pulmonary disease (COPD), may require pressure support to increase their ventilation during sleep and normalize nocturnal ventilation and the oxygen saturation (SpO2) profile. This chapter will examine the current knowledge on CPAP and bilevel ventilation in OSA, and the likely increase in the use of telemedicine in the management of OSA patients.

1. Continuous Positive Airway Pressure (CPAP)

The literature on CPAP in OSA is quite extensive, and the reader interested in a historical perspective is referred to a recent paper published by Colin Sullivan, who invented it (Sullivan, 2018).

Currently, there is a strong and established trend to use automatic CPAP rather than CPAP at a fixed pressure in the treatment of OSA. Automatic CPAP machines are commonly used to determine the therapeutic pressure, based on the analysis of data recorded by the device over a few nights, thus preventing the high cost of in-laboratory traditional titration. Alternatively, automatic CPAP can be prescribed without any titration, and the respiratory physician can modify the CPAP mode from automatic to fixed CPAP at the first clinical visit shortly after initation of treatment. Automatic CPAP devices have the advantage of requiring less strict follow-up, especially in patients undergoing bariatric surgery who would need frequent pressure adjustments during progressive weight loss. There are also some disadvantages, for example leaks from the mask during automatic CPAP can be associated with discomfort due to excessive flow of air while the machine tries to reach the therapeutic pressure. However, leaks were not shown to be associated with CPAP mode, but increased with increasing therapeutic pressure (Lebret et al., 2019). Finally, some studies suggest that fixed CPAP pressure might be more effective in reducing sympathetic hyperactivity (Patruno et al., 2007; Patruno et al., 2014) or preventing deterioration of renal function in OSA patients (Marrone et al., 2018). Randomized controlled trials are ongoing to assess whether fixed and automatic CPAP differ as clinical outcomes are concerned (Triptow et al., 2019).

The main problem associated with CPAP treatment for OSA is the variable adherence to treatment. The minimum of CPAP use that defines a patient as being compliant to CPAP is 4 hours/night for at least 70% of the nights. Sleepy and/or symptomatic patients accept CPAP treatment more easily than asymptomatic OSA patients (Gagnadoux et al., 2016). Conversely, lean patients with OSA and insomnia usually show poor CPAP adherence (Eysteinsdottir et al., 2017).

CPAP should be used every night, and only a minority of patients can resolve OSA by other means, i.e., mandibular advancement device, upper airway surgery, or weight loss. Some studies examined the adherence to treatment at 10 years after prescription (Zampogna et al., 2020; Tsuyumu et al., 2020). Major predictors of continued use were: hours of use in the first month of treatment, body mass index (BMI), and use of nasal rather than face mask. CPAP was still used after 10 years of treatment in 56% and 42% of the patients in the studies by Zampogna et al., and Tsuyumu et al., respectively. Other studies identified psychological profiles associated with a high risk of CPAP discontinuation (Pelletier-Fleury et al., 2020).

Technological improvements over decades have not been successful in improving CPAP adherence, as it had been hoped in the past. Current CPAP devices are smaller in size and much less noisy than old devices, many mask models are available, and mask are softer and lightweight compared to the past, with improved comfort; nevertheless, a significant percentage of patients do not tolerate CPAP and stop using it. Good adherence in the first month of treatment, and improvement in symptoms remain the best predictors of prolonged CPAP use.

Technological advancement has been at least partly successful for OSA in women, since CPAP devices with dedicated algorithms specifically developed for female patients are available. Since premenopausal women develop more often partial than complete upper airway collapse during sleep, this algorithm is effective against inspiratory flow limitation, and mean therapeutic pressure is lower than with traditional automatic CPAP (McArdle et al., 2015).

Availability of data on CPAP use collected by telemedicine has allowed to describe some patterns, i.e., great users (17%), good users (32.8%), low users (22.7%) and slow decliners (27.5%) (Babbin et al., 2015). Such data are very relevant for clinicians, since assessment of adherence to CPAP in different clinical phenotypes of OSA patients could suggest CPAP prescription to patients with a good likelihood of success, and reinforced motivating interventions for patients unlikely to accept treatment. Many research projects are ongoing to reshape the definition of OSAS, its clinical presentations, and the best therapeutic options for each phenotype, including drug treatment according to physiological phenotypes of OSA (Eckert, 2018). When the results of this process will be established, OSAS treatment will be personalized, and CPAP treatment possibly restricted to those patients who would benefit most from it (Bonsignore et al., 2017).

2. Bilevel Ventilation

Bilevel ventilation has evolved over the years, from simple ventilators to be used in the S/T mode, to more sophisticated machines with automatic algorithms. Such evolution has increased the use of automatic bilevel ventilation, which exists in different models. The simplest one is an automatic CPAP with a fixed pressure support, variable between 4 and 10 cmH_2O. Other devices allow to set a range of expiratory and inspiratory pressures, and a range of pressure support, with the machine graduating the latter according to the degree of upper airway inspiratory limitation and/or decreased airflow. In cases of poor tolerance to CPAP, switching to automatic bilevel ventilation was associated with improvement in adherence according to a recent analysis of a large database (Benjafield et al., 2019).

Autobilevel devices are especially useful when OSA is associated with sleep hypoventilation and additional pressure is required to normalize ventilation during sleep. This typically occurs in patients with OSA and COPD (overlap syndrome) or with moderate-severe obesity. In a study by our group in consecutive patients undergoing CPAP titration for OSA, titration was considered successful in the case of sleep-disordered breathing resolution (apnea–hypopnea index <10/hr) with cumulative time at SaO_2 < 90% (CT90%) <10% and/or improved daytime arterial blood gases at the end of titration. The majority of OSA patients (268/356, 75%) were successfully titrated with CPAP, whereas in the remaining patients (n=88) autobilevel ventilation was successful in 70 patients and failed in the remaining 18. Failure of automatic bilevel ventilation was independently associated with baseline body mass index >40 kg/m^2 (odds ratio 6.16, confidence interval 1.50–25.17, $p = 0.011$) and CT90% >42% (odds ratio 5.87, confidence interval 1.39–24.83, $p = 0.016$). Adherence to ventilatory treatment at follow-up was about 5 h/night, and similar in the CPAP and automatic bilevel groups (Baiamonte et al., 2018). These data suggest that extreme obesity and occurrence of moderate-severe hypoventilation at baseline can be better treated by using devices capable of a higher performance than automatic bilevel devices. As for patients' feedback, satisfaction in those who tried both devices was higher with automatic bilevel ventilation than with CPAP, but these data are hard to interpret since full resolution of respiratory nocturnal events was not obtained with the latter treatment (Baiamonte et al., 2018).

Obesity hypoventilation syndrome (OHS) has been traditionally managed with noninvasive ventilation rather than with CPAP, because occurrence of hypercapnia during wakefulness was interpreted as secondary to inability to increase ventilation during either day or night. Recent data from the Pickwick randomized controlled trial on patients with uncomplicated OSA and OHS have shown a good response to CPAP treatment, with resolution of hypercapnia a little slower but overall similar to that obtained with bilevel ventilation (Masa et al., 2018). Although the clinical presentation of OHS is variable, with about half of the patients being admitted to hospital for acute respiratory failure and often discharged home on bilevel ventilation, the Pickwick study is important from a clinical point of view because CPAP is cheaper and easy to use than bilevel ventilation. Additional studies, however, are currently collecting data to further explore the best therapeutic approach for OHS.

3. The Role of Telemedicine in the Management of OSA

Since the start of the lockdown for COVID-19, the clinical activity regarding patients with suspected or diagnosed sleep disordered breathing (SDB), and home titration of positive airway pressure (PAP) treatment, has stopped due to need to limit access of patients to the hospital, and the risk of droplet dispersion associated with the use of PAP/NIV (Schiza et al., 2020). According to a multicenter European study, a minority of Sleep Centers used Telemedicine (TM) regularly during the COVID-19 epidemic, mostly to monitor adherence to treatment rather than for full clinical management (Grote et al., 2020).

The high prevalence of SDB in the population is associated with long waiting lists, further lengthened during the emergency caused by COVID-19. Telemedicine is a potentially useful option (Bonsignore et al., 2017; Suarez-Giron et al., 2019; Bruyneel, 2019), but it is not yet included among the services provided by many European National Health Systems (Schiza et al., 2020), although such attitude is expected to change in the near future. A paradigm shift in Sleep Medicine practice after the COVID-19 pandemic has been foreseen, not only for SDB, but also for other sleep disorders (Irfan et al., 2020). Telemedicine will be at the center of such paradigm shift, and may represent the major innovation in Sleep Medicine in the years to come.

The interest in TM for the management of patients with SDB has progressively grown, with identification of advantages and drawbacks (Verbraecken et al., 2016). Studies have mostly addressed questions regarding the role of TM in monitoring adherence to PAP treatment, or follow-up at the initiation of treatment for SDB, but overall advantages over traditional management were small, as the results of TM management were comparable to, and costs were slightly lower than the usual sleep laboratory-centered management (Isetta et al., 2015; Turino et al., 2019). The COVID-19 pandemic has dramatically raised the issue of safety, changing the balance in favor of TM with regard to many medical conditions, including SDB.

A recent review has summarized the results of RCTs on the effects of TM during home CPAP treatment as adherence is concerned (Bruyneel, 2019). While results were on average similar in the TM or usual care arms, or slightly in favor of TM, one study reported higher patient satisfaction with usual care and concern by the patients for privacy issues (Turine et al., 2019). In Asian patients, adherence to PAP treatment tended to increase and sleep quality improved in the group receiving TM during the first month (Chumpangern et al., 2021). There could be problems in implementing TM services in different countries, because of different cultural background, local legislation, and systems of home care. The Spanish Society of Respiratory Medicine has recently released a comprehensive document on TM use in patients on home CPAP or noninvasive ventilation (Montserrat Canal et al., 2020), which is the first official document by a Scientific European Society on this matter, and will likely be followed by other National documents in the near future.

Further development are possible in the evolution of TM. Instead of limited programs on specific aspects, such as treatment initiation and remote control of CPAP pressure, or monitoring adherence to treatment, a comprehensive e-Health program, including teleconsultation, educational programs for patients, and feedback regarding their overall care satisfaction, would be well suited for both clinicians, technicians and patients, especially for uncomplicated OSA patients (Murphie et al., 2019). There are several barriers to be overcome, for example in elderly patients who may not be familiar with advanced smartphone use, or in economically disadvantaged patients. On the other hand, active involvement of patients via web-based systems is highly advisable, and may improve the relationship between patients and health personnel (Hwang, 2016; Hostler et al., 2017). Further development is expected by application of Artificial Intelligence to the sleep field (Kuziemsky et al., 2019).

Conclusion

Positive airway pressure treatment remains the mainstay of OSA treatment, but the future promises significant advancement. On one hand, development of new drugs to treat specific physiologic phenotypes of OSA will be of relief, especially in patients poorly tolerant to CPAP or bilevel ventilation. On the other hand, technological applications such as TM and e-Health will move the field towards a Virtual Sleep Laboratory, thus limiting costs while keeping a high level of care. This change in paradigm will take some time, and considerable educational effort for health professionals, but will eventually result in major improvement for the patients, and inspire new research taking advantage of the new tools.

References

Babbin, S. F., Velicer, W. F., Aloia, M. S., Kushida, C. A. (2015). Identifying Longitudinal Patterns for Individuals and Subgroups: An Example with Adherence to Treatment for Obstructive Sleep Apnea. *Multivariate Behav Res*, 50(1): 91-108.

Baiamonte, P., Mazzuca, E., Gruttad'Auria, C. I., Castrogiovanni, A., Marino, C., Lo Nardo, D., Basile, M., Algeri, M., Battaglia, S., Marrone, O., Gagliardo, A., Bonsignore, M. R. (2018). Use of autobilevel ventilation in patients with obstructive sleep apnea: An observational study. *J Sleep Res*, 27(6): e12680.

Benjafield, A. V., Pépin, J. L., Valentine, K., Cistulli, P. A., Woehrle, H., Nunez, C. M., Armitstead, J., Malhotra, A. (2019). Compliance after switching from CPAP to bilevel for patients with non-compliant OSA: big data analysis. *BMJ Open Respir Res*, 6(1): e000380.

Bonsignore, M. R., Suarez Giron, M. C., Marrone, O., Castrogiovanni, A., Montserrat, J. M. (2017). Personalised medicine in sleep respiratory disorders: focus on obstructive sleep apnoea diagnosis and treatment. *Eur Respir Rev*, 26(146):170069.

Bruyneel, M. (2019). Telemedicine in the diagnosis and treatment of sleep apnoea. *Eur Respir Rev*, 28(151): 180093.

Chumpangern, W., Muntham, D., Chirakalwasan, N. (2021). Efficacy of a telemonitoring system in continuous positive airway pressure therapy in Asian obstructive sleep apnea. *J Clin Sleep Med*, 17(1): 23-29.

Cistulli, P. A., Sullivan, C. E. (2019). In search of a good fit: CPAP therapy mask selection for obstructive sleep apnoea. *Respirology*, 24(3): 199-200.

Eckert, D. J. (2018). Phenotypic approaches to obstructive sleep apnoea - New pathways for targeted therapy. *Sleep Med Rev*, 37:45-59.

Eysteinsdottir, B., Gislason, T., Pack, A. I., Benediktsdottir, B., Arnardottir, E. S., Kuna, S. T., Björnsdottir, E. (2017). Insomnia complaints in lean patients with obstructive sleep apnea negatively affect positive airway pressure treatment adherence. *J Sleep Res*, 26(2): 159-165.

Gagnadoux, F., Le Vaillant, M., Paris, A., Pigeanne, T., Leclair-Visonneau, L., Bizieux-Thaminy, A., Alizon, C., Humeau, M. P., Nguyen, X. L., Rouault, B., Trzepizur, W., Meslier, N.; Institut de Recherche en Santé Respiratoire des Pays de la Loire Sleep Cohort Group. (2016). Relationship between OSA Clinical Phenotypes and CPAP treatment outcomes. *Chest*, 149(1): 288-290.

Grote, L., McNicholas, W. T., Hedner, J.; ESADA collaborators. (2020). Sleep apnoea management in Europe during the COVID-19 pandemic: data from the European Sleep Apnoea Database (ESADA). *Eur Respir J*, 55(6): 2001323.

Hostler, J. M., Sheikh, K. L, Andrada, T. F, Khramtsov, A., Holley, P. R., Holley, A. B. (2017). A mobile, web-based system can improve positive airway pressure adherence. *J Sleep Res*, 26(2): 139-146.

Hwang, D. (2016). Monitoring progress and adherence with positive airway pressure therapy for obstructive sleep apnea: the roles of telemedicine and mobile lealth applications. *Sleep Med Clin*, 11(2): 161-171.

Kuziemsky, C., Maeder, A. J., John, O., Gogia, S. B., Basu, A., Meher, S., Ito, M. (2019). Role of Artificial Intelligence within the telehealth domain. *Yearb Med Inform*, 28(1): 35-40.

Irfan, M., Khalil, W., Iber, C. (2020). Practicing sleep medicine amidst a pandemic: a paradigm shift. *J Clin Sleep Med*, 16(8):1405-1408.

Isetta, V., Negrín, M. A., Monasterio, C., Masa, J. F., Feu, N., Álvarez, A., Campos-Rodriguez, F., Ruiz, C., Abad, J., Vázquez-Polo, F. J., Farré, R., Galdeano, M., Lloberes, P., Embid, C., de la Peña, M., Puertas, J., Dalmases, M., Salord, N., Corral, J., Jurado, B., León, C., Egea, C., Muñoz, A., Parra, O., Cambrodi, R., Martel-Escobar, M., Arqué, M., Montserrat, J. M., Spanish Sleep Network. (2015). A Bayesian cost-effectiveness analysis of a telemedicine-based strategy for the management of sleep apnoea: a multicentre randomised controlled trial. *Thorax*, 70(11): 1054-1061.

Lebret, M., Rotty, M. C., Argento, C., Pepin, J. L., Tamisier, R., Arbib, F., Jaffuel, D., Molinari, N., Borel, J. C. (2019). Comparison of auto- and fixed-continuous positive airway pressure on air leak in patients with obstructive sleep apnea: data from a randomized controlled trial. *Can Respir J,* 2019:6310956.

Marrone, O., Cibella, F., Pépin, J. L., Grote, L., Verbraecken, J., Saaresranta, T., Kvamme, J. A., Basoglu, O. K., Lombardi, C., McNicholas, W. T., Hedner, J., Bonsignore, M. R., ESADA Network. (2018). Fixed but not autoadjusting positive airway pressure attenuates the time-dependent decline in glomerular filtration rate in patients with OSA. *Chest*, 154(2): 326-334.

Masa, J. F., Mokhlesi, B., Benítez, I., Gomez de Terreros, F. J., Sánchez-Quiroga, M. Á., Romero, A., Caballero-Eraso, C., Terán-Santos, J., Alonso-Álvarez, M. L., Troncoso, M. F., González, M., López-Martín, S., Marin, J. M., Martí, S., Díaz-Cambriles, T., Chiner, E., Egea, C., Barca, J., Vázquez-Polo, F. J., Negrín, M. A., Martel-Escobar, M., Barbe, F., Corral, J.; Spanish Sleep Network. (2019). Long-term clinical effectiveness of continuous positive airway pressure therapy versus non-invasive ventilation therapy in patients with obesity hypoventilation syndrome: a multicentre, open-label, randomised controlled trial. *Lancet*, 393(10182):1721-1732.

McArdle, N., King, S., Shepherd, K., Baker, V., Ramanan, D., Ketheeswaran, S., Bateman, P., Wimms, A., Armitstead, J., Richards, G., Hillman, D., Eastwood, P. (2015). Study of a novel APAP algorithm for the treatment of obstructive sleep apnea in women. *Sleep*, 38(11): 1775-1181.

Modica DM, Marchese D, Lorusso F, Speciale R, Saraniti C, Gallina S. Functional Nasal Surgery and Use of CPAP in OSAS Patients: Our Experience. *Indian J Otolaryngol Head Neck Surg*. 2018 Dec;70(4): 559-565.

Montserrat Canal, J. M., Suárez-Girón, M., Egea, C., Embid, C., Matute-Villacís, M., de Manuel Martínez, L., Orteu, Á., González-Cappa, J., Tato Cerdeiras, M., Mediano, O. (2020) Spanish Society of Pulmonology and Thoracic Surgery positioning on the use of telemedicine in sleep-disordered breathing and mechanical ventilation. *Arch Bronconeumol*, July 6:S0300-2896(20)30190-3, e-pub ahead of print.

Murphie, P., Little, S., McKinstry, B., Pinnock, H. (2019). Remote consulting with telemonitoring of continuous positive airway pressure usage data for the routine review of people with obstructive sleep apnoea hypopnoea syndrome: A systematic review. *J Telemed Telecare*, 25(1):17-25.

Patruno, V., Aiolfi, S., Costantino, G., Murgia, R., Selmi, C., Malliani, A., Montano, N. (2007). Fixed and autoadjusting continuous positive airway pressure treatments are not similar in reducing cardiovascular risk factors in patients with obstructive sleep apnea. *Chest*, 131(5): 1393-1399.

Patruno, V., Tobaldini, E., Bianchi, A. M., Mendez, M. O., Coletti, O., Costantino, G., Montano, N. (2014). Acute effects of autoadjusting and fixed continuous positive airway pressure treatments on cardiorespiratory coupling in obese patients with obstructive sleep apnea. *Eur J Intern Med*, 25(2): 164-168.

Pelletier-Fleury, N., Le Vaillant, M., Goupil, F., Paris, A., Pigeane, T., Gagnadoux, F., Meslier, N.; IRSR sleep cohort group. (2020). Risk-seeking attitude in health and safety domain is associated with CPAP discontinuation in patients with OSA-a multicenter prospective cohort study. *Sleep*, 2020 Aug 24:zsaa156, e-pub ahead of print.

Sabil, A., Le Vaillant, M., Stitt, C., Goupil, F., Pigeanne, T., Leclair-Visonneau, L., Masson, P., Bizieux-Thaminy, A., Humeau, M. P., Meslier, N., Gagnadoux, F. (2020). A CPAP data-based algorithm for automatic early prediction of therapy adherence. *Sleep Breath*, 2020 Sep 25. doi: 10.1007/s11325-020-02186-y. Epub ahead of print.

Schiza, S., Simonds, A., Randerath, W., Fanfulla, F., Grote, L., Montserrat, J., Pepin, J. L., Verbraecken, J., Bonsignore, M. R. (2020) Sleep laboratories reopening and COVID-19: A consensus of European experts. *Eur Respir J* in press, accepted Nov 3, 2020, doi: 10.1183/13993003.02722-2020.

Suarez-Giron, M., Bonsignore, M. R., Montserrat, J. M. (2019). New organisation for follow-up and assessment of treatment efficacy in sleep apnoea. *Eur Respir Rev*, 28(153): 190059.

Sullivan, C. E., Issa, F. G., Berthon-Jones, M., Eves, L. (1981). Reversal of obstructive sleep apnoea by continuous positive airway pressure applied through the nares. *Lancet*, 1(8225): 862-865.

Sullivan, C. E. (2018). Nasal positive airway pressure and sleep apnea. Reflections on an experimental method that became a therapy. *Am J Respir Crit Care Med*, 198(5): 581-587.

Treptow, E., Pepin, J. L., Bailly, S., Levy, P., Bosc, C., Destors, M., Woehrle, H., Tamisier, R. (2019). Reduction in sympathetic tone in patients with obstructive sleep apnoea: is fixed CPAP more effective than APAP? A randomised, parallel trial protocol. *BMJ Open*, 9(4): e024253.

Tsuyumu, M., Tsurumoto, T., Iimura, J., Nakajima, T., Kojima, H. (2020). Ten-year adherence to continuous positive airway pressure treatment in patients with moderate-to-severe obstructive sleep apnea. *Sleep Breath*, 24(4): 1565-1571.

Turino C, de Batlle J, Woehrle H, Mayoral A, Castro-Grattoni AL, Gómez S, Dalmases M, Sánchez-de-la-Torre M, Barbé F. (2017). Management of continuous positive airway pressure treatment compliance using telemonitoring in obstructive sleep apnoea. *Eur Respir J*, 49(2): 1601128.

Verbraecken, J. (2016). Telemedicine applications in sleep disordered breathing: Thinking out of the box. *Sleep Med Clin*, 11(4): 445-459.

In: Advances in Sleep Apnea
Editors: F. Lorusso et al.
ISBN: 978-1-53619-758-7

Chapter 10

ADVANCES IN THE ROLE OF ORAL DEVICES IN THE TREATMENT OF OSAS

V. Panzarella, P. Spinuzza, G. La Mantia, G. Campisi and G. Giuliana*

Department of Surgical, Oncological and Oral Sciences, University of Palermo, Palermo, Italy

ABSTRACT

Over the past years, a novel direction in dentistry, named 'Dental Sleep Medicine,' has been increasingly developed. The objective is to find an effective remedy for the treatment of Obstructive Sleep Apnoea Syndrome (OSAS) through the use of various Oral Appliances (OAs). These appliances can be used alternatively or in conjunction with the Continuous Positive Airway Pressure (CPAP), depending on the degree of OSAS and patient compliance.

The various OAs available and discussed in the medical literature differ from each other based on the patency mechanism of the airways. Furthermore, OAs determine not only an improvement of the respiratory flow, but also the improvement of cardiovascular system of patient, as well as the general

* Corresponding Author's Email: giovanna.giuliana@unipa.it.

improvements of the quality of life. The use of OA reduces the risk of hypertension, cardiovascular and cerebrovascular diseases, that are common with patients with OSAS.

The purpose of this Chapter is to provide a review of medical literature in order to evaluate the different types of OAs, their characteristics, use and effects and to provide a guidance for an effective multidisciplinary management of OSAS treatment.

INTRODUCTION

Early publications on Oral Appliances (OAs) for Obstructive Sleep Apnea Syndromes (OSAS) aimed to find alternative treatments to surgical procedures or treatment with Continuous Positive Airway Pressure (CPAP).

Oral appliances for the treatment of upper airway obstruction were first addressed in the literature in 1923 by Pierre Robin, who described respiratory failure during sleep caused by pharyngeal obstruction in children with micrognathia and glossoptosis. This was the first clear demonstration of how anatomical oropharyngeal anomalies can induce a narrowing of the airways that hinders breathing during sleep. In this key contribution, Robin laid the foundation for understanding the role of pharyngeal obstruction in the pathogenesis of sleep apnea.

Pierre Robin also recommended the use of a monobloc appliance with the aim of achieving a functional advancement of the mandible, bringing it to the maximum degree of protrusion. At the same time this appliance avoids a posterior slipping of the tongue (glossoptosis) during the supine position, typical of children with mandibular hypoplasia.

Another 50 years went by to obtain the first news about the use of oral appliances for the treatment of snoring and OSAS; with this regard, a tongue holding and a mandibular advancement device were proposed.

The evidence base supporting the role of oral appliances in OSAS management has gradually evolved over the last 30 years, reaching the point where OAs has been increasingly recognized as a viable and effective treatment option for many patients.

Substantial progress in this field has been achieved, particularly in the last decade, through rigorous research that has assessed the effectiveness and efficiency of OAs therapy, and in particular of mandibular advancement appliances. The first randomized controlled trials of OAs were published in 1996 by Clark et al. and Ferguson et al. In 2001, Mehta et al. published the first placebo-controlled study on the efficacy of OA treatment with results comparable to CPAP treatment.

On consequence, a number of further studies have been generated including rigorous clinical trial designs, comparisons with placebo treatment, more rigorous treatment outcome evaluations, direct comparisons to gold standard therapy (i.e., CPAP) and a growing focus on general health.

Randomized controlled trials have shown that OA not only leads to an improvement in polysomnographic and symptomatic values, including snoring, daytime somnolence, but also in neuropsychological and cardiovascular endpoints.

The purpose of any OSAS treatment is to prevent the occurrence of a complete or partial collapse of the upper airways during sleep. OA was associated with a reduction in the apnea-hypopnea index (AHI) to normal levels (<5/h) in 36-50% of patients and up to 70% of patients achieving an AHI <10/h.

Classification and Use of Oral Appliances

Appliances for the treatment of OSAS are different in adults and in children.

In patients of developmental age, appliances have the ability to modify and guide the growth of craniofacial skeletal structures. Since the alteration of these structures are risk factors for OSAS, their correction could allow the resolution of the disease.

On the other hand, the anatomical structures are fully defined and structured in adults, and thus they cannot be modified except surgically. As a consequence, the patency of the airways during sleep can be allowed by the positioning of oral appliances, which guarantees a momentary resolution of the pathology, allowing the passage of air during sleep.

Given that the purpose of OSAS treatment by OAs is different in patients of developmental age compared to adults, a breakdown of oral appliances used with particular attention to use and management is proposed below, depending on age.

Devices used with particular attention to use and management are proposed below, depending on age.

Oral Appliances (OAs) in Adult Patients

In the literature, the most studied and proposed OAs in adult patients can be classified according to the mechanism of action.

The main OAs are the Tongue Retaining Devices (TRDs), the Soft Palate Lift (SPLs) and the Mandibular Advancement Devices (MADs).

The first are currently much less employed and investigated than MADs. The latter is considered as the most standard choice of treatment for patients presenting simple snoring mild or mild-moderate OSAS, low body mass index and with increased upper airway resistance syndrome. MADs are also recommended as the last treatment option in patients who do not respond or reject CPAP, patients with a high surgical risk and patients with a deficient response to surgical treatment.

Tongue Retaining Device (TRD)

TRDs (Figure 1) were first described in 1982. They are among the first appliances designed to reduce snoring and apnea in adult patients.

TRD consist of a soft elastic bulb in which the tip of the tongue can be sucked in and held in place by negative pressure. It can be performed or made to measure from tongue and tooth casts using a soft copolymer. A mandibular protrusion of between 50% and 75% can be achieved when making the device. This advancement distance is reduced if the patient reports pain, while it is increased if the main symptoms remain unchanged after a 3-week trial.

This "suction effect" on the tongue determines its protrusion during sleep and favors an increase in the tension of the walls of the pharynx through an increase in diameter in the lateral and antero-posterior direction.

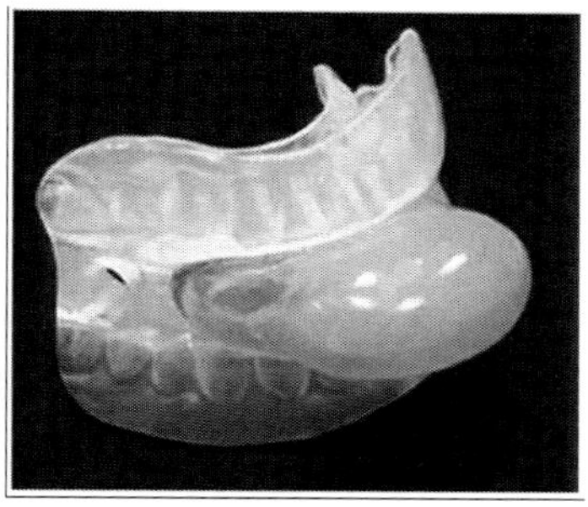

Figure 1. Tongue Retaining Device (TRD).
Courtesy of dental technician Antonio Licandro, Laboratorio Ortodontico Licandro.

The most frequent side effects reported by patients are related to size of the device and to aesthetic reasons, considering the unique design. TRD can also cause severe tissue irritation due to the vacuum effect required.

Since there is little evidence in the literature of their efficacy and as their use is related to severe discomforts in patients, they can be considered an option in edentulous subjects or subjects with reduced protrusion capacity, always in the absence of increased nasal resistance, considering the intrinsic characteristics of the device.

Soft Palate Lift (SPL)

The first SPLs (Figure 2) were described in literature by Gibbons and Bloomer in 1958. Gonzalez, Aranson and Lang used it for the first time in patients with neurological handicaps.

The palatal lifting device consists of a front portion with hooks that anchor on the teeth, and a resin back portion that extends to the palatine veil. At the beginning of the treatment, the construction of the device foresees that only the anterior portion of the veil is affected by the resin posterior portion, then, when the individual starts to tolerate the device, the posterior portion is gradually extended until it reaches the area of the veil dimple.

The SPL, as the name says, moves the soft palate upwards and backwards in order to lift it and avoid the closure of the airways with the peripheral pharyngeal tissues, improving the passage of air and increasing the superior pharyngeal dimensions.

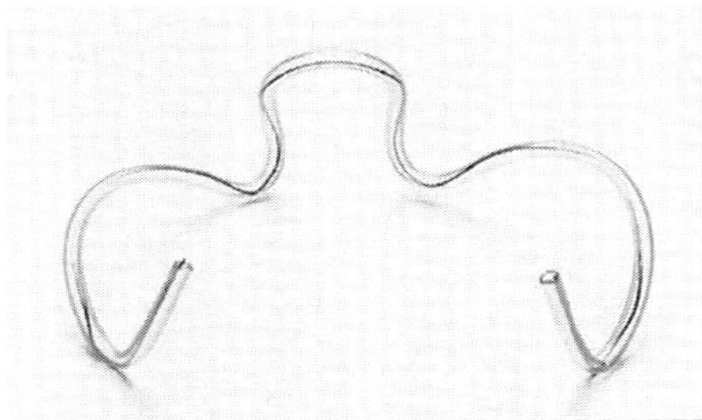

Figure 2. Soft Palate Lift (SPL).
Courtesy of dental technician Antonio Licandro, Laboratorio Ortodontico Licandro.

It is also used in cases of cleft palate, myasthenia gravis, bulbar poliomyelitis, cerebral palsy and soft palate injuries (e.g., tonsillectomy and maxillary resection).

SPLs have the advantage of not compromising the physiology and position of the tongue, thanks to the positioning of the device on the upper jaw. The use of this device increases the patency of the airway, evaluated in tele-radiography, by approximately 3 mm.

However, this kind of device cannot be used in cases where there is inadequate retention, cases where the soft palate cannot be moved or where patients are not compliant.

The side effect most commonly reported by the patients is discomfort due to the stimulation of the vomiting reflex; however, in a short period of time, the patient tends to get used to the device.

SPLs are considered an optional treatment for patients who cannot tolerate MADs or TRDs; however, literature research has revealed only a few reports describing the treatment of OSAS patients with SPLs.

Mandibular Advancement Device (MAD)

The mandibular advancement devices (MADs) were first applied between the late 1980s and early 1990s. After several cases series and controlled clinical trials, to date it was possible to assume that, despite the considerable variety of MAD designs, there is a strong evidence in the literature about their effectiveness on the treatment of bronchopathy and of mild and moderate OSAS.

There are different classifications of mandibular feeding appliances according to different parameters. In relation to the material (soft or rigid resin) or to the manufacturing technique we can distinguish MADs in:

- universal (made with soft resin so that the patient can deform it by making both arches adhere well);
- preformed (they adapt domestically simply by heating them and giving the shape of the occlusion);
- individual (made by the clinician according to the shape of the patient's arches).

The latter type of luminaire can further be categorized as:

- not adjustable, in which the degree of jaw advancement cannot be modified;
- adjustable, which can be adjusted in protrusion.

Non-adjustable MADs are monobloc appliances built on the patient's individual impressions and consisting of two jaws, one maxillary and the other mandibular, joined in a protruding position decided by the clinician at the beginning of therapy that can no longer be changed. It is therefore necessary to know from the beginning the maximum advancement achievable. If it is necessary to increase the degree of protrusion during therapy, it is inevitable to take the patient's fingerprints and ask the laboratory to make a new device, causing a further waste of time for the clinician and money for the patient.

On the other hand, the adjustable MADs allow you to decide the advancement based on the patient's needs and to obtain the maximum benefit more easily with just one device.

More significant reductions in sleepiness in patients with adjustable MAD than in non-adjustable have been described. However, according to the literature, there is no statistical difference between the two types of device as regards the reduction of the Apnea Hypopnea Index (AHI). However, according to the literature, there is no statistical difference between the two types of devices with regards to the reduction of the Apnea Hypopnea Index (AHI). Fleetham et al., in fact, taking into account the reduction in AHI and symptomatic resolution, obtained a positive result of 61% in adjustable devices and 48% in non-adjustable devices.

The first results on the effectiveness of MAD were reported in the *New England Journal of Medicine* by Peter George, who published an article on an acrylic monobloc device with retention hooks on dental elements, named Nocturnal Airway Patency Appliance (NAPA) (Figure 3, 4).

The first successes achieved with this device led, some years later, to the creation of hybrid appliances which, in addition to the mandibular advancement, were intended to physically support the soft palate by means of resin or metal handles, or to increase the passage of air and give space to the tongue through the construction of large anterior respiratory fissures.

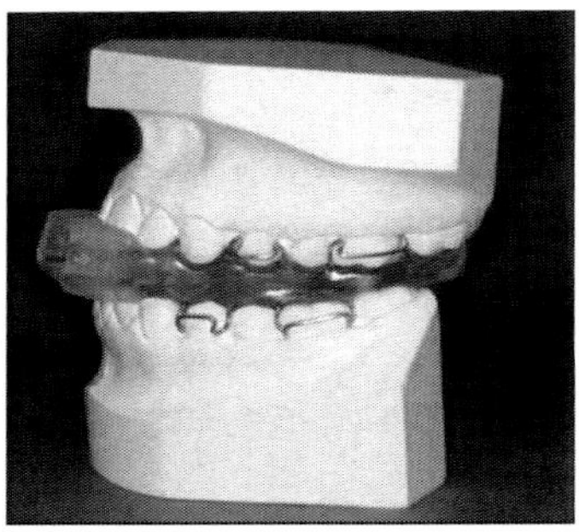

Figure 3. Nocturnal Airway Patency Appliance (NAPA). Lateral view. Courtesy of dental technician Antonio Licandro, Laboratorio Ortodontico Licandro.

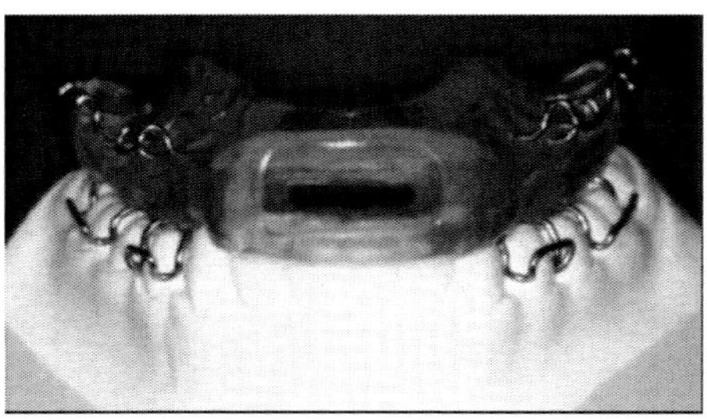

Figure 4. Nocturnal Airway Patency Appliance (NAPA). Frontal view. Courtesy of dental technician Antonio Licandro, Laboratorio Ortodontico Licandro.

As an alternative to the monobloc appliances, difficult to advance from the initial therapeutic protrusion, the first bimaxillary appliances were born, designed with different degrees of freedom for the lateral and vertical movements of the jaw, which, to date, are undoubtedly the most used. Over time, numerous propulsion mechanisms have been created, evaluated and compared.

In the early 1990s, Alan Lowe, professor and director of the Division of Orthodontics at the Canadian University of British Columbia, proposed the Klearway, the first gradually advancing device using an expansion screw in the center of the upper splint. The screw can be activated by 0.25 mm at a time and allows a range of movement in the antero-posterior direction of 11 mm. The device is made of a thermo-active acrylic, which allows an easy insertion on the arches after being in contact with hot water and returns rigid to the mouth temperature: the aim of this material is to guarantee a good anchorage and minimize the risk of dental movements.

A few years later, Thorton introduced the TAP (Thornton Adjustable Positioner) (Figure 5), a device in which the two splints are connected together by a single front hook that snaps onto a bar or a special housing in the lower splint. The mechanism has a minimum freedom for the opening movements of the mouth but guarantees a discreet freedom of movement in a lateral direction (especially in its versions with the bar on the lower splint.

Over the years the various devices proposed in literature have become less and less bulky, seeking ever greater comfort for the patient. Greater freedom of movement for the jaw when opening was achieved by the MAD who used a HERBST type propulsion mechanism, with one metal and telescopic arm per side.

IST (Intraoral Snoring-Therapy appliance), SomnoDent, Narval, OrthoApnea are examples of these devices.

In the version designed by Dr. Hinz, IST (Intraoral Snoring-Therapy appliance), the length of the arm can be increased with an adjustable mechanism. There is a version in which the direction of the telescopic arm can be reversed (reverse connecting rod), with the aim of increasing the mandibular protrusion rate when the mouth is opened.

TAP® and IST® are made of heat-printable sheets, which allow for minimum space requirements, especially for the tongue, and do not include hooks for anchoring. Other appliances that allow maximum freedom for the opening movement are those that use inclined slides of the Twin-Block type as propulsion mechanism.

The evolution of the latter mechanism, designed by Richard Palmisano in the early 2000s, is the SomnoDent (Figure 6).

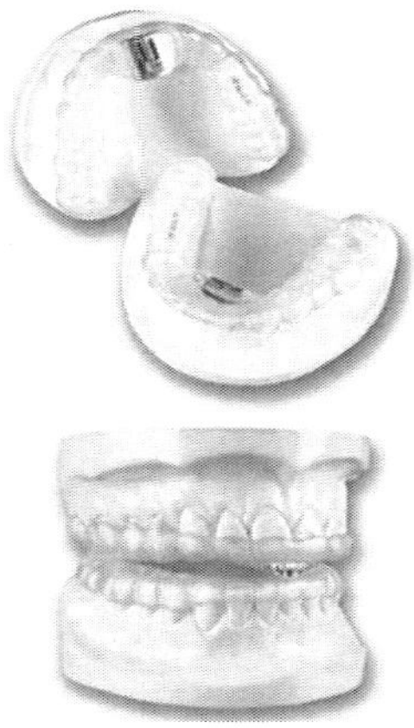

Figure 5. Thornton Adjustable Positioner (TAP). Type 3.
Courtesy of dental technician Antonio Licandro, Laboratorio Ortodontico Licandro.

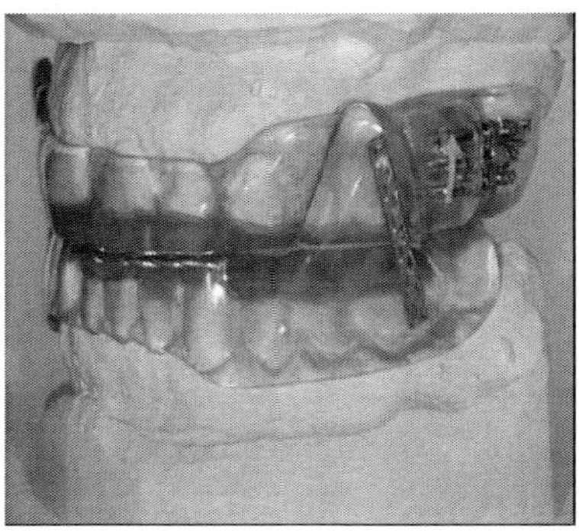

Figure 6. SomnoDent.
Courtesy of dental technician Antonio Licandro, Laboratorio Ortodontico Licandro.

This device has two vestibular fins on the sides of the lower splint made with an inclination of 17 degrees, which rest on the two inclined planes positioned on the upper splint and which can be advanced gradually by 0.1 mm per activation thanks to an expansion screw sunk into the resin. The only activation of the expansion screw provides 6 mm of progressive advancement range. SomnoDent can be constructed with a hot molded resin that covers the internal surface of the device, guaranteeing excellent comfort and high retention without the use of hooks and retaining the possibility of being lowered. The lack of a mechanism connecting the two splints and the evolution of the material make this device suitable also for patients with complete edentulousness of the upper arch. Narval CC is a bimaxillary device made of biocompatible polymer with CAD/CAM (Computer Aided Design/Computer Aided Manufacturing) technology that uses connectors able to achieve a gradual advancement of 0.5 mm at a time. OrthApnea uses a front reverse rod advance mechanism to allow a slight freedom of opening the mouth and induces the protraction of the jaw when opening the mouth.

The mechanism of action by which MADs increase patency in the upper airway is not yet fully clear, but studies using three-dimensional imaging techniques and sleep endoscopy have provided important indications. The desire to fully understand the mechanisms responsible for the increased patency of the first airways stems from the need to be able to select patients eligible for dental therapy. The greatest difficulty in precisely defining the action that the appliances exert on the airways is the difference in size of the pharynx between sleep and wakefulness Magnetic Resonance Imaging (MRI) with the patient awake and the patient asleep (propofol-induced sleep), a reduction in the mean surface area of approximately 75.5%. Mandibular advancement appliances achieve an anterior inferior movement of the jaw, increasing the caliber of the upper airway. This movement stabilizes and fixes the mandible and hyoid bone, preventing post-rotation of these structures during decubitus. The hourly rotation of the jaw and the increase in the vertical dimension activate the genioglossus muscle, which produces a more anterior and superior location of the tongue, preventing the collapse of the airways.

There is also an increase in the activity of the pharyngeal dilator muscles, increasing their longitude and improving their contractility.

A study carried out by Johal et al. (2007) concludes that the use of mandibular advancement appliances significantly increases the electromyographic activity of the genioglossus, genioid and masticatory muscles. A greater impact is produced in the velopharyngeal area, although its action affects all segments of the pharynx. Initially there is an increase in stiffness and elevation of the space between the anterior and posterior pillars of the pharynx. The soft palate moves ventrally, increasing the caliber of the lateral walls and the velopharyngeal area and decreasing the frequency of snoring.

The functional advancement of the mandible induces changes in the position of the hyoid bone to a more anterior position, creating a situation of balance of the suprahyoid muscles, which favors an increase in the volume and permeability of the airways. Some authors argue that there is a dose-dependent effect, since increasing the degree of mandibular advancement improves the patient's clinical situation.

To sum up the mandibular propulsion. It induces:

- an increase in the velopharyngeal diameter, especially in its lateral portion, due to the anatomical contiguity between the mandible, tongue and tonsillar pillars (palatopharyngeal muscle and palatoglossal muscle);
- an increase in the tone of the muscles of the base of the tongue, which moves away from the posterior wall of the pharynx, with a consequent reduction in the tendency to verticalization;
- the protraction of the hyoid bone and the stabilization of the epiglottis, with a consequent increase in the hypopharyngeal diameter.

The result of these actions is an overall increase in the posterior air space at the retrolingual level (hypopharyngeal) and an increase in the pharyngeal diameter at the retropalatal level (velopharyngeal), especially in the lateral sense. The hypothesis on the effect of the downward distraction of the mandible on the patency of the airways is that they affect the increase in the diameter of the velopharynx, due to the traction that the depression exerts on the upper constrictor of the pharynx and the increase in the action on the tone of the palatoglossal muscle. The response of muscle tone to protrusion is not always predictable and may lead to insufficient normalization of the airway caliber.

Further studies have shown that the use of MAD also determines changes in the position of the dental elements and jaw bones. This is influenced by the length of time the appliance is used and the amount of protrusion and vertical opening that the appliance produces, since the lower the degree of opening, the less overbite is recorded.

Regarding the effectiveness of MADs, there is a limitation of not being able to objectively measure the use of these devices, unlike what happens with CPAP. Although there are not many studies on the subject, some authors describe in the literature a level of patient collaboration similar to that achieved with CPAP treatment.

In 2011 a Task Force of the European Respiratory Society (ERS) published a report with the aim of summarizing the evidence on the effectiveness of all non-CPAP therapies. The conclusions of the ERS produced the recommendation for the use of MADs for the treatment of mild and moderate OSAS as an alternative to CPAP and for the treatment of severe OSAS in patients who do not tolerate CPAP.

Furthermore, through polysomnographic registers, MADs have demonstrated their effectiveness in improving sleep structure by decreasing the AHI index, improving nocturnal gas exchange and allowing a greater amount of deep and REM sleep and decreasing the number of arousals.

Comparing these results with the treatment of choice (CPAP), the latter is better. However, considering some subjective parameters, such as excessive daytime sleepiness or patients' quality of life, the results appear controversial: while some authors found significant differences in favor of CPAP, other authors found no differences in the two treatments.

For the treatment of snoring, MADs are very effective, with an elimination of snoring in 50% of cases and a significant reduction in 90-100% of patients as well as an improvement in sleep quality. Finally, comparing the effectiveness of MAD with certain techniques such as

Uvulo-Palato-Pharyngo-Plasty (UPFP), it is clear that there are no significant differences compared to AHI, gas exchange or excessive daytime sleepiness at 6 months of treatment. Furthermore, when evolution is taken into account, the differences in favor of MAD are appreciated as they appear to be able to maintain their long-term effectiveness.

According to the current indications of the Italian Society of Dental Sleep Medicine (SIMSO), it is accepted that MAD can be used in patients with simple rhonchopathy, in cases of mild OSAS and in selected cases of moderate OSAS. With regard to patients with severe OSAS, some authors consider the level of severity not influential in the selection of treatment with MAD. However, there are cases in the literature of patients with severe OSAS who, thanks to the use of oral appliances, have reduced the alteration of AHI.

Moreover, in patients in whom the treatment of UPFP has not worked, MADs manage to improve clinical symptoms in more than 50% of cases.

In addition to the above indications, in order to achieve the best possible result for the individual patient MADs can be combined with positional therapy; CPAP; or with surgical therapy.

For this reason, the Italian guidelines (SIMSO) for the treatment of adult patients with OSAS underline the importance that the dentist expert in sleep medicine is able to manage the patient in collaboration with other specialists, in case the single therapy with MAD is not sufficient to treat the patient.

The side effects of MAD are generally of a mild transitory nature and tend to decrease after an initial period of adaptation. Adjustable mandibular advancement patterns allow this period to be progressive and, therefore, the side effects and possible rejection of the treatment appear to be minor. The most frequent symptoms relate to mandibular pain, excess salivation, xerostomia and bruxism.

A very common adverse effect is pain in the temporomandibular region. It appears upon awakening, after withdrawing the MAD and remains for a certain period of time.

The doubt is that these appliances can create joint pathology in the long term even in healthy patients. However, studies have shown that after two years of treatment with MAD no joint pathology has occurred.

There are also a number of skeletal and facial contraindications that could influence a positive outcome in MAD treatment: reduced anterior facial height; large anterior skull base; increased maxillary longitude; reduced mandibular plane; short soft palate; absence of nasal problems; grade I and II Mallampati; mandibular protrusion greater than 5-7 mm; normal proportions between the diameter of the airway of the soft palate and tongue.

Oral Appliances (OAs) in Pediatric Patients

Although the published work on OSAS therapy with oral appliances mainly concerns adult patients, it can be considered to be effective also in pediatric age. However, the treatment of OSAS in pediatric age differs substantially from the treatment of adults, as it is based on a different philosophy consisting in orthodontic treatment. A recent systematic review of the literature points out that the success of pediatric OSAS orthodontic treatment is linked to airway expansion, and polysomnographic clinical evidence after orthodontic treatment suggests that orthodontic treatment improves airway patency. Since the treatment of pediatric OSAS is closely related to orthodontic treatment, it is necessary to carefully investigate craniofacial dimorphisms, which can be risk factors for the onset of OSAS, leading to a reduction in the airways.

The craniofacial dimorphisms that can lead to a reduction of the airways are transverse palate reduction, mandibular retroposition or both.

These dimorphisms are resolved by expansion of the palate and mandibular advancement respectively.

The palatal expansion device increases nasal volume, stimulates growth of the maxillary complex and improves nasal ventilation in the OSAS child.

Mandibular advancement appliances (MAD), on the other hand, facilitate the lowering of the jaw, reduce airway collapse and stimulate the dilatory muscles of the airways.

Maxillary Expansion (ME)

Maxillary expansion (ME) is an orthopedic appliance that aimed, through the use of a mobile or fixed device called ‘maxillary or palatal expander’ (Figure 7-8), at increasing the maxillary transversal width by acting both on the median palatine suture, resulting in diastasis, and on the peri-mascellar and peri-zygomatic sutures. The first to talk about this device was Angell in 1860 with the article "treatment of irregularities of the permanent or adult teeth" where he described the increase in the transverse diameter of the upper arch two weeks after using the expander.

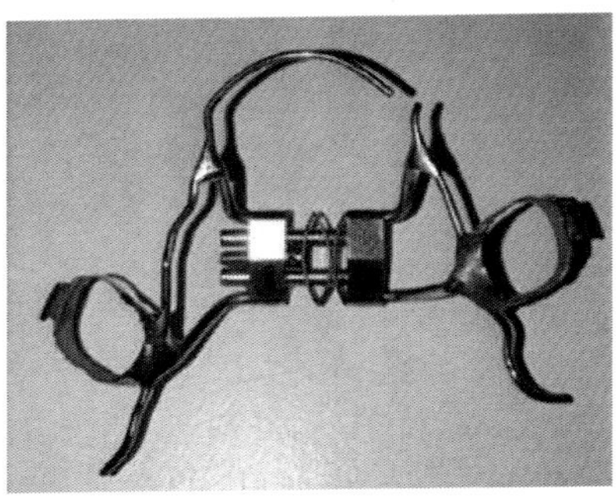

Figure 7. Fixed Maxillary Expansion (ME).
Courtesy of dental technician Deiana Giuseppe, Laboratorio Deiana Ortodonzia.

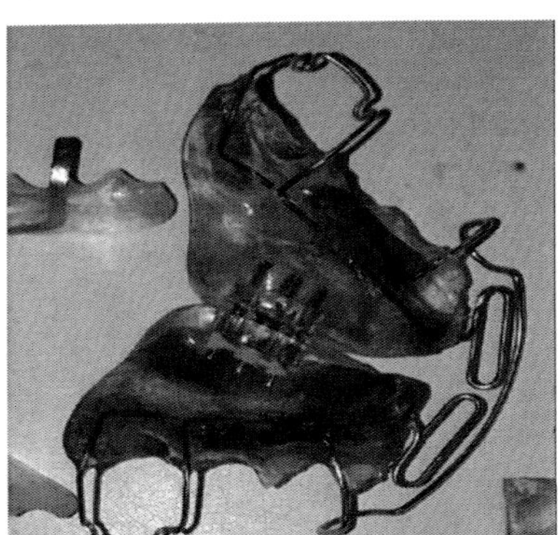

Figure 8. Mobile Maxillary expansion (ME).
Courtesy of dental technician Deiana Giuseppe, Laboratorio Deiana Ortodonzia.

The expander consists of 2 or 4 bands, respectively for molars and premolars, welded by means of metal arms to a median screw. Two types of expander, Haas type and Hyrax type are described in the literature. These differ in the presence or absence of an acrylic pad in correspondence to the palate. The Haas expander has this acrylic pad so that the expansion force is distributed between the posterior teeth and the palatal vault. The Haas expander has this acrylic pad so that the expansion force is distributed between the posterior teeth and the palatal vault. The Hyrax type expander does not include acrylic and presumably discharges the force to the jawbone only through the teeth supporting the braces.

The three potential ways in which the expander helps patients with OSAS are: (1) changes in the nasal airway, (2) changes in the oropharyngeal airway and (3) changes in mandibular position and growth. Maxillary expansion may be associated with increases in nasal space, reduction in nasal resistance and subsequent improvement in respiratory patterns. A study by McNamara and colleagues concluded that orthopedic maxillary expansion provides a stable and significant increase in upper airway volume in the maxillary and nasopharyngeal regions. A recent metanalysis, showed that after expansion, taking into account recurrence, there is an increase in amplitude of +2.21 mm at the level of the maxillary basal bone and +1.55 mm at the level of the nasal cavities. A further benefit of the expander to the oropharyngeal spaces is the change of the resting lingual posture, which, after expansion, is more relieved. This condition favor patients with OSAS since a more backward lingual posture is a risk factor for the collapse of the upper airways during sleep.

In order to obtain beneficial effects on the treatment of OSAS, Villa et al. concluded that orthodontic treatment with maxillary expander should be started as soon as the first symptoms of OSAS appear, and in any case before the palato-median suture fusion occurs (around puberty), i.e., before the completion of the permanent dentition. Some et al. suggest that chronological age is not a reliable predictor of suture patency after age 11.

The side effects associated with the maxillary expander are minimal and are mainly represented by the consequences of attempted expansion beyond the period of fusion of the intra- and intermaxillary sutures, or more commonly by the discomfort the patient may experience after activation of the expansion screw. This discomfort tends to disappear after a few days of expansion and depends on the activation protocol, in fact a rapid expansion protocol causes greater discomfort than a slow protocol.

Mandibular Advancement Device (MAD)

Mandibular advancement devices (MADs) in pediatric OSAS find their use in corrections of second dentoskeletal classes, improving not only craniofacial dysmorphism but also OSAS symptoms. As shown in the study by Ma Yanyan et al. 2019, the meta-analysis of two high-quality RCTs showed evidence of support for MAD treatment in pediatric OSAS patients, and analysis of the subgroups of these RCTs suggested that MAD therapy may be effective for mild to severe patients before the end of the pubertal peak.

Furthermore, class II correction using functional appliances during childhood could help to eliminate adaptive changes in the upper airway and OSAS predisposing factors, thus reducing the risk of OSAS development in adulthood.

When analyzing subjects with Class II mandibular retrusion, the position of the mandible is often retroposed with respect to the base of the skull and this can cause narrowing of the palate and adaptations in the soft palate. Decreased space between the cervical spine and the mandibular body can lead to a posterior position of the tongue and soft palate, thus increasing the chances of impaired respiratory function during the day and possibly causing respiratory problems during sleep such as snoring, upper airway resistance syndrome and obstructive sleep apnea syndrome.

The treatment of pediatric OSAS with MAD, therefore, aims to correct the retrognathic jaw by redirecting its growth to a more advanced position and stimulating it in a passive or active way through the use of a functional device. There are different types of functional appliances, such as twin-block, activator, Herbst, Frankel-II, Bionator (Figure 9-10).

These appliances are made of acrylic resin on plaster models of individual impressions. Made in the laboratory, they are applied and adapted by the dentist, but are easily removable by the child whenever necessary, such as for hygiene or meals. They are of different conformation, but all of them, once applied in the mouth of the young patient, interpose themselves to the antagonistic dental jaws. This involves on the one hand the loss of interocclusal relations generated by malocclusion and, on the other hand, a repositioning of the jaw according to the therapeutic programme decided by the dentist. In addition to individual mandibular advancement appliances, there are also preformed plastic appliances that, as indicated by several studies, improve the comfort of children with OSAS, thus favoring their adherence to treatment. These appliances are inserted in the frontal part of the oral cavity and have niches for housing the dental elements of both arches.

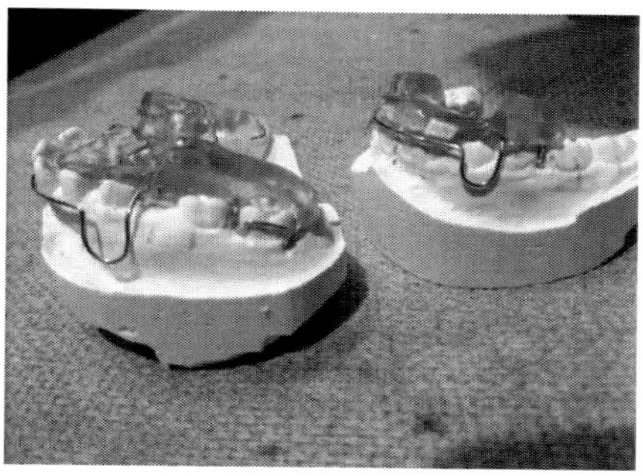

Figure 9. Twin-Bloch. Courtesy of dental technician Deiana Giuseppe, Laboratorio Deiana Ortodonzia.

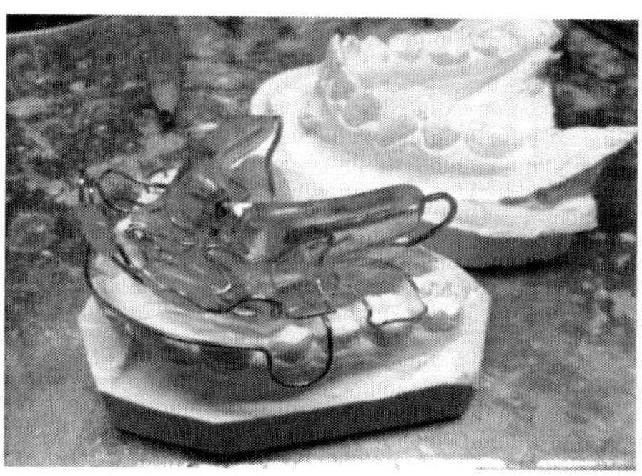

Figure 10. Mandibular Advancer.
Courtesy of dental technician Deiana Giuseppe, Laboratorio Deiana Ortodonzia.

Their action induces an advancement of the bite. The advantage of these plastic appliances is also the ability to combine orthodontic therapy with myofunctional therapy aimed at restoring intra and extraoral muscle balance and restoring normal nasal ventilation.

All the mandibular advancement appliances in the child, both individual and preformed models, although similar in structure and in some therapeutic aspects to the MAD for the adult, do not involve an indefinite mandibular advancement for OSAS purposes. They are intended to correct on the three planes of space (sagittal, horizontal and frontal) the mandibular malposition that the individual case presents.

The mandibular repositioning also involves a different lingual posture, since the tongue is largely inserted on the mandible, and the widening of the upper respiratory tract, particularly at the oropharyngeal level, with a consequent decrease in resistance and contrast to the occurrence of apnea.

It should be stressed that the application phase of these appliances in the child does not constitute a prosthetic-like therapy to be undergone for life, as in the case of the adult's MAD, but simulates and anticipates the structural and mandibular posture changes that the orthodontist expects to make in the following technical stages. Another advantage of these appliances is their absolute reversibility, which makes this approach free of any biological risk. Moreover, the child who responds positively to the therapy begins to improve dramatically from the first weeks of application of the device, even if the result is artificially linked to the presence of the device itself in the mouth. There is no consensus in the literature on the time of daily use and the total duration of treatment with MADs, however, it has been found that a longer daily use could advance the jaw faster and longer usage time could lead to a more stable and favorable muscle function against airway collapse. The consolidation of the result is, routinely, entrusted to the orthodontic follow-up, which, on the other hand, has the necessarily long technical times inherent in this therapy, which cannot ignore the peaks in growth of the bone bases and the eruption times of the permanent teeth.

When MADs are used in children with a skeletal and dental class, only as OSAS therapy, prolonged use can cause adverse dental and facial changes, so it should only be recommended that the device be used during sleep and close monitoring by the orthodontist.

CONCLUSION

Thanks to the transversal beneficial effects, the use of oral appliances has also found a role in the multidisciplinary management of OSAS.

Oral appliances used for OSAS, as reported by Walker et al. 2000, determine, in fact, not only an improvement in the respiratory flow, but also in the quality of life, analyzed through three parameters: vitality, contentment and sleep. These parameters are assessed through a questionnaire one year after treatment with OASs, and it is significant to see how there is an improvement in these as well as in polysomnographic variables.

Another beneficial effect of OAs, widely described, concerns the cardiovascular system. OSAS is an independent risk factor for hypertension and cardiovascular and cerebrovascular diseases including coronary heart disease, heart failure and stroke.

Cardio-vascular improvements were observed with a reduction in blood pressure following treatment with OAs, and in particular MADs, to a degree similar to CPAP.

A recent metanalysis reported that CPAP was associated with a systolic blood pressure reduction of 2.5 mm Hg and diastolic blood pressure reduction of 2.0 mm Hg, similarly MAD was associated with a reduction in systolic blood pressure of 2.1mm Hg and diastolic blood pressure of 1.9mmHg. There was no significant difference between CPAP and MAD. In terms of intermediate markers of cardiovascular health (biomarkers, heart rate variability, arterial stiffness, endothelial function), the effects of OASs are not yet well delineated, as most studies in the literature are very small and short-term and have heterogeneous designs.

Finally, it has been confirmed that OAs, like CPAP, are effective in improving arterial oxygen saturation (SaO2). With MADs this improvement is due to a non-linear dose dependent mechanism to the degree of advancement.

The efficacy of MAD may be associated with that of CPAP; however, it depends on a better tolerability of MAD than CPAP resulting in a similar overall attenuation of OSAS. Several studies have then described a good efficacy of the combined MAD and CPAP therapy that would lead to achieving an optimal therapeutic dose and to shorten significantly the duration of the advancement protocol. However, these studies are difficult to standardize given the high variability of tolerance and the individual response to treatment.

Despite the greater compliance for OAs, the occurrence of good results is limited in certain cases, such as some cases of severe OSAS in which the percentage of outcome is lower compared to mild and moderate cases; patients with poor progress mandibular; excessive overbite; dental and/or periodontal problems and patients with temporomandibular joint disease.

To be more efficient OASs therapy requires, therefore, a multidisciplinary approach, involving a sleep doctor and dentist with expertise in managing sleep disorders.

It is thanks to the development of a multidisciplinary vision of the pathology that a new branch of dentistry, named Dental sleep Medicine, has developed in recent years has increasingly developed.

Its purpose is to find an effective option for treating OSAS through the use of OASs. These appliances can be used alternatively or in conjunction with CPAP, depending on the degree of OSAS and patient compliance.

Patient preference is a key component in treatment and plays a vital role in therapy acceptance, device use, and outcomes. In fact, OASs are especially recommended for patients with OSAS who cannot tolerate CPAP therapy.

The American Academy of Sleep Medicine and the American Academy of Dental Sleep Medicine in 2015 created a guideline for clinical practice of the use of OAS that recommends continuous monitoring of follow-up, if appropriate, by both sleep doctors and dentists.

To date, however, it is necessary to improve undergraduate and postgraduate training in oral sleep medicine in order to guide a more effective multidisciplinary management of OSAS treatment and acquire new ideas and useful tools that can improve the quality of sleep and therefore of the life of the subject with OSAS.

REFERENCES

American Sleep Disorders Association Standards of Practice Committee. Practice parameters for the treatment of snoring and obstructive sleep apnea with oral appliances. *Sleep.* 1995; 18: 511-3.25.

Abad, F. et al. (2007). Dispositivos orales en el tratamiento del síndrome de apnea-hipopnea del sueño [Oral devices in the treatment of sleep apnea-hypopnea syndrome]. *Rev Patol Respir,* 10(1):16-21.

Almeida, F. R. de, Lowe, A. A., Sung, J. O., Tsuiki, S., and Otsuka, R. (2006). Long-term sequellae of oral appliance therapy in obstructive sleep apnea patients: Part 1. Cephalometric analysis. *American Journal of Orthodontics and Dentofacial Orthopedics: Official Publication of the American Association of Orthodontists, Its Constituent Societies, and the American Board of Orthodontics,* 129(2): 195–204. https://doi.org/10.1016/j.ajodo.2005.10.001

Angelieri, F., Cevidanes, L. H. S., Franchi, L., Gonçalves, J. R., Benavides, E., and McNamara, J. A. (2013). Midpalatal suture maturation: Classification method for individual assessment before rapid maxillary expansion. *American Journal of Orthodontics and Dentofacial Orthopedics: Official Publication of the American Association of Orthodontists, Its Constituent Societies, and the American Board of Orthodontics,* 144(5): 759–769. https://doi.org/10.1016/j.ajodo.2013.04.022.

Arens, R., and Marcus, C. L. (2004). Pathophysiology of upper airway obstruction: A developmental perspective. *Sleep,* 27(5): 997–1019. https://doi.org/10.1093/sleep/27.5.997.

Barnes, M., McEvoy, R. D., Banks, S., Tarquinio, N., Murray, C. G., Vowles, N., and Pierce, R. J. (2004). Efficacy of positive airway pressure and oral appliance in mild to moderate obstructive sleep apnea. *American Journal of Respiratory and Critical Care Medicine,* 170(6): 656–664. https://doi.org/10.1164/rccm.200311-1571OC.

Barthlen, G. M., Brown, L. K., Wiland, M. R., Sadeh, J. S., Patwari J., and Zimmerman, M. (2000). Comparison of Three Oral Appliances for Treatment of Severe Obstructive Sleep Apnea Syndrome. *Sleep Medicine* 1(4):299–305. doi: 10.1016/s1389-9457(00)00030-7.

Battagel, J. M., and Kotecha, B. (2005). Dental side-effects of mandibular advancement splint wear in patients who snore. *Clinical Otolaryngology: Official Journal of ENT-UK; Official Journal of Netherlands Society for Oto-Rhino-Laryngology & Cervico-Facial Surgery*, 30(2): 149–156. https://doi.org/10.1111/j.1365-2273.2004.00944.x

Bear, S. E., and Priest, J. H. (1980). Sleep apnea syndrome: Correction with surgical advancement of the mandible. *Journal of Oral Surgery (American Dental Association: 1965)*, 38(7): 543–549.

Bernkopf, E., and Insalaco, G. (2006). Occlusal treatment for obstructive sleep apnea. *Rassegna Di Patologia Dell'Apparato Respiratorio*, 21: 240–247.

Blanco, J., Zamarrón, C., Abeleira Pazos, M. T., Lamela, C., and Suarez Quintanilla, D. (2005). Prospective evaluation of an oral appliance in the treatment of obstructive sleep apnea syndrome. *Sleep & Breathing = Schlaf & Atmung*, 9(1): 20–25. https://doi.org/10.1007/s11325-005-0003-4.

Bloch, K. E., Iseli, A., Zhang, J. N., Xie, X., Kaplan, V., Stoeckli, P. W., and Russi, E. W. (2000). A randomized, controlled crossover trial of two oral appliances for sleep apnea treatment. *American Journal of Respiratory and Critical Care Medicine*, 162(1): 246–251. https://doi.org/10.1164/ajrccm.162.1.9908112.

Bondemark, L. (1999). Does 2 years' nocturnal treatment with a mandibular advancement splint in adult patients with snoring and OSAS cause a change in the posture of the mandible? *American Journal of Orthodontics and Dentofacial Orthopedics: Official Publication of the American Association of Orthodontists, Its Constituent Societies, and the American Board of Orthodontics*, 116(6): 621–628. https://doi.org/10.1016/s0889-5406(99)70196-4

Bratton, D. J., Gaisl, T., Wons, A. M., and Kohler, M. (2015). CPAP vs Mandibular Advancement Devices and Blood Pressure in Patients with Obstructive Sleep Apnea: A Systematic Review and Meta-analysis. *JAMA*, 314(21): 2280–2293. .https://doi.org/10.1001/jama. 2015.16303.

Cartwright, R. D.,and Samelson, C. F. (1982). The effects of a nonsurgical treatment for obstructive sleep apnea. The tongue-retaining device. *JAMA*, 248(6): 705–709.

Chan, A. S. L., Phillips, C. L., and Cistulli, P. A. (2009). Obstructive sleep apnea - an update. *Internal Medicine Journal*, 40(2):102–106. https://doi.org/10.1111/j.1445-5994.2009.02069.x.

Chan, A. S., Sutherland, K., Schwab, R. J., Zeng, B., Petocz, P., Lee, R. W., Darendeliler, M. A., and Cistulli, P. A. (2010). The effect of mandibular advancement on upper airway structure in obstructive sleep apnea. *Thorax*, 65(8): 726–732. https://doi.org/10.1136/thx. 2009.131094.

Cistulli, P. A., Ferguson, K. A., and Lowe, A. (2011) Oral appliances for sleep-disordered breathing. In: Kryger M. H., Roth T., Dement W. C., eds. *Principles and practice of sleep medicine.* Elsevier Saunders, 2011:1261-77.

Clark, G. T., Blumenfeld, I., Yoffe, N., Peled, E. and Lavie, P. (1996). A crossover study comparing the efficacy of continuous positive airway pressure with anterior mandibular positioning devices on patients with obstructive sleep apnea. *Chest*, 109(6): 1477–1483. https://doi.org/10.1378/chest.109.6.1477.

Clark, W. J. (1988). The twin block technique. A functional orthopedic appliance system. *American journal of orthodontics and dentofacial orthopedics: official publication of the American Association of Orthodontists, its constituent societies, and the American Board of Orthodontics*, 93(1): 1–18. https://doi.org/10.1016/0889-5406(88) 90188-6.

Cozza, P., Polimeni, A., and Ballanti, F. (2004). A modified monobloc for the treatment of obstructive sleep apnea in paediatric patients. *European Journal of Orthodontics*, 26(5): 523–530. https://doi.org/ 10.1093/ejo/26.5.523

de Vries, G. E., Wijkstra, P. J., Houwerzijl, E. J., Kerstjens, H. A. M., and Hoekema, A. (2018). Cardiovascular effects of oral appliance therapy in obstructive sleep apnea: A systematic review and meta-analysis. *Sleep Medicine Reviews*, 40: 55–68. https://doi.org/10. 1016/j.smrv.2017.10.004

Deane, S. A., Cistulli, P. A., Ng, A. T., Zeng, B., Petocz, P., and Darendeliler, M. A. (2009). Comparison of mandibular advancement splint and tongue stabilizing device in obstructive sleep apnea: A randomized controlled trial. *Sleep*, 32(5): 648–653. https://doi.org/10.1093/sleep/32.5.648.

Dispositivos de avance mandibular (DAM) en el tratamiento del SAHS [Mandibular advancement devices (MAD) in the treatment of SAHS]. (2005). *Archivos de Bronconeumología*, 41: 68–74. https://doi.org/10.1016/s0300-2896(05)70755-9.

El-Solh, A. A., Moitheennazima, B., Akinnusi, M. E., Churder, P. M., and Lafornara, A. M. (2011). Combined oral appliance and positive airway pressure therapy for obstructive sleep apnea: A pilot study. *Sleep & Breathing=Schlaf & Atmung*, 15(2): 203–208. https://doi.org/10.1007/s11325-010-0437-1.

Engleman, H. M., McDonald, J. P., Graham, D., Lello, G. E., Kingshott, R. N., Coleman, E. L., Mackay, T. W., and Douglas, N. J. (2002). Randomized crossover trial of two treatments for sleep apnea/hypopnea syndrome: Continuous positive airway pressure and mandibular repositioning splint. *American Journal of Respiratory and Critical Care Medicine*, 166(6): 855–859. https://doi.org/10.1164/rccm.2109023.

Faria, A. C., Garcia, L. V., Santos, A. C. D., Diniz, P. R. B., Ribeiro, H. T., and Mello-Filho, F. V. (2012). Comparison of the area of the pharynx during wakefulness and induced sleep in patients with obstructive sleep apnea (OSA). *Brazilian Journal of Otorhinolaryngology*, 78(1): 103–108. https://doi.org/10.1590/s1808-86942012000100016.

Ferguson, K. A., Ono, T., Lowe, A. A., al-Majed, S., Love, L. L., and Fleetham, J. A. (1997). A short-term controlled trial of an adjustable oral appliance for the treatment of mild to moderate obstructive sleep apnea. *Thorax*, 52(4): 362–368.

Ferguson, K. A., Ono, T., Lowe, A. A., Keenan, S. P., and Fleetham, J. A. (1996). A randomized crossover study of an oral appliance vs nasal-continuous positive airway pressure in the treatment of mild-moderate obstructive sleep apnea. *Chest*, 109(5): 1269–1275. https://doi.org/10.1378/chest.109.5.1269.

Fleetham, J. A., Ferguson, K. A., Lowe, A. A., and Ryan, C. F. (1996). Oral appliance therapy for the treatment of obstructive sleep apnea. *Sleep*, 19(10 Suppl): S288-290. https://doi.org/10.1093/sleep/19.suppl_10.s288.

Fransson, A. M. C., Tegelberg, A., Svenson, B. A. H., Lennartsson, B., and Isacsson, G. (2002). Influence of mandibular protruding device on airway passages and dentofacial characteristics in obstructive sleep apnea and snoring. *American Journal of Orthodontics and Dentofacial Orthopedics: Official Publication of the American Association of Orthodontists, Its Constituent Societies, and the American Board of Orthodontics*, 122(4): 371–379. https://doi.org/10.1067/mod.2002.125993.

García, E. A., González, A. M., and Pérez, J. de la C. (2010). Eficacia y efectos adversos de los aparatos intraorales en el tratamiento de la apnea obstructiva del sueño [Efficacy and adverse effects of intraoral devices in the treatment of obstructive sleep apnea]. *Científica dental: Revista científica de formación continuada*, 7(2 (MAY-AGO)): 19–26.

Gasparini, G., Azzuni, C., Rinaldo, F., Cervelli, D., Marianetti, T., Sferrazza, A., and Pelo, S. (2013). OSAS treatment with oral appliance: Assessment of our experience through the use of a new device. *European Review for Medical and Pharmacological Sciences*, 17: 385–391.

George, P. T. (2001). Selecting sleep-disordered–breathing appliances: Biomechanical considerations. *The Journal of the American Dental Association*, 132(3): 339–347. https://doi.org/10.14219/jada.archive.2001.0177.

Ghazal, A., Jonas, I. E., and Rose, E. C. (2008). Dental side effects of mandibular advancement appliances—A 2-year follow-up. *Journal of Orofacial Orthopedics = Fortschritte Der Kieferorthopadie: Organ/Official Journal Deutsche Gesellschaft Fur Kieferorthopadie*, 69(6): 437–447. https://doi.org/10.1007/s00056-008-0811-9.

Ghodke, S., Utreja, A. K., Singh, S. P., and Jena, A. K. (2014). Effects of twin-block appliance on the anatomy of pharyngeal airway passage (PAP) in class II malocclusion subjects. *Progress in Orthodontics*, 15: 68. https://doi.org/10.1186/s40510-014-0068-3.

Gibbons, P., and Bloomer, H. (1958). A supportive-type prosthetic speech aid. *Journal of Prosthetic Dentistry*, 8(2): 362–369. https://doi.org/10.1016/0022-3913(58)90169-0.

Gonzalez, J. B., and Aronson, A. E. (1970). Palatal lift prosthesis for treatment of anatomic and neurologic palatopharyngeal insufficiency. *The Cleft Palate Journal*, 7: 91–104.

Gotsopoulos, H., Chen, C., Qian, J., and Cistulli, P. A. (2002). Oral appliance therapy improves symptoms in obstructive sleep apnea: A randomized, controlled trial. *American Journal of Respiratory and Critical Care Medicine*, 166(5): 743–748. https://doi.org/10.1164/rccm.200203-208OC

Halicioğlu, K., and Kiki, A. (2012). Subjective symptoms of RME patients treated with three different screw activation protocols: A randomised clinical trial. *Australian Orthodontic Journal*, 28: 225–231.

Hammond, R. J., Gotsopoulos, H., Shen, G., Petocz, P., Cistulli, P. A., and Darendeliler, M. A. (2007). A follow-up study of dental and skeletal changes associated with mandibular advancement splint use in obstructive sleep apnea. *American Journal of Orthodontics and Dentofacial Orthopedics: Official Publication of the American Association of Orthodontists, Its Constituent Societies, and the American Board of Orthodontics*, 132(6): 806–814. https://doi.org/10.1016/j.ajodo.2005.08.047.

Hoekema, A., Stegenga, B., and De Bont, L. G. M. (2004). Efficacy and co-morbidity of oral appliances in the treatment of obstructive sleep apnea-hypopnea: A systematic review. *Critical Reviews in Oral Biology and Medicine: An Official Publication of the American Association of Oral Biologists*, 15(3): 137–155. https://doi.org/10.1177/154411130401500303.

Iftikhar, I. H., Hays, E. R., Iverson, M.-A., Magalang, U. J., and Maas, A. K. (2013). Effect of Oral Appliances on Blood Pressure in Obstructive Sleep Apnea: A Systematic Review and Meta-analysis. *Journal of Clinical Sleep Medicine : JCSM : Official Publication of the American Academy of Sleep Medicine*, 9(2): 165–174. https://doi.org/10.5664/jcsm.2420.

Iwasaki, T., Saitoh, I., Takemoto, Y., Inada, E., Kanomi, R., Hayasaki, H., and Yamasaki, Y. (2012). Improvement of nasal airway ventilation after rapid maxillary expansion evaluated with computational fluid dynamics. *American Journal of Orthodontics and Dentofacial Orthopedics: Official Publication of the American Association of Orthodontists, Its Constituent Societies, and the American Board of Orthodontics*, 141(3): 269–278. https://doi.org/10.1016/j.ajodo.2011.08.025.

Jena, A. K., Singh, S. P., and Utreja, A. K. (2010). Sagittal mandibular development effects on the dimensions of the awake pharyngeal airway passage. *The Angle Orthodontist*, 80(6): 1061–1067. https://doi.org/10.2319/030210-125.1.

Johal, A., Gill, G., Ferman, A., and McLaughlin, K. (2007). The effect of mandibular advancement appliances on awake upper airway and masticatory muscle activity in patients with obstructive sleep apnea. *Clinical Physiology and Functional Imaging*, 27(1): 47–53. https://doi.org/10.1111/j.1475-097X.2007.00714.x.

Johnston, C. D., Gleadhill, I. C., Cinnamond, M. J., Gabbey, J., and Burden, D. J. (2002). Mandibular advancement appliances and obstructive sleep apnea: A randomized clinical trial. *European Journal of Orthodontics*, 24(3): 251–262. https://doi.org/10.1093/ejo/24.3.251.

Kato, J., Isono, S., Tanaka, A., Watanabe, T., Araki, D., Tanzawa, H., and Nishino, T. (2000). Dose-dependent effects of mandibular advancement on pharyngeal mechanics and nocturnal oxygenation in patients with sleep-disordered breathing. *Chest*, 117(4): 1065–1072. https://doi.org/10.1378/chest.117.4.1065.

Kyung, S. H., Park, Y. C., and Pae, E. K. (2005). Obstructive sleep apnea patients with the oral appliance experience pharyngeal size and shape changes in three dimensions. *The Angle orthodontist*, 75(1): 15–22. https://doi.org/10.1043/0003-3219(2005)075<0015:OSAPWT>2.0.CO;2.

Lang, B. R. (1967). Modification of the palatal lift speech aid. *The Journal of Prosthetic Dentistry*, 17(6): 620–626. https://doi.org/10.1016/0022-3913(67)90134-5.

Levrini, L., Sacchi, F., Milano, F., Polimeni, A., Cozza, P., Bernkopf, E., Segù, M., Zucconi, M., Vicini, C., and Brunello, E. (2016). Italian recommendations on dental support in the treatment of adult obstructive sleep apnea syndrome (OSAS). *Annali Di Stomatologia*, 6(3–4): 81–86. https://doi.org/10.11138/ads/2015.6.3.081

Liu, T., Li, W., Zhou, H., and Wang, Z. (2017). Verifying the Relative Efficacy between Continuous Positive Airway Pressure Therapy and Its Alternatives for Obstructive Sleep Apnea: A Network Meta-analysis. *Frontiers in neurology*, 8: 289. https://doi.org/10.3389/fneur.2017.00289.

Lo Giudice, A., Spinuzza, P., Rustico, L., Messina, G., and Nucera, R. (2020). Short-term treatment effects produced by rapid maxillary expansion evaluated with computed tomography: A systematic review with meta-analysis. *Korean Journal of Orthodontics*, 50(5): 314–323. https://doi.org/10.4041/kjod.2020.50.5.314

Lorusso F, Dispenza F, Modica DM, Gallina S. The Role of Modified Expansion Sphincter Pharyngoplasty in Multilevel Obstructive Sleep Apnea Syndrome Surgery. *Int Arch Otorhinolaryngol.* 2018 Oct; 22(4):432-436.

Lorusso, F., Dispenza, F., Martinciglio, G., Battaglia, A., Gallina, S. Postural changes in patients undergoing hyoid surgery for OSAS. *EuroMediterranean Biomedical Journal*, 2017; 12(29):140-143.

Lowe, A. A. (1990). The Tongue and Airway. *Otolaryngologic Clinics of North America*, 23(4): 677–698. https://doi.org/10.1016/s0030-6665(20)31245-7.

Machado-Júnior, A. J., Signorelli, L. G., Zancanella, E., and Crespo, A. N. (2016). Randomized controlled study of a mandibular advancement appliance for the treatment of obstructive sleep apnea in children: A pilot study. *Medicina Oral, Patologia Oral Y Cirugia Bucal*, 21(4): e403-407. https://doi.org/10.4317/medoral.21072.

Marklund, M., Braem, M. J. A., and Verbraecken, J. (2019). Update on oral appliance therapy. *European Respiratory Review*, 28(153): 190083. https://doi.org/10.1183/16000617.0083-2019.

Marklund, M., Franklin, K., Sahlin, C., and Lundgren, R. (1998). The effect of mandibular advancement device on apneas and sleep in patients with OSAS. *Chest*, 113: 707–713. https://doi.org/10.1378/chest.113.3.707.

Marklund, M., Persson, M., and Franklin, K. A. (1998). Treatment success with a mandibular advancement device is related to supine-dependent sleep apnea. *Chest*, 114(6): 1630–1635. https://doi.org/10.1378/chest.114.6.1630.

Marklund, M., Stenlund, H., and Franklin, K. A. (2004). Mandibular advancement devices in 630 men and women with obstructive sleep apnea and snoring: Tolerability and predictors of treatment success. *Chest*, 125(4): 1270–1278. https://doi.org/10.1378/chest.125.4.1270

Marklund, M., Verbraecken, J., and Randerath, W. (2012). Non-CPAP therapies in obstructive sleep apnea: Mandibular advancement device therapy. *European Respiratory Journal*, 39(5): 1241–1247. https://doi.org/10.1183/09031936.00144711.

Maspero, C., Giannini, L., Galbiati, G., Kairyte, L., and Farronato, G. (2015). Upper airway obstuction in class II patients. Effects of Andresen activator on the anatomy of pharingeal airway passage. Cone beam evalution. *Stomatologija*, 17(4): 124–130.

McNamara, J. A., Lione, R., Franchi, L., Angelieri, F., Cevidanes, L. H., Darendeliler, M. A., and Cozza, P. (2015). The role of rapid maxillary expansion in the promotion of oral and general health. *Progress in Orthodontics*, 16:33. https://doi.org/10.1186/s40510-015-0105-x.

McNamara, J. A., Brudon, W. L. (2001). *Orthodontics and dentofacial orthopedics*. Ann Arbor (MI): Needham Press, Inc, p. 211–31.

Mehta, A., Qian, J., Petocz, P., Darendeliler, M. A., and Cistulli, P. A. (2001). A randomized, controlled study of a mandibular advancement splint for obstructive sleep apnea. *American Journal of Respiratory and Critical Care Medicine*, 163(6): 1457–1461. https://doi.org/10.1164/ajrccm.163.6.2004213.

Meier-Ewert, K., and Brosig, B. (1987). Treatment of Sleep Apnea by Prosthetic Mandibular Advancement. In J. H. Peter, T. Podszus, P. von Wichert (Eds.), *Sleep Related Disorders and Internal Diseases* (pp. 341–345). Springer. https://doi.org/10.1007/978-3-642-72560-9_37.

Menn, S. J., Loube, D. I., Morgan, T. D., Mitler, M. M., Berger, J. S., and Erman, M. K. (1996). The mandibular repositioning device: Role in the treatment of obstructive sleep apnea. *Sleep*, 19(10): 794–800. https://doi.org/10.1093/sleep/19.10.794.

Millman, R. P., Rosenberg, C. L., Carlisle, C. C., Kramer, N. R., Kahn, D. M., and Bonitati, A. E. (1998). The efficacy of oral appliances in the treatment of persistent sleep apnea after uvulopalatopharyngoplasty. *Chest*, 113(4): 992–996. https://doi.org/10.1378/chest.113.4.992.

Monasterio, C., Navarro, A., Brinquis, T., Estopà, R., and Manresa, F. (2000). Eficacia de una prótesis de avance mandibular en el tratamiento del síndrome de apneas obstructivas del sueño [Efficacy of a mandibular advancement prosthesis in the treatment of obstructive sleep apnea syndrome]. *Archivos de Bronconeumología*, 36(7): 371–376. https://doi.org/10.1016/S0300-2896(15)30136-8.

Nazarali, N., Altalibi, M., Nazarali, S., Major, M. P., Flores-Mir, C., and Major, P. W. (2015). Mandibular advancement appliances for the treatment of paediatric obstructive sleep apnea: A systematic review. *European Journal of Orthodontics*, 37(6): 618–626. https://doi.org/10.1093/ejo/cju101.

O'Sullivan, R. A., Hillman, D. R., Mateljan, R., Pantin, C., and Finucane, K. E. (1995). Mandibular advancement splint: An appliance to treat snoring and obstructive sleep apnea. *American Journal of Respiratory and Critical Care Medicine*, 151(1): 194–198. https://doi.org/10.1164/ajrccm.151.1.7812552.

Oliveira De Felippe, N. L., Da Silveira, A. C., Viana, G., Kusnoto, B., Smith, B., and Evans, C. A. (2008). Relationship between rapid maxillary expansion and nasal cavity size and airway resistance: Short- and long-term effects. *American Journal of Orthodontics and Dentofacial Orthopedics: Official Publication of the American Association of Orthodontists, Its Constituent Societies, and the American Board of Orthodontics*, 134(3): 370–382. https://doi.org/10.1016/j.ajodo.2006.10.034

Ozbek, M. M., Memikoglu, U. T. T., Altug-Atac, A. T., and Lowe, A. A. (2009). Stability of maxillary expansion and tongue posture. *The Angle Orthodontist*, 79(2): 214–220. https://doi.org/10.2319/010908-12.1.

Pantin, C. C., Hillman, D. R., and Tennant, M. (1999). Dental side effects of an oral device to treat snoring and obstructive sleep apnea. *Sleep*, 22(2): 237–240. https://doi.org/10.1093/sleep/22.2.237.

Perez, C. V., de Leeuw, R., Okeson, J. P., Carlson, C. R., Li, H.-F., Bush, H. M., and Falace, D. A. (2013). The incidence and prevalence of temporomandibular disorders and posterior open bite in patients receiving mandibular advancement device therapy for obstructive sleep apnea. *Sleep & Breathing = Schlaf & Atmung*, 17(1): 323–332. https://doi.org/10.1007/s11325-012-0695-1.

Phillips, C. L., Grunstein, R. R., Darendeliler, M. A., Mihailidou, A. S., Srinivasan, V. K., Yee, B. J., Marks, G. B., and Cistulli, P. A. (2013). Health outcomes of continuous positive airway pressure versus oral appliance treatment for obstructive sleep apnea: A randomized controlled trial. *American Journal of Respiratory and Critical Care Medicine*, 187(8): 879–887. https://doi.org/10.1164/rccm.201212-2223OC.

Premkumar, S. (2011). Clinical application of palatal lift appliance in velopharyngeal incompetence. *Journal of the Indian Society of Pedodontics and Preventive Dentistry*, 29: S70-3. https://doi.org/10.4103/0970-4388.90746.

Ramar, K., Dort, L. C., Katz, S. G., Lettieri, C. J., Harrod, C. G., Thomas, S. M., and Chervin, R. D. (2015). Clinical Practice Guideline for the Treatment of Obstructive Sleep Apnea and Snoring with Oral Appliance Therapy: An Update for 2015. *Journal of Clinical Sleep Medicine: JCSM: Official Publication of the American Academy of Sleep Medicine*, 11(7): 773–827. https://doi.org/10.5664/jcsm.4858.

Rider, E. A. (1988). Removable Herbst appliance for treatment of obstructive sleep apnea. *Journal of clinical orthodontics : JCO*, 22(4): 256–257.

Ringqvist, M., Walker-Engström, M. L., Tegelberg, A., and Ringqvist, I. (2003). Dental and skeletal changes after 4 years of obstructive sleep apnea treatment with a mandibular advancement device: A prospective, randomized study. *American Journal of Orthodontics and Dentofacial Orthopedics: Official Publication of the American Association of Orthodontists, Its Constituent Societies, and the American Board of Orthodontics*, 124(1): 53–60. .https://doi.org/10.1016/s0889-5406(03)00240-3

Robertson, C., Herbison, P., and Harkness, M. (2003). Dental and occlusal changes during mandibular advancement splint therapy in sleep disordered patients. *European Journal of Orthodontics*, 25(4): 371–376. https://doi.org/10.1093/ejo/25.4.371.

Robin, P. (1934). Glossoptosis due to atresia and hypotrophy of the mandible. *American Journal of Diseases of Children*, 48(3): 541–547. https://doi.org/10.1001/archpedi.1934.01960160063005.

Robin, P. (1994). A fall of the base of the tongue considered as a new cause of nasopharyngeal respiratory impairment: Pierre Robin sequence, a translation. 1923. *Plastic and Reconstructive Surgery*, 93(6):1301–1303.

Rodríguez-Lozano, F. J., Sáez-Yuguero, M. del R., Linares Tovar, E., and Bermejo Fenoll, A. (2008). Sleep apnea and mandibular advancement device. Revision of the literature. *Medicina Oral, Patologia Oral Y Cirugia Bucal*, 13(9): E549-554.

Rose, E. C., Staats, R., Virchow, C., and Jonas, I. E. (2002). Occlusal and skeletal effects of an oral appliance in the treatment of obstructive sleep apnea. *Chest*, 122(3): 871–877. https://doi.org/10.1378/chest.122.3.871.

Ryan, C. F., Love, L. L., Peat, D., Fleetham, J. A., and Lowe, A. A. (1999). Mandibular advancement oral appliance therapy for obstructive sleep apnea: effect on awake calibre of the velopharynx. *Thorax*, 54(11): 972–977. https://doi.org/10.1136/thx.54.11.972.

Sanner, B. M., Heise, M., Knoben, B., Machnick, M., Laufer, U., Kikuth, R., Zidek, W., and Hellmich, B. (2002). MRI of the pharynx and treatment efficacy of a mandibular advancement device in obstructive sleep apnoa syndrome. *European Respiratory Journal*, 20(1): 143–150. https://doi.org/10.1183/09031936.02.00268902

Schaefer, K. S., Taylor, T. D. (2000). Clinical application of the palatal lift. In: Taylor TD, editor. *Clinical Maxillofacial Prosthetics*. Chicago, Ill, USA: Quintessence Publication, pp. 133–43.

Schmidt-Nowara, W. W., Meade, T. E., and Hays, M. B. (1991). Treatment of snoring and obstructive sleep apnea with a dental orthosis. *Chest*, 99(6): 1378–1385. https://doi.org/10.1378/chest.99.6.1378.

Schmidt-Nowara, W., Lowe, A., Wiegand, L., Cartwright, R., Perez-Guerra, F., and Menn, S. (1995). Oral appliances for the treatment of snoring and obstructive sleep apnea: A review. *Sleep*, 18(6): 501–510. https://doi.org/10.1093/sleep/18.6.501.

Soll, B. A., and George, P. T. (1985). Treatment of obstructive sleep apnea with a nocturnal airway-patency appliance. *The New England journal of medicine*, 313(6): 386–387. https://doi.org/10.1056/NEJM198508083130612.

Sutherland, K., Deane, S. A., Chan, A. S. L., Schwab, R. J., Ng, A. T., Darendeliler, M. A., and Cistulli, P. A. (2011). Comparative Effects of Two Oral Appliances on Upper Airway Structure in Obstructive Sleep Apnea. *Sleep*, 34(4): 469–477.

Sutherland, K., Vanderveken, O. M., Tsuda, H., Marklund, M., Gagnadoux, F., Kushida, C. A., and Cistulli, P. A. (2014). Oral appliance treatment for obstructive sleep apnea: An update. *Journal of Clinical Sleep Medicine: JCSM: Official Publication of the American Academy of Sleep Medicine*, 10(2): 215–227. https://doi.org/10.5664/jcsm.3460.

Tan, Y. K., L'Estrange, P. R., Luo, Y. M., Smith, C., Grant, H. R., Simonds, A. K., Spiro, S. G., and Battagel, J. M. (2002). Mandibular advancement splints and continuous positive airway pressure in patients with obstructive sleep apnoa: A randomized cross-over trial. *European Journal of Orthodontics*, 24(3): 239–249. https://doi.org/10.1093/ejo/24.3.239.

Tan, Y. K., L'Estrange, P. R., Grant, H. R., Smith, C., Simonds, A. K., and Spiro, S.G. (1998) A randomised crossover study of continuous positive airway pressure (CPAP) vs mandibular advancement splint (MAS) in mild and moderate obstructive sleep apnea (OSA). *Thorax,* 53(Suppl 4):A4.

Tasker, C., Crosby, J., and Stradling, J. (2002). Evidence for persistence of upper airway narrowing during sleep, 12 years after adenotonsillectomy. *Archives of Disease in Childhood*, 86(1): 34–37. https://doi.org/10.1136/adc.86.1.34.

Ueda, H., Almeida, F. R., Lowe, A. A., and Ruse, N. D. (2008). Changes in occlusal contact area during oral appliance therapy assessed on study models. *The Angle Orthodontist*, 78(5): 866–872. https://doi.org/10.2319/100107-470.1.

Villa, M. P., Bernkopf, E., Pagani, J., Broia, V., Montesano, M., and Ronchetti, R. (2002). Randomized controlled study of an oral jaw-positioning appliance for the treatment of obstructive sleep apnea in children with malocclusion. *American Journal of Respiratory and Critical Care Medicine*, 165(1): 123–127. https://doi.org/10.1164/ajrccm.165.1.2011031.

Villa, M. P., Rizzoli, A., Rabasco, J., Vitelli, O., Pietropaoli, N., Cecili, M., Marino, A., and Malagola, C. (2015). Rapid maxillary expansion outcomes in treatment of obstructive sleep apnea in children. *Sleep Medicine*, 16(6): 709–716. https://doi.org/10.1016/j.sleep.2014.11.019.

Wagner, A. G., and Price, R. R. (1987). An intraoral device to prevent snoring. *General Dentistry*, 35(3): 212–213.

Walker-Engström, M. L., Wilhelmsson, B., Tegelberg, A., Dimenäs, E., and Ringqvist, I. (2000). Quality of life assessment of treatment with dental appliance or UPPP in patients with mild to moderate obstructive sleep apnea. A prospective randomized 1-year follow-up study. *Journal of Sleep Research*, 9(3): 303–308. https://doi.org/10.1046/j.1365-2869.2000.00210.x.

Walker-Engström, M.-L., Ringqvist, I., Vestling, O., Wilhelmsson, B., and Tegelberg, A. (2003). A prospective randomized study comparing two different degrees of mandibular advancement with a dental appliance in treatment of severe obstructive sleep apnea. *Sleep & Breathing = Schlaf & Atmung*, 7(3): 119–130. https://doi.org/10.1007/s11325-003-0119-3.

Walker-Engström, M. L., Tegelberg, A., Wilhelmsson, B., and Ringqvist, I. (2002). 4-year follow-up of treatment with dental appliance or uvulopalatopharyngoplasty in patients with obstructive sleep apnea: A randomized study. *Chest*, 121(3): 739–746. https://doi.org/10.1378/chest.121.3.739.

Wang, X., Gong, X., Yu, Z., Gao, X., and Zhao, Y. (2015). Follow-up study of dental and skeletal changes in patients with obstructive sleep apnea and hypopnea syndrome with long-term treatment with the Silensor appliance. *American Journal of Orthodontics and Dentofacial Orthopedics: Official Publication of the American Association of Orthodontists, Its Constituent Societies, and the*

American Board of Orthodontics, 147(5): 559–565. https://doi.org/10.1016/j.ajodo.2015.01.013.

Yanyan, M., Min, Y., and Xuemei, G. (2019). Mandibular advancement appliances for the treatment of obstructive sleep apnea in children: A systematic review and meta-analysis. *Sleep Medicine*, 60: 145–151. https://doi.org/10.1016/j.sleep.2018.12.022.

Zhang, C., He, H., and Ngan, P. (2013). Effects of twin block appliance on obstructive sleep apnea in children: A preliminary study. *Sleep & Breathing=Schlaf & Atmung*, 17(4): 1309–1314. https://doi.org/10.1007/s11325-013-0840-5.

In: Advances in Sleep Apnea
Editors: F. Lorusso et al.
ISBN: 978-1-53619-758-7

Chapter 11

ADVANCES IN THE ROLE OF NASAL SURGERY IN THE TREATMENT OF OSAS

Pierluigi Ortenzio, Onofrio Guzzo, Francesco Lorusso, Salvatore Gallina and Federico Sireci*
Unit of Otolaringology,
Department of Experimental Biomedicine
and Clinical Neurosciences, Policlinico Paolo Giaccone,
University of Palermo, Palermo, Italy

ABSTRACT

Nasal surgery is a useful therapeutic strategy for lowering nasal resistance, ameliorating sleep-disordered breathing, and improving sleep quality and daytime sleepiness in OSAS.

Nasal surgery is to be meant in a wider perspective of a multilevel surgical approach for OSAS patient.

In this chapter we highlighted the state of the art on surgical techniques aimed at the treatment of nasal and nasopharyngeal pathologies implicated in the pathophysiology of OSAS, like valve

* Corresponding Author's Email: federicosireci@hotmail.it.

collapse, septal deviation, turbinate hypertrophy, chronic rhinosinusitis and adenoid hypertrophy.

Keywords: OSAS, Valve collapse, septoplasty, turbinate hypertrophy, endoscopic sinus surgery, adenoidectomy

INTRODUCTION

Obstructive sleep apnoea (OSA) is established as a spectrum of signs and symptoms arising from obstruction of airflow somewhere in the nasopharyngeal, oropharyngeal and/or hypopharyngeal regions. This obstruction occurs during sleep state and arises from the collapse of the upper airway coupled with muscle tone relaxation.

OSA is included in a wider spectrum of disorders termed sleep disordered breathing (SDB) that range from simple snoring, defined as noisy breathing during sleep, to upper ways resistance syndrome (UARS), snores who have daytime somnolence but have normal hypopnoea/apnoea index. OSAS patients are characterized by snoring, subjective symptoms, daytime sleepiness and abnormal apnoea/hypopnoea index.

In this chapter we will focus our attention on nasal obstruction in sleep-disordered breathing, providing a "state of the art" view upon the role played by nasal surgery in the treatment of OSA.

The Role of Nasal Surgery in OSAS

One of the common sites of airflow obstruction in patients with OSA is the nasal complex. Nasal airflow obstruction can also be seen in many subsets of the population without any evidence of OSA, so diagnosing nasal airflow issues in patients with OSA should not be a surprise. The most common sites of airflow obstruction within the nasal complex include external and internal nasal valve areas, nasal tip, nasal septum, and nasal turbinates. Mucosal hypertrophy, as a result of environmental insults such as pollen, pollution, and seasonal allergies can also contribute to this airflow deficit. It is also known that the anterior nasal cavity has more effect on nasal airway resistance than the posterior one because the smallest part of the airway is located anteriorly at the level of the internal nasal valve.

Airway resistance is proportional to the length of the airway and inversely proportional to the fourth power of the radius. As a result, a very small change in the size of the nasal airway can determine a very huge increase in nasal airway resistance. Secondarily, any kind of nasal obstruction is responsible of the shift from laminar airflow to turbulent airflow. This is the most important effect of increasing resistance (nasal obstruction itself) and can be regarded as 'primum movens' of deriving vibrations in oral cavity, such as uvula, soft palate, tonsils, base of tongue, epiglottis and pharyngeal wall. This physical mechanism give rise to snoring and inferior airways obstructions.

Effective surgical treatment for obstructive sleep apnea/hypopnea syndrome (OSAHS) must be designed to eliminate collapsible soft tissue in the upper airway without interfering with normal function. Creation of a non-collapsible airspace and reduction of airway resistance enables maintenance of adequate airflow with normal inspiratory effort. This translates into elimination or reduction of apneic/hypopneic episodes during sleep, control of symptoms and further minimizes ongoing multi-system damage in OSAHS patients. OSAHS is often caused by multiple levels of obstruction and therefore requires multilevel treatment. From this point of view, we could say that single level surgery cannot be the only treatment for most of OSAHS patient. Surgical interventions on the nose, tongue and oral cavity must be meant as complementary procedures, each of them with his own "specific weight." Multi-level pre-operative assessment is a well-practice appliable not only to severe conditions but must be a part of standard clinical evaluation of OSAHS patients. In this perspective we will show in this chapter the importance of rating nasal obstruction and the essential role of nasal surgery. Therefore, nasal surgery is to be meant as pivotal, but not primary, in the armamentarium of OSAS's surgery.

Nasal obstruction may cause sleep disordered breathing in many ways, including increasing upper airway resistance, provoking sleep onset and sleep maintenance insomnia, worsening sleep fragmentation, increased work of breathing, and unstable oral breathing. It is also responsible of worsening of apnoea/hyponoea index (AHI), leading to a depression of central respiratory drive. Finally, one could safely say that nasal obstruction is involved as a major driver in the pathogenesis of SDB and of all its manifestations.

As the nose is the primary route of entry for air that will ultimately be inhaled into the lungs, maintaining, creating and providing a smooth laminar flow of air into the lower airway is crucial. The nose needs to be opened for patients who require nasal continuous positive airway pressure (CPAP) mask in order to splint and open their airway during sleep. Hence, the indications for nasal surgery in OSA are listed below:

1. Significant/Symptomatic Nasal Pathology: reversible or reactive nasal pathologies (like inflammatory allergic rhinosinusitis, nasal polyps, and/or infective sinusitis) are associated with sleep-disordered breathing. General principles of surgery, combined with long-term medical therapy, should be instituted in patients with SDB. In addition, an awareness of options to maximize the effectiveness of positive airway pressure (e.g., appropriate humidification, adjunctive sprays, etc.) and avoid exacerbation of underlying mucosal disease is important.
2. Significant Structural/Anatomic Nasal Pathology: it is well accepted that nasal surgery for obstructive or functional nasal deficits should be performed when it would improve the patient's OSA and/or increases compliance of other OSA treatments. Septoplasty, functional rhinoplasty and nasal valve surgery are potential procedures to consider in patients with OSA and snoring.
3. As Part of Multi-level Surgery Treatment Modality to Improve SDB: nasal surgery is generally part of the surgical armamentarium used to treat sleep apnoea, as part of a multi-level surgical plan. Nasal surgery facilitates other treatments for SDB, rather than being a treatment modality in and of itself. However, a significant treatment effect may be achieved in reduction of snoring, improvement in daytime symptoms, or even reduction in markers of OSA severity [e.g., apnoea - hypopnea index (AHI)].

4. Failed Tolerance/Efficacy of CPAP/Oral Appliance Use Patients with OSA on CPAP or MAS with poor compliance due to a blocked nose and/or nasal pathology should be considered for nasal surgery in order to improve device compliance. Objective measurements of nasal resistance confirm that nasal obstruction not only decreases device tolerance but also increase treatment efficacy.

Effects of Nasal Surgery on OSAS

Most authors would agree that nasal surgery, as a single site procedure, would not significantly impact sleep apnoea severity.

Pang et al. in a recent nonrandomized trial of 745 OSA patients found out that combining nose surgery in multilevel surgery improves surgical success (level of evidence IIc). 160 subjects underwent palate and/or tongue surgery without nasal surgery, the remaining 575 subjects underwent palate and/or tongue surgery with nasal surgery. They found significant difference between the two groups in mean postoperative AHI (nose group 13.5 ± 10.2, no nose group 17.1 ± 16.0), in mean postoperative ESS (Epworth Sleep Scale) (nose group was 5.3 ± 3.2, no nose group was 6.7 ± 2.8), and in success rate of surgery (nose group 68.2%, no nose group 55.0%).

A meta-analysis by Wu et al. of total 18 articles found that isolated nasal surgery applied to OSA patients did significantly improves both AHI and ESS, but the improvement of AHI is slightly, confirming what already suggested by Li et al. in a previous study. In this previous meta-analysis was highlighted that effectiveness of nasal surgery is statistically significant in reducing daytime sleepiness and snoring, but no efficacy was found when considering objective parameters. Similarly Ishii et al. showed in a systematic review a significant improvement in the pooled results of both Epworth Sleepiness Scale (ESS; difference 3.53, 95% confidence interval [CI] [0.64, 6.23]) and Respiratory Disturbance Index (RDI; 11.06, 95% CI [5.92, 16.19]) scores with isolated nasal surgery. There was no significant improvement in the Apnea Hypopnea Index (AHI) in the random effects model (4.83, 95% CI [–1.6, 11.62]).

A recent meta-analysis, including 19 studies and 896 patients, with the aim of determine if isolated nasal and sinus surgery in patients with and without OSA could improve sleep quality after surgery, found a significant improvement in subjective sleep parameters and reduction of daytime sleepiness. No significant improvement on objective parameters like AHI were showed.

As showed above, it is shared by all authors that more studies are needed in other to demonstrate the benefits of nasal surgery as a stand-alone surgery in OSAS patients.

1. Valve Collapse Surgery

1.1. Introduction

The nasal valve was first described by Mink in the 1920s and its role in the pathophysiology of nasal obstruction is well-described.

The nasal valve can be subdivided into internal and external components and it constitutes the narrowest point of the nasal airway. The internal nasal valve (INV) refers to the area defined by the nasal septum medially, the upper lateral cartilages superolaterally, and the head of the inferior turbinate inferiorly. The cross-sectional area of the nasal ala, or opening of the nasal vestibule, defines the external nasal valve (ENV).

Nasal valve collapse is a common cause of functional upper airway obstruction that leads to varying difficulty with nasal inspiration, diminished exercise tolerance, and significant decreases in quality of life. Nasal valve collapse can be innate to patient anatomy, iatrogenic as a sequela of rhinoplasty (it's the most common cause of nasal valve dysfunction), congenital, or traumatic, but regardless of cause, causes significant patient distress.

The nasal valve provides the greatest resistance to airflow in the nose; this rate limitation is an important feature as the airflow must not exceed the capacity of the nose to humidify and warm the inspired air and, when compromised, can lead to nasal valve collapse with significant functional deficiencies with worsened quality of life. As the airflow increases through the nasal valves, negative pressure is produced, which leads to collapse of the nasal valve and lateral wall. Because of velocity of airflow inherently creating negative pressure within the nasal valve, iatrogenic narrowing or loss of lateral wall support reliably leads to significant supra-alar pinching and eventual obstruction.

Nasal valve clinical assessment includes history taking in order to identify etiologic causes and also the physical examination.

Assessing patient nasal airflow at rest and on inspiration is paramount to determine the presence and severity of nasal valve collapse. It's possible with the Cottle maneuver and modified Cottle maneuver. The Cottle maneuver is a lateral distraction of the cheek away from the airway, is a rather nonspecific test and almost uniformly shows improvement in breathing without specificity for site of obstruction. With the modified Cottle maneuver patients are asked if the exaggerated nasal breathing impacts their nasal obstruction. A cotton swab or cerumen loop can then be placed through the nasal vestibule to support the lateral wall cartilage to see if this provides improvement in their airway. If they have improvement with this maneuver, nasal valve collapse can be consdered a source of their nasal obstruction.

Defining the degree of nasal obstruction is an important outcome measure. The NOSE questionnaire, a validated quality-of-life assessment instrument, allows standardization of the symptoms of nasal obstruction in assessing functional improvements.

Once a diagnosis of nasal valve collapse is made and the cause is determined, appropriate management can be discussed with the patient. There are several nonsurgical options as well as a wide array of surgical maneuvers to improve nasal valve collapse. Nonsurgical management focuses on stenting or providing external support to the nasal valve and lateral wall. Surgical maneuvers focus more on widening the nasal valve and providing support with cartilage grafts.

1.2. Nonsurgical Management of Nasal Valve Collapse

For patients who are poor surgical candidates or hesitant about surgery, there are nonsurgical management options for nasal valve collapse like nasal strips and internal dilators.

In addition, minimally invasive treatments have been developed for internal nasal valve collapse and to bolster lateral wall support. The Latera implant (Spirox Inc, Redwood City, CA, USA) can be placed in the office percutaneously through the vestibular skin on each side or the affected side of lateral wall collapse. The implant is made of an absorbable polymer material that will resorb over a period of approximately 18 months leaving a fibrous capsule in place that may provide additional support after the implant has dissolved. The Latera device is initially marked with a positioning device and inserted endonasally stenting the internal valve and lateral wall. It is important for the proximal aspect of the implant to remain above the alar crease with the distal aspect situated over the ipsilateral nasal bone. Local anesthesia is more than adequate for anesthesia during implantation and is highly effective. The implant is then loaded into the device and implanted into the previously marked plane taking care to insert above the alar crease and over the ipsilateral nasal bone.

Although the implant has only recently become available, preliminary clinical studies have shown improvement in nasal obstruction and reduction in NOSE scores. Not only does the device have an impact on the internal nasal valve but also possibly on the external valve as well. The risks are minimal and include extrusion, minor bleeding, and low risk of infection.

Although nonsurgical devices can be very successful in properly selected patients, surgical correction of nasal valve collapse is oftentimes required and various methods can lead to excellent results in functional and aesthetic rhinoplasty.

1.3. Surgical Management of the Internal Nasal Valve

There are multiple surgical options available to open the internal nasal valve to improve breathing and also to alter the aesthetic appearance of the nose at the middle nasal vault. This can be accomplished by traditional spreader grafts, spreader flaps, butterfly grafts, and with additional support by batten grafts. Regardless of the method, the goal is to expand the nasal valve area. The most commonly used method to improve obstruction at the internal nasal valve is spreader graft placement.

Spreader grafts can be placed endonasally or via an external approach and various autologous grafting materials can be used, most commonly from septal or costal cartilage.

The grafts are placed either into a submucosal pocket placed at the apex of the internal nasal valve, or between the upper lateral cartilage and dorsal septum in the correspondence of the soft tissue between themselves.

The length of the spreader grafts is dependent on the goals of reconstruction: sometimes the grafts need be extended underneath the nasal bones to provide support and maintain nasal bone position; other times the grafts need to be extended caudally for stabilization of a caudal septal extension graft. Because of the ability to alter length and width of the grafts, the spreader graft allows for the greatest versatility and is the preferred method of middle vault reconstruction.

Spreader flaps are less frequently used due to the thin nature of the upper lateral cartilage, but in certain patients can be appropriate. The spreader flap is crafted entirely from the upper lateral cartilage.

Butterfly grafts, commonly harvested from the concha due to the natural curvature and flexibility of the cartilage, can also be used to stent open the internal nasal valve.

1.3.1. Surgical Management of the External Valve/Lateral Wall

Collapse of the lateral wall as it relates to nasal obstruction can be due to weakness of the lower lateral cartilage, cephalic malposition of the lower lateral cartilage, or concavity, all of which can be inherent to the patient anatomy or iatrogenic.

Traditional reductive rhinoplasty with cephalic trim and dome sutures often leads to weakness of the lateral wall as well as concavity of the lateral crus, creating an unappealing aesthetic result and nasal valve obstruction. In the case of a concave or weak lateral crus, the strut grafts can be placed to provide additional support to the lateral wall as well as flatten out the concavity of the lateral crus. These grafts have the additional benefit of tip refinement and caudal rotation of the lateral crus.

Alternatively, in cephalic malpositioned lower lateral cartilages, repositioning is often required. Lateral crural repositioning begins with an open septorhinoplasty approach using hydrodissection with local anesthetic agent to assist in the dissection of the lateral crura from the underlying vestibular skin and eventual release of the crura from its most lateral attachments. Once the lateral crura is released, it is repositioned into a more caudal orientation after suturing lateral crural strut grafts to the undersurface of the lateral crura.

Septal cartilage is preferred. The lateral crural strut graft is fashioned with an angled medial edge and with the longer margin being placed just under the dome to increase its front projection. A 5-0 PDS suture is used to secure the graft to the overlying lateral crura. Lateral crural repositioning can be further supplemented by domal sutures. The angle of the dome suture should be oriented so it is closer to the caudal margin medially and directed toward the cephalic margin laterally. Then, creation of the lateral pocket for the placement of the lateral crural strut graft is made along the alar groove or just caudal to it. Furthermore, splinting of the nasal sidewall with clear plastic splints ensures a correct cicatrization and positioning of the cartilagous.

Although proper management of the lateral wall and the apex of the internal nasal valve are essential for patency of the nasal airway, the septum and inferior turbinate also play a role in nasal valve obstruction.

2. Septoplasty

2.1. Introduction

Septal deviation is one of the most common causes of nasal obstruction and a prevalent problem among the general population. The nasal septum is an integral support structure of the nose. Deviation or deformity of the septum can cause nasal obstruction, the most common complaint in the average rhinologic practice. When conservative medical management is unsuccessful in relieving symptoms of obstruction, surgical intervention to correct the septal deformity is indicated. Septoplasty is a cornerstone of the otolaryngologist's practice ranking as the third most common head and neck operation, with approximately 260,000 cases performed each year Although most often performed to fix structural deformities resulting in nasal obstruction, surgical correction of a deviated nasal septum may also be indicated in other cases including recurrent epistaxis, sinusitis, obstructive sleep apnoea, and facial pain/headaches secondary to septal spurs contacting the lateral nasal wall (Sluder syndrome). Septoplasty may also play a complementary role to improve nasal access during endoscopic sinus surgery (ESS) and endoscopic orbital procedures.

The three main approaches used to perform septoplasty include the traditional open endonasal approach, the endoscopic approach and the external open or open septorhinoplasty approach. First described by Freer and Killian in the early twentieth century, the traditional approach to address a deviated nasal septum involves direct visualization using headlight illumination and a nasal speculum. Alternatively, endoscopic septoplasty, which was initially described by Lanza and colleagues in 1991, involves the use of rigid endoscopes for visualization and targeted correction of any deformities. Both techniques can be used to address nasal septal deviations and have been shown to have similar functional outcomes. The external open approach is often used to address markedly caudally deviated septa with external nasal deformities.

2.1.1. Preoperative Considerations

A thorough preoperative workup is essential for maximizing the potential for benefit and minimizing the risk of complication. Patients' interviews include an analysis of symptomatic severity. Different scale questionnaires can be routinely administered to the patient such as Nasal Obstructive Symptom Evaluation (NOSE) or Rhinoplasty Health Inventory and Nasal Outcomes. Patients with scaled NOSE scores of less than 30 are classified as "mild" obstruction and are unlikely to be operative candidates. Remarkable ananmnestic facts include a history of maxillofacial trauma or previous nasal surgery, autoimmune disease, drug use, bleeding disorders, use of anticoagulants or systemic steroids. Hence, it is of outmost importance that the surgeon determines if the patient currently or previously used vasoconstrictive nasal sprays or illicit drugs intranasally in order to assess the preoperative risk of septal perforation. Photodocumentation of nasal form with standard rhinoplasty views is recommended, although not required of septoplasty patients.

Preoperative physical examination consisting of a full head and neck inspection, anterior rhinoscopy with a nasal speculum in order to visualize the nasal septum, as well as the nasal valves. Flexible or rigid nasal endoscopy can complement anterior rhinoscopy. Mucosal status, as well as the size of the turbinates must be taken into account. Some key findings to note on examination are: location, degree, and direction of septal deviation (ie, parallel or perpendicular to plane of the septum); presence of posterior nasal spurs, which occur with abnormal bony growth under the posterior QC extension; presence of septal perforation; degree of inferior turbinate hypertrophy; presence of internal nasal valve stenosis (assessed with the modified Cottle manoeuvre); any internal valve narrowing or lateral wall insufficiency which, if present, is noted and graded; the degree of tip support; presence of any external deformities of the nose, especially dorsal and caudal deviations.

2.2. Surgical Techniques

The modern septoplasty has evolved into a more conservative procedure than the initially described SMR technique and involves resection of the targeted area of the deviated septum and may include modification and/or replacement of a cartilage graft. Despite its variations, each septoplasty technique is based on the fundamental principles of intact flap elevation, mucosal preservation, careful reapproximation, and preservation of dorsal and caudal supporting struts.

2.2.1. Traditional Septoplasty

The traditional septoplasty is typically performed under general anesthesia using nasal speculums and headlight illumination for visualization. The nasal mucosa is decongested using topical epinephrine, oxymetazoline, or 4% cocaine. Lidocaine 1% with

1:100,000 epinephrine is then injected along the septum bilaterally in a subperichondral plane in an anterior to posterior fashion until the mucosa is well blanched. After adequate time for vasoconstriction, either a Killian or hemi-transfixion incision is made using a 15 blade extending through the mucosa and perichondrium but sparing the cartilage itself. The side of the incision depends on surgeon preference and experience. The Killian incision is placed approximately 1 to 2 cm posterior to the caudal septal margin and is useful when the septal deviation involves only the middle to posterior part of the septum. It does not provide adequate access to the anterior septum and is, thus, not used for caudal septal deviations. Alternatively, the hemi-transfixion incision, which is made at the caudal border of the septum, allows adequate exposure and is used when the caudal portion of the septum is involved. A curved elevator (Cottle or Freer elevator) is then used to dissect within a subperichondral plane and elevate the perichondrium and mucosa from the cartilage. The dissection is continued broadly over and beyond the septal deformity, with caution during flap elevation along the septal deviation or spur to avoid tearing the mucosa at these sites. After the ipsilateral flap is elevated, the Cottle elevator or a 15 blade is used to incise the cartilage anterior to the site of the deviation and the contralateral flap is elevated. An adequate so-called "L-strut" is preserved to prevent loss of external nasal support and subsequent external deformity (saddle nose). Once both mucoperichondral flaps are elevated, the Cottle elevator, scissors, True-cut forceps, or Jansen Middleton forceps can be used to incise the cartilage superiorly and inferiorly to isolate the segment of deviated septum. The remaining deformity is then grasped using forceps, separated from its posterior attachment using a rotational movement in an anterior-posterior axis, and finally removed. Any remaining posterior bony deviation can be subsequently resected using True-cut or Jansen Middleton forceps. If the deviated segment of the septum is wide, modifications of cartilage with cartilaginous scoring or weakening incisions can be used to minimize the extent of resected septal cartilage; alternatively, the removed cartilage can be morselized and replaced. Once the septal deformity is resected, the mucoperichondral flaps are reapproximated and the initial mucosal incision is closed using an absorbable suture. A quilting stitch, nonabsorbable packing, or secured nasal splints are usually placed bilaterally to compress the flaps together. In the end patients start antibiotics therapy with Staphylococcus aureus coverage as prophylaxis for toxic shock syndrome secondary to nasal packing. Nasal packing or splints are removed in the clinic 3 to 5 days postoperatively.

2.2.2. Endoscopic Septoplasty

Endoscopic septoplasty is very similar to the traditional approach. Instead of a nasal speculum and headlight, rigid nasal endoscopes are used for illumination and visualization throughout the procedure. Often performed in conjunction with ESS, endoscopic septoplasty requires similar instrumentation and set up as these procedures. Under visualization using a 0° endoscope, the nasal mucosa is decongested and anesthetized as described with the traditional technique. A more posteriorly positioned modified Killian incision is made for complex or broad-based deviations, whereas a mucosal incision immediately anterior to or over the deformity is made for focal deviations or isolated septal spurs. Using a Cottle elevator, flaps are then elevated in a subperichondral or subperiosteal plane as previously described over the deviated cartilage or bone. The septal cartilage is then incised, leaving at least 1 cm of caudal and dorsal strut for nasal support. The inferior turbinate concha and middle turbinate axilla are reliable landmarks; placing the mucosal incision at or posterior to the conchal line and at or inferior to the axillary line, will result in adequate L-strut preservation. The mucoperichondral flap is then raised on the contralateral side, and the cartilaginous and/or osseous deformity is resected similarly to the traditional approach. Some investigators have also described using the powered microdebrider to remove the deviated septum. As with the nasal speculum in the traditional approach, the endoscope is used throughout the procedure in endoscopic septoplasty and can be placed between mucosal flaps and within the nasal cavity to ensure adequate resection of the septal deviation. Once this is completed, the mucosal flaps are repositioned and the mucosal incision and dead space created are closed with an absorbable suture. A quilting suture, nasal splints, or packing can be used as previously described.

2.2.3. Traditional versus Endoscopic Technique

Although studies comparing endoscopic septoplasty with the traditional technique have shown similar outcomes, surgical results, and comparable operative times, endoscopic technique provides several advantages over the open approach. By providing superior visualization of tissue planes with optimal illumination and magnification, the endoscopic approach allows to surgeon a more accurate evaluation of nasal anatomy and gives him more precision in debris and small fragments removal. The endoscopic approach may also be helpful for submucoperichondral flap elevation during revision cases in which tissue planes are less obvious. In addition, the use of the endoscope may enhance the experience of residents and fellows and enables better teaching, as it projects the procedure onto a monitor. Limitations of the endoscopic technique arise when operating very anteriorly in the nose where the nostril is not adequately available to support the endoscope (so-called "free handing"). For this reason, caudal deflections are often considered a relative contraindication to the endoscopic.

Thus, indications for the endoscopic approach include more posterior deviations of the septum without involvement of the caudal septum. In addition, as it is performed using similar instrumentation to ESS, endoscopic septoplasty can be performed in conjunction with ESS, if necessary, for improved access to the sinuses.

Endoscopic septoplasty is contraindicated for caudal deviations or crooked nose and the traditional open technique is preferred in cases of caudal septal deviations or severe septal deviations. Ultimately, the location and severity of the septal deformity along with surgeon experience and preference will play an important role in the selection of the septoplasty technique. Surgeons may opt to use a combined approach to take advantage of the unique benefits offered by each approach.

Complications that can occur after septoplasty are nearly identical for both the traditional and endoscopic approaches. Persistent nasal obstruction is the most common complication, followed by septal perforation and external nasal deformity. Septal perforations may result from unrepaired opposing mucoperichondral tear or vascular compromise of mucosa after postoperative hematoma or abscess. Risk of nasal deformities, such as tip ptosis or saddle nose deformity, which usually result from over-resection of the caudal septum or loss of dorsal nasal support, can be minimized by maintaining an adequate L-strut during septoplasty. Other possible complications include epistaxis, septal hematoma, septal abscess, synechiae formation, and injury to the nasopalatine nerve with subsequent dental pain (usually temporary) and hypesthesia. Patients should be instructed to avoid the use of medications that can increase the risk of bleeding and to avoid strenuous activity and heavy lifting in the immediate postoperative period. Nasal packing, stents, and quilting sutures are thought to decrease the risk of postoperative bleeding and hematoma formation. Major complications, such as cerebrospinal fluid leak, unilateral blindness, and death, are extremely rare. In general, overall complication rates reported with endoscopic septoplasty are similar to those reported in the literature for traditional septoplasty.

2.3. Septoplasty and OSA

Most authors recognise that surgical treatment of nose in OSA treatment is pivotal, but not primary. In other word nose surgery as a single operative site has minimal effect in both subjective and objective parameters taken into account when evaluating OSA. Very few literature can be found when considering, among surgical nose armamentarium, septoplasty alone. The status of current evidence for the effectiveness of septoplasty is unclear.

Recently Moxness and Nordgard in an observational cohort study evaluated the outcomes of septoplasty with and without inferior turbinate reduction in patients with OSA. They found a significant reduction in the apnea-hypopnea index (AHI) only in the group that had septoplasty with turbinate reduction (17.4, (SD 14.4) – 11.7, (SD 8.2), $p < 0.01$). This effect was significantly better than in the group treated with septoplasty alone. Other objective parameters remained unchanged. Subjective assessments obtained with a postoperative questionnaire showed an equally positive effect on diurnal sleepiness and nasal obstruction in both groups, and a better effect on sleep quality in the combined treatment group.

Van Egmond et al. made a systematic review in order to evaluate the effectiveness of septoplasty with concurrent turbinate surgery versus septoplasty alone, for nasal obstruction due to a deviated nasal septum in adults. Five studies described both subjective and objective outcomes; six studies reported one or the other. Although outcomes generally improved after treatment, eight out of nine studies on subjective measures and five out of seven studies on objective measures found no additional benefit of turbinate surgery.

What is surprising is that, despite the routine application of septoplasty in clinical practice, the current body of evidence does not support firm conclusions on its effectiveness.

3. Endoscopic Sinus Surgery

Endonasal endoscopic sinus surgery (ESS) is the standard procedure for surgery of most paranasal sinus diseases. Appropriate frame conditions provided, the respective procedures are safe and successful. These prerequisites encompass appropriate technical equipment, anatomical oriented surgical technique, proper patient selection, and individually adapted extent of surgery. The range of endonasal sinus and Skull Base Surgery, operations has dramatically increased during the last 20 years and reaches from partial uncinectomy to pansinus surgery with extended surgery of the frontal (Draf type III), maxillary (grade 3–4, medial maxillectomy, prelacrimal approach) and sphenoid sinus. In addition, there are operations outside and beyond the paranasal sinuses.

The development of surgical technique is still constantly evolving. The concept of functional endoscopic sinus surgery (FESS) is based on the rational that disturbed mucociliary clearance and narrow areas of the ostiomeatal unit can be considered as the origins of recurrent and chronic rhinosinusitis. The concept of conventional FESS that is known and established since many years aims at treating inflammatory diseases of the maxillary and frontal sinus and the anterior ethmoid by resecting anatomical and/or inflammatory disturbing factors in the ostiomeatal unit and at the same time preserving the marginal mucosa and avoiding an extensive radical intervention.

Today, FESS is the gold standard of surgical therapy of chronic rhinosinusitis. The extent of appropriate surgery, however, is still variable in actual concepts of FESS. Similarly, CRS is a multifactorial and includes many subtypes that can be managed through different approaches. Disturbed ventilation and drainage of the paranasal sinuses due to obstruction of the ostiomeatal unit are certainly important in part of the patients with CRS while others have a diffuse inflammatory process that is predominant and/or other factors contribute to persisting inflammation.

There is no universal classification of sinus operations even if it was desirable, already with regard of quality management. Different classifications have been elaborated, among them especially the classification of frontal sinus drainages (according to Draf) has been widely accepted. Details of such a classification would be: uncinectomy (infundibulotomy), maxillary sinus fenestration/maxillary sinus surgery, anterior ethmoidectomy, posterior ethmoidectomy, sphenoid sinus fenestration/ sphenoid sinus surgery, frontal sinus drainage/frontal sinus surgery type I-III, and pansinus surgery. Only an intervention that includes middle meatal antrostomy, anterior and posterior ethmoidectomy, opening of the sphenoid sinus, and frontal sinus drainage type IIa should be called "pansinus operation."

3.1. FESS and OSAS

Individuals with chronic rhinosinusitis (CRS) are known to experience sleep disruption and sleep-disordered breathing (SDB), including Obstructive Sleep Apnea (OSA). Chronic rhinosinusitis with nasal polyps (CRSwNP), a severe inflammatory status of sinonasal mucosa, may have a role in SDB, but the involvement of CRS in the clinical presentation of OSA is still unclear. The etiology of sleep dysfunction in CRS is multifactorial. Although CRS patients usually experience nasal obstruction, it has been suggested that CRS is associated with the release of proinflammatory cytokines, which may also result in sleep impairment. Sukato et al. conducted a meta-analysis regarding the effect of FESS on obstructive sleep apnoea syndrome (OSAS).They discovered only 7 studies showing that FESS could benefit sleep quality and possibly improve apnoea hypopnea index (AHI), although the results displayed high heterogeneity among studies.

Uz et al., recently found a significant improvement in rhinomanometric nasal resistance, apnea-hypopnea index (AHI), minimal oxygen saturation (SaO2), and quality of life scores following polypectomy in 22 patients with CRSwNP by functional endoscopic sinus surgery. Another study reported an improvement of sleep quality in CRS patients who underwent FESS, except those with severe OSAS; moreover, a preoperative lower AHI has been enlightened as the only significant predictor of post-FESS OSAS outcome.

More research is needed to establish whether or not FESS could improve global sleep problems in CRS patients.

4. Turbinate Hypertrophy Surgery

4.1. Introduction

Inferior turbinate hypertrophy is the most common cause of chronic nasal obstruction. When conservative medical treatment options fail in patients with inferior turbinate hypertrophy, reduction of the inferior turbinate can be performed using surgical techniques.

An ideal procedure for turbinate reduction should be performed with minimal discomfort or adverse reactions and should preserve the physiologic function of the turbinate, such as regulation of humidification and temperature of inspired air. All the current techniques have potential short and long-term complications such as bleeding and atrophic rhinitis. No technique is perfect, and the main goal of turbinate surgery should be the preservation of mucosal surfaces with reduction of submucosal tissue. The variety of surgical techniques available indicates the lack of consensus on the optimal technique.

4.2. Radiofrequency Ablation (RFA)

Radiofrequency tissue reduction is a surgical procedure that uses radiofrequency heating to induce submucosal tissue destruction, leading to the reduction of tissue volume. This energy induces ion agitation within the tissue, which increases the local temperature and causes a thermal lesion that should occur in the deep mucosa without damaging the surface. The healing process secondarily induces fibrosis with wound contraction, leading to tissue volume reduction. Radiofrequency ablation is an efficient, easily applicable technique, which does not lead to serious complications in the treatment of the nasal obstruction caused by inferior turbinate hypertrophy.

A sub-specialization of RFA is the Temperature-controlled radiofrequency inferior turbinate ablation (TCRFA), which uses a feedback system to control thermal injury and achieve precise volumetric heating to induce specific scar formation. However, it requires costly single-use proprietary consumables. Comparable volumetric tissue heating may be achieved for a fraction of the cost by adjusting the power settings on traditional monopolar electrosurgery devices that use low-cost needle tips.

4.3. Laser Treatment

Laser treatments includes:

- CO2 (10,600 nm)
- Diode (805/810/940 nm)
- Argon-ion (488/514 nm)
- KTP (532 nm)
- Nd:YAG (1,064 nm)
- Ho:YAG (2,080 nm)

Laser surgery of inferior turbinates can be performed as an outpatient procedure under local anesthesia. Due to a minimally invasive and controllable coagulation and ablation of soft tissue, almost no complications or bleedings are observed during the operation or postoperatively. Depending on the chosen parameters (power, energy) and the application modalities (contact, non-contact, superficial, interstitial) laser treatment of hyperplastic inferior nasal turbinates achieved comparable or better results than most of the conventional techniques for turbinate surgery like conchotomy, electrocautery, cryotherapy, chemical cauterization, and vidian neurectomy. More invasive (radical) operative methods, such as inferior turbinoplasty, submucous turbinectomy, lateral outfracture, partial and total turbinectomy, seemed to be more effective than laser surgery in the long-term.

4.3.1. Diode Laser

The diode laser (λ = 980 nm) is one of the most safe, minimally invasive, portable and least expensive of the lasers available for turbinate surgery, makes it possible for turbinate reduction to be performed under topical anesthesia within a short period of time with excellent patient acceptance and can be performed on a day care basis under local anesthesia.

The mean operation time is 3 min per turbinate and no nasal packing is necessary. Both subjective and objective evaluations show significant improvement. VAS (Visual Analogic Scale) scores improve, the mean MCA2 (Minimal Cross Area of head of the inferior turbinate and cavernous body of the nasal septum), MCA3, and V2-5 (the volume of the nasal cavity between 2 to 5 cm from the tip of the nosepiece) measured with acoustic rhinometry increase significantly 1 year after surgery. In the first year after surgery, patients report marked improvements in nasal breathing.

In a study of Parida PK at all, patients were followed up at 1 week, 1, 3 and 6 months postoperatively. During each follow up visit, symptoms were analysed (nasal obstruction, rhinorrhoea, sneezing, headache, hyposmia and snoring were reassessed by VAS score). Difference between preoperative and postoperative VAS score was statistically significant. All patients had significant symptomatic improvement which started from 1 week postoperatively and persisted throughout the follow up period.

4.4. Microdebrider-Assisted Inferior Turbinoplasty (MAIT)

Microdebrider-assisted inferior turbinoplasty is a minimally invasive method for reducing inferior turbinate size and maintaining mucosal integrity. It has the advantages of a short healing time, only a mild decrease in mucociliary clearance, only minor postoperative problems, and a good functional outcome.

Microdebrider-assisted partial turbinoplasty is more effective and satisfactory then coblation-assisted partial turbinoplasty in long-term relief of nasal obstruction and reduction in mucosal volume of anterior head of inferior turbinate.

A study demonstrates that all the examined techniques decreased the VAS score for the severity of nasal obstruction statistically significantly. There was no deterioration found in the symptoms of crusting, nasal discharge, and sneezing, nor in mucociliary function in any of the groups. All the three techniques increased the non-decongested total V2-5 cm values and decreased the decongested total V2-5 cm values statistically significantly. The V2-5 cm change (%) values decreased statistically significantly in the RFA, diode laser, and the MAIT groups following the operations, the mean changes being -57 percentage points (pp), -53 pp, and -73 pp respectively.

All three techniques decreased the severity of nasal obstruction significantly in the one-year follow-up. Although submucosal fibrosis seemed to increase, all the techniques increased the anterior nasal cavity volume significantly. Inferior turbinate contractility decreased to the normal level from the preoperative congested state following the surgery with every examined technique.

5. Adenoidectomy

5.1. Introduction

Adenotonsillar hypertrophy is the leading cause for obstructive sleep apnea syndrome (OSAS) in children. Traditional adenoidectomy is performed by the cold curettage technique. This approach was well applied for decades, and was recognized as useful. However, some complications were observed, such as the difficulty in total resection, injuries to the soft tissues of the Eustachian tube orifice, the posterior wall of the epipharynx and the soft palate, and bleeding during and after the operation. In order to improve these problems, new procedures have been developed.

In this section we will focus on adenoid hypertrophy and the state of art of its surgical treatment, which is rapresented by Endoscopic-assisted Coblation Adenoidectomy and Microdebrider-assisted Adenoidectomy.

5.2. Endoscopic-Assisted Coblation Adenoidectomy

Plasma adenoidectomy is performed using the Procise XP Wand system, designed for ablation and dissection of soft tissue, which is malleable to reach the adenoid.

Power level is set to 7-8 for ablation of adenoids, and to 3 for coagulation, depending on surgeon's preference as judged by the adenoid volume. A paediatric nasal endoscope 0° short, 2.7 mm diameter is connected to a video camera for direct visualization of the rhinopharynx.

A McIvory mouth gag is placed with a properly sized paediatric tongue depressor. The superior portion of the rhinopharynx and the opening to the Eustachian tubes is accessed with the Procise XP Wand malleable, double curved.

Using a 0° nasal endoscope, the size of the adenoid is identified and the border to be reached is assessed. The correct double curve of the Procise Wand is chosen such that it is able to reach all the rhinopharynx areas. Foot pedal ablation is activated when the wand is close to the inferior edge of the adenoid, avoiding direct contact. The wand in the rhinopharynx is carefully inserted and removed without injury to uvula or soft palate.

Endoscopic check of all compartments is performed to ensure removal of all adenoid tissue.

The absence of any bleeding or mucosal damage is verified. If necessary, bleeding areas are coagulated with the wand by pressing directly on the bleeder for 2-3 seconds.

The main advantages observed with coblation adenoidectomy, compared with the cold curettage technique are:

- the lack of bleeding (abundant bleeding with cold curettage)
- provides a direct endoscopic view of the adenoid (blind surgery or mirror view with traditional cold curettage)
- the ability to reach all the areas of the rhinopharynx up to the Eustachian tube opening (the cranial part of the rhinopharynx cannot be reached with curettage)
- lower risk of residual adenoid tissue after coblator surgery
- fewer complications (no cutting blade with coblation adenoidectomy)
- adjacent structures such as the tubes, nasal and pharyngeal mucosa are carefully preserved. For this reason, coblation adenoidectomy, as reported by others, is associated with less postoperative neck pain than curette/cautery adenoidectomy.
- it is suitable for patients of all ages, although the decrease of pain intensity and duration is important in paediatric patients
- a reduction in the use of post-operative drug and loss of working days for parents due to faster post- surgical healing (as shown by the days reporting pain, analgesic days, liquid diet days, absent from school days)
- the ability to use a single instrument to ablate and coagulate tissue, with significant improvement of patient recovery compared to cold curettage
- Histological examination of the rhinopharygeal mucosa sections revealed in the coblation group, a fibrosis type healing with a low presence of lymphocytes infiltrating the lamina propria, which is compatible with more stable and definitive control of the adenoid hypertrophy. Recurrence is more likely to occur after traditional cold curette treatment, which is followed by a marked lymphocyticinfiltration.

- Respiratory outcomes after endoscopic coblator adenoidectomy, are within the normal range and stable, with no risk of recurrence or persistence of adenoid tissue. Instead the persistence of adenoid tissue is the main reason for high nasal resistance values in the cold curettage group of patients.

The main disadvantages of an endoscopic technique compared with traditional cold curettage is the need to have a complete set-up for paediatric endoscopy in the operating theatre, the time for preparation and to obtain decongestion of nasal cavity with patties, in addition to a specific learning curve in paediatric endoscopy.

5.3. Microdebrider Assisted Adenoidectomy

The microdebrider is a powered cutting device that precisely removes tissue while avoiding inadvertent mucosal trauma. The term "powered instrumentation" refers to motor-driven tools that deliver continuous suction and cutting. The main benefit of microdebrider adenoidectomy is its ability to provide precise, rapid, and complete removal of the adenoid tissue in a safe manner, without injury to the pharyngobasilar fascia.

The main advantages observed with Microdebrider assisted adenoidectomy, compared with the cold curettage technique are:

- Shorter intra-operative time
- Lack of bleeding
- Complete remotion of adenoids
- Less pain
- Better recovery rates

Though conventional adenoidectomy is a quick and a simple procedure but it is a crude and a blind procedure too. Besides known complications such as injury to eustachian tube orifice and pharyngeal musculature, there is high percentage of residual tissue remaining after this procedure. This residual tissue can lead to a combination of potential problems, including peritubaric obstruction, bacterial reservoirs and hyperplasia of the remnants with the persistence of obstructive symptoms; all these aspects highlight the importance of addressing a complete removal of the adenoid tissue. To overcome the drawbacks of the above mentioned procedure, the need for endoscopic assisted microdebrider adenoidectomy and coblation assisted adenoidectomy came into existence.

Conclusion

Obstructive sleep apnoea (OSA) is established as a spectrum of signs and symptoms arising from obstruction of airflow. One of the common sites of airflow obstruction in patients with OSA is the nasal complex. Effective surgical treatment for obstructive sleep apnea/hypopnea syndrome (OSAHS) must be designed to eliminate collapsible soft tissue in the upper airway without interfering with normal function. OSAHS is often caused by multiple levels of obstruction and therefore requires multilevel treatment. From this point of view, we could say that single level surgery cannot be the only treatment for most of OSAHS patient. Surgical interventions on the nose, tongue and oral cavity must be meant as complementary procedures, each of them with his own "specific weight". Multi-level pre-operative assessment is a well-practice appliable not only to severe conditions but must be a part of standard clinical evaluation of OSAHS patients. Nasal surgery as a stand-alone surgery in OSAS patients is to be meant as pivotal, but not primary, in the armamentarium of OSA's surgery. Nonetheless more studies are needed to understand how and in what measure nasal surgical procedures can be applied to OSAS patients together with other surgical possibilities.

References

Bidaye, R., N. Vaid, and K. Desarda, Comparative analysis of conventional cold curettage versus endoscopic assisted coblation adenoidectomy. *J Laryngol Otol*, 2019. 133(4): p. 294-299.

Bonaparte, J. P. and R. Campbell, A prospective cohort study assessing the clinical utility of the Cottle maneuver in nasal septal surgery. *J Otolaryngol Head Neck Surg*, 2018. 47(1): p. 45.

Cabibi D, Speciale R, Lorusso F. Recurrent ossifying fibroma of the maxillary sinus in an adult patient. *Pathologica* 2013; 105(1):11–14.

Cakli, H., et al., Diode laser treatment of hypertrophic inferior turbinates and evaluation of the results with acoustic rhinometry. *Eur Arch Otorhinolaryngol*, 2012. 269(12): p. 2511-7.

Di Rienzo Businco, L., et al., Paediatric adenoidectomy: endoscopic coblation technique compared to cold curettage. *Acta Otorhinolaryngol Ital*, 2012. 32(2): p. 124-9.

Epstein, L. J., et al., Clinical guideline for the evaluation, management and long-term care of obstructive sleep apnea in adults. *J Clin Sleep Med*, 2009. 5(3): p. 263-76.

Friedman, M., et al., Effect of improved nasal breathing on obstructive sleep apnea. *Otolaryngol Head Neck Surg*, 2000. 122(1): p. 71-4.

Getz, A .E. and P. H. Hwang, Endoscopic septoplasty. *Curr Opin Otolaryngol Head Neck Surg*, 2008. 16(1): p. 26-31.

Haight, J. S. and P. Cole, The site and function of the nasal valve. *Laryngoscope*, 1983. 93(1): p. 49-55.

Harju, T. and J. Numminen, The effect of inferior turbinate surgery on nasal symptoms and inferior turbinate contractility. *Am J Otolaryngol*, 2020. 42(1): p. 102778.

Hong, C. J., et al., Open versus endoscopic septoplasty techniques: A systematic review and meta-analysis. *Am J Rhinol Allergy*, 2016. 30(6): p. 436-442.

Hwang, P. H., et al., Endoscopic septoplasty: indications, technique, and results. *Otolaryngol Head Neck Surg*, 1999. 120(5): p. 678-82.

Ishii, L., et al., Does Nasal Surgery Improve OSA in Patients with Nasal Obstruction and OSA? A Meta-analysis. *Otolaryngol Head Neck Surg*, 2015. 153(3): p. 326-33.

Janda, P., et al., Laser treatment of hyperplastic inferior nasal turbinates: a review. *Lasers Surg Med*, 2001. 28(5): p. 404-13.

Jiang, R. S. and K. L. Liang, The Influence of Functional Endoscopic Sinus Surgery on Sleep Related Outcomes in Patients with Chronic Rhinosinusitis. *Int J Otolaryngol*, 2019. 2019: p. 7951045.

Kshirsagar, R. S., et al., Electrosurgery Turbinate Reduction Revisited: Can Comparable Volumetric Heating be Achieved without Feedback Control? *Lasers Surg Med*, 2020.

Lanza, D. C., D. W. Kennedy, and P. J. Koltai, Applied nasal anatomy & embryology. *Ear Nose Throat J*, 1991. 70(7): p. 416-22.

Lee, J. Y. and J. D. Lee, Comparative study on the long-term effectiveness between coblation- and microdebrider-assisted partial turbinoplasty. *Laryngoscope*, 2006. 116(5): p. 729-34.

Li, H. Y., et al., Critical appraisal and meta-analysis of nasal surgery for obstructive sleep apnea. *Am J Rhinol Allergy*, 2011. 25(1): p. 45-9.

Lo Casto A, Lorusso F, Lombardo F, Speciale R. Secondary septal mucocele diagnosed by MRI and CBCT and treated surgically. *B-ENT.* 2014;10(3):221-225.

Lorenz, K. J. and H. Maier, [Microdebrider-assisted inferior turbinoplasty. Minimally invasive technique for the treatment of nasal airway obstruction caused by enlarged turbinates]. *HNO*, 2013. 61(3): p. 240-9.

Lorusso F, Dispenza F, Modica DM, Gallina S. The Role of Modified Expansion Sphincter Pharyngoplasty in Multilevel Obstructive Sleep Apnea Syndrome Surgery. *Int Arch Otorhinolaryngol.* 2018; 22: p. 432-436.

Lorusso F, Dispenza F, Saraniti C, Sireci F, Modica DM, Gallina S. Sleep disordered breathing: evaluation of dynamic patterns of the upper airways in obese subjects. *Otorinolaringologia* 2014; 64:57–64.

Lorusso F, Verro B, Dispenza F, Gallina S. Respiratory epithelial adenomatoid hamartoma: an unusual case report. *Otorinolaringologia*. 2020; 70:86-90.

Mahato, N. B., D. Regmi, and M. Bista, Diode Laser Reduction of Symptomatic Inferior Turbinate Hypertrophy. *JNMA J Nepal Med Assoc*, 2018. 56(214): p. 958-962.

Mandavia, R., N. Mehta, and V. Veer, Guidelines on the surgical management of sleep disorders: A systematic review. *Laryngoscope*, 2020. 130(4): p. 1070-1084.

Mickelson, S. A., Nasal Surgery for Obstructive Sleep Apnea Syndrome. *Otolaryngol Clin North Am*, 2016. 49(6): p. 1373-1381.

Migueis, D. P., et al., Obstructive sleep apnea in patients with chronic rhinosinusitis with nasal polyps: a cross-sectional study. *Sleep Med*, 2019. 64: p. 43-47.

Modica, D. M., et al., Functional Nasal Surgery and Use of CPAP in OSAS Patients: Our Experience. *Indian J Otolaryngol Head Neck Surg*, 2018. 70(4): p. 559-565.

Most, S. P. and S. F. Rudy, Septoplasty: Basic and Advanced Techniques. *Facial Plast Surg Clin North Am*, 2017. 25(2): p. 161-169.

Moxness, M. H. and S. Nordgard, An observational cohort study of the effects of septoplasty with or without inferior turbinate reduction in patients with obstructive sleep apnea. *BMC Ear Nose Throat Disord*, 2014. 14: p. 11.

Mularczyk, C., D. L. Walner, and K. K. Hamming, Coblation versus microdebrider in pediatric adenoidectomy. *Int J Pediatr Otorhinolaryngol*, 2018. 104: p. 29-31.

Nakata, S., et al., Effects of nasal surgery on sleep quality in obstructive sleep apnea syndrome with nasal obstruction. *Am J Rhinol*, 2008. 22(1): p. 59-63.

Pang, K. P., B. W. Rotenberg, and B. T. Woodson, *Advanced surgical techniques in snoring and obstructive sleep apnea*. 2013: Plural Publishing.

Pang, K. P., et al., Does nasal surgery improve multilevel surgical outcome in obstructive sleep apnea: A multicenter study on 735 patients. *Laryngoscope Investigative Otolaryngology*. n/a(n/a).

Parida, P. K., et al., Diode laser turbinate reduction in the treatment of symptomatic inferior turbinate hypertrophy. *Indian J Otolaryngol Head Neck Surg*, 2013. 65(Suppl 2): p. 350-5.

Samra, S., et al., Surgical Management of Nasal Valve Collapse. *Otolaryngol Clin North Am*, 2018. 51(5): p. 929-944.

San Nicolo, M., et al., Absorbable Implant to Treat Nasal Valve Collapse. *Facial Plast Surg*, 2017. 33(2): p. 233-240.

Shah, J., C. R. Roxbury, and R. Sindwani, Techniques in Septoplasty: Traditional Versus Endoscopic Approaches. *Otolaryngol Clin North Am*, 2018. 51(5): p. 909-917.

Sireci, F., et al., Cerebrospinal Fluid Leak Following Nasal Packing for Epistaxis. *J Craniofac Surg*, 2019. 30(8): p. 2536-2538.

Sireci, F., et al., Nasal packing in sphenopalatine artery bleeding: therapeutic or harmful? *Eur Arch Otorhinolaryngol*, 2017. 274(3): p. 1501-1505.

Stewart, M. G., et al., Outcomes after nasal septoplasty: results from the Nasal Obstruction Septoplasty Effectiveness (NOSE) study. *Otolaryngol Head Neck Surg*, 2004. 130(3): p. 283-90.

Sukato, D. C., et al., Endoscopic Sinus Surgery Improves Sleep Quality in Chronic Rhinosinusitis: A Systematic Review and Meta-analysis. *Otolaryngol Head Neck Surg*, 2018. 158(2): p. 249-256.

Uz, U., et al., The evaluation of pattern and quality of sleep in patients with chronic rhinosinusitis with nasal polyps. *Auris Nasus Larynx*, 2017. 44(6): p. 708-712.

van Egmond, M., et al., Septoplasty versus non-surgical management for nasal obstruction due to a deviated nasal septum in adults: A modelling study of cost-effectiveness. *Clin Otolaryngol*, 2019. 44(1): p. 53-62.

Villwock, J. A. and R. B. Kuppersmith, Diagnostic Algorithm for Evaluating Nasal Airway Obstruction. *Otolaryngol Clin North Am*, 2018. 51(5): p. 867-872.

Wang, M., et al., Effect of nasal and sinus surgery in patients with and without obstructive sleep apnea. *Acta Otolaryngol*, 2019. 139(5): p. 467-472.

Weber, R. K. and W. Hosemann, Comprehensive review on endonasal endoscopic sinus surgery. *GMS Curr Top Otorhinolaryngol Head Neck Surg*, 2015. 14: p. Doc08.

Wu, J., et al., Apnea-hypopnea index decreased significantly after nasal surgery for obstructive sleep apnea: A meta-analysis. *Medicine* (Baltimore), 2017. 96(5): p. e6008.

In: Advances in Sleep Apnea
Editors: F. Lorusso et al.
ISBN: 978-1-53619-758-7

Chapter 12

Advances in the Role of Pharyngeal Surgery in the Treatment of OSAS

Angelo Immordino, Salvatore Gallina, Federico Sireci and Francesco Lorusso*
Department of Otolaryngology, Head and Neck Surgery, Policlinico Paolo Giaccone University of Palermo, Palermo, Italy

Abstract

The American Academy of Sleep Medicine and the American Academy of Otolaryngology–Head and Neck Surgery recommend surgery as an option for the treatment of OSAS, when non-invasive treatments such as CPAP or oral appliances have not been successful or are not tolerated.

A gradual and logical approach must be taken into account when a patient seeks a surgical solution, and it is a fundamental requirement that the patient find a surgeon who understands both the pathophysiology of sleep apnea and anatomy of the upper airways (UA) to guarantee the best chances of success.

The surgical options aim to solve the obstructive problem according to two ways, the first is the reduction of the content, and then acts through the volumetric reduction of soft tissues at the

* Corresponding Author's Email: dott.francescolorusso@gmail.com.

level of UA, most often at the level of palate, uvula, tonsils, adenoids and tongue. The second option aims at enlarging the container, and therefore on more complex interventions to adapt the bony structures of the skull.

The soft palate in the snore-surgery is the anatomical site on which most of the attention has always been concentrated since it is responsible for most of the phenomena of snoring and most of the obstructive ones and has undergone the greatest innovations.

The rationale for palatal surgery is to reduce volume and stiffen a structure that vibrating with the passage of air causes snoring and collapsing causes an obstruction of the UA.

In general, interventions on the palate can be broadly divided into two groups, the first is represented by interventions that have the aim of reduce snoring, and in this case are less invasive surgeries, as the goal is that of stiffening the palate and reducing the excess mucosa that vibrating causes snoring.

The second group consists of interventions that have the aim of reducing above the snoring especially the apnoic episodes, so they are interventions that have a greater invasiveness, since they must stiffen and reconstitute the functionality of a segment of the UA.

INTRODUCTION

Oropharyngeal surgery is the richest chapter of snoring and OSAS surgery. In fact, the oropharynx represents the topographical passage region from the nasal to the oral tract of the upper airways and is characterized by a considerable amount of soft tissues which make this area subject to both vibratory and obstructive phenomena.

Some studies have highlighted a particular correlation between obesity and greater susceptibility to the development of OSAS: the almost constant presence of anatomical and functional alterations of the oropharyngeal district in this particular population would make it more susceptible to the development of obstructive phenomena with a greater involvement of the male sex.

The objectives of the snoring and OSAS surgery at this level are therefore the stabilization of these structures by reduction or complete ablation of the tissues responsible for the obstruction from which the phenomena of RERA, hypopneas and apneas derive, and the reduction of snoring. If in the past the surgeons tended to apply more demolitive surgical techniques, today the goals can be achieved through more conservative techniques such as the remodeling of the velo-uvular unit with conservation of both the soft palate and the uvula, the posterior palate space expansion and the stiffening, anteriorization and stabilization of the soft palate. The ablation or volumetric reduction of the palatine tonsils still remain, however, often essential steps in most cases.

Tonsil Surgery

Child's Tonsillar Ronco-Surgery

Tonsillar hypertrophy is the main cause of OSAS and snoring in the pediatric population. The age of less than three years, neurological and maxillofacial comorbidity are to be assessed with care and caution for an increased post-operative risk and for a greater share of failures. The opportunity for post-operative monitoring in pediatric intensive care units should be considered in this group of patients.

Tonsillotomy or Tonsillar Volumetric Reduction

Tonsillotomy consists in reducing the volume of the tonsils, with preservation of their capsule, which can be performed with various instruments such as coblator, microdebrider, radiofrequency. This technique appears to be burdened with a lower risk of post-operative bleeding. But it presents the risk of recurrence of hypertrophy.

Tonsillectomy

Tonsillectomy consists in the complete removal of the tonsil with its capsule, it can be performed with cold techniques or with hot techniques. These latter techniques are burdened from a slightly higher risk of post-operative late hemorrhage 2-4%, compared to 1-2% of cold techniques.

The almost total disappearance of night snoring after adenotonsillectomy in children is widely known, but there are only a few studies to prove it.

The work of Hultcranz et al. Is interesting in this regard that in a randomized study compared the effectiveness on tonsillectomy and tonsillotomy snoring after one year, showing a 9.5% recurrence of snoring in the group of patients undergoing tonsillotomy, suggesting a possible relapse hypertrophy. Adenotonsillectomy is considered the first line treatment in the treatment of pediatric OSAS.

Brietzke in his meta-analysis has shown how obesity is a fundamental factor in the determinism of the presence of post-surgical OSAS residue. Finding an AHI > 5 sleep events/hour in 59% of obese children subjected to adenotonsillectomy. And highlighting as predisposing factors in the maintenance of a post-operative high AHI age > 7 aa, the presence of asthma and a severe preoperative OSAS, in all these cases the child must undergo post-operative polysomnography, to evaluate the possible presence of residual OSAS.

In an attempt to reduce post-operative pain, various devices have been developed, which in most cases aim to achieve the simplicity of a tonsillectomy with hot instruments while maintaining contained temperatures of use. From this point of view we conducted a comparative study between tonsillectomy for cold dissection and tonsillectomy with Molecular Quantum Resonance, results showed a saving in surgical time and a significant reduction in intra-operative bleeding, although not having significant results with regard to post-operative pain that was substantially overlapping.

Adult's Tonsillar Surgery

The hypertrophic palatine tonsil is a significant obstacle at the VAS level, easily eliminated with relatively rudimentary surgery, but usually this is not sufficient to completely solve the snoring and OSAS problem. As evidenced by Tzifa and coll. tonsillectomy in children does not reduce the risk of becoming snoring adults. Rarely in the surgical treatment of snoring and OSAS is it limited only to tonsillectomy, but when this procedure is performed within a multisite procedure the contribution of tonsillar time to overall success appears to be relevant. This is also due to the fact that an important tonsillar hypertrophy is rare in the adult subject, but when this happens the tonsillectomy has a success rate similar to that of the pediatric age.

Tonsillar Volumetric Reduction Radio-Frequencies

The principle consists in the submucosal application of low frequency radio waves. It is used as an interstitial treatment, with an electrode that is inserted into the soft tissue of the tonsil creating a thermal lesion that causes necrosis and is followed by successive cicarizial processes. As a consequence, the soft tissue shrinks and stiffens.

Palatal Surgery

The first plastic coded intervention of the soft palate was described for the first time by Ikematsu in 1963, since then numerous interventions have been proposed that aim to reduce the excess components of the soft palate tissue, without compromising the swallowing and phonatory functions. The palatoglossus muscle (anterior palatal pillar) contains within it neuro-muscular spindles, playing an important role in swallowing and therefore must be preserved together with the muscle of the uvula. While the glossopharyngeal muscle (posterior palatal pillar) has no neuro-muscular spindles, therefore, it can be partially dissected without hindering swallowing or the possibility of a future nasal ventilatory therapy (nCPAP). In fact, an excessive resection of the palatal musculature creates serious difficulties in the application of nCPAP due to oral venting. A fundamental prerequisite of palatal surgery is the implementation of techniques that make it possible to maintain CPAP in any case as a therapeutic alternative in the event of failure. Indications and contraindications are similar for all palatal interventions to reduce apnea.

Indications for palatal surgery

- Hypertrophic and elongated uvula (dolico-mega-uvula)
- Palatine Ptosis
- Thick palate
- Tonsillar hypertrophy

- Restricted oropharyngeal isthmus
- Plication of the pharyngeal walls
- BMI <30
- AHI <20 or simple snoring

Contraindications to treatment with palatal surgery

- Obesity: exclusive palatal intervention with BMI > 30 is contraindicated
- severe OSAS, AHI > 30 also 20 according to some authors
- Retrognathia or micrognathia (usually lingual back obstruction)
- Severe occlusal or temporomandibular joint dysfunction (oral opening <3 cm)
- High distance between the hyoid and lower edge of the jaw

Relative contraindications of palatal surgery

- Professional use of the voice
- Wind instrument players
- Scuba diving activities (possible problems of tubal compensation)
- Professional use of taste

Absolute contraindications of palatal surgery

- Cleft palate
- Short palate
- Insufficient oral opening, interdental distance <3 cm (small operating field)
- Severe chronic cardiac or pulmonary disorders
- Severe neurological or psychiatric disorders requiring pharmacological treatment
- High anesthetic risk
- Alcoholism
- Sedative abuse
- Skull facial anomalies

Is possible to classify the oropharyngeal district surgery into tissue ablation techniques, now almost abandoned, non-ablative tissue reduction techniques, circular resection techniques, parasagittal section techniques, segmental resection techniques and flaps, stiffening techniques, lateral widening techniques and front suspension techniques. It is also possible to classify the surgical procedures into minor procedures and major procedures: the former can also be performed under local anesthesia, the latter require narcosis. The minor procedures are usually, but not always, aimed at the treatment of snoring, while the latter are more frequently used for the treatment of obstructive sleep apnea.

Uvulectomy and Single-Stage Snare Dissection Uvulopalatoplasty (SUPP)

In the history of snoring and OSAS surgery uvuloplasty have played an important role. However, few results have been reported in the literature regarding uvulectomy and Single-stage snare dissection uvulopalatoplasty (SUPP) as exclusive surgical strategies. The uvulectomy is quick, easy to perform and low cost procedure and involves the removal or shortening of the uvula both by traditional cutting technique and by CO_2 laser technique. SUPP, on the other hand, is performed with a snare-wire loop for tonsil and allows the section of the uvular base with a small portion of the soft palate.

In literature there are no reported complications such as swallowing difficulties or post-surgical velo-pharyngeal dysfunctions, probably this is due to the fact that the loop of the snare-wire, during its closing phase, follows the lower margins of the tensor and levator muscles of palatine veil, minimizing their damages. However, it was noted that patients undergoing uvuloplasty with snoring of velar origin develop a snoring of non-velar origin, therefore these surgical practices are currently not recommended.

Punctate Diathermy

Palatal flutter is a recognized source of noise production in people who snore, and many authors have postulated that this can be reduced by stiffening the soft palate. In 1995 Whinney and coll. suggested a procedure, carried out under general anaesthesia, consisting in diathermocoagulation of the palatal muscles by infixion. This technique provides Ten to 15 penetrations of the palatal muscles trough the mucosa to achieve a stiffening of the soft palate. This procedure, used in the past for the treatment of simple snoring, was almost abandoned as it was considered an excessively painful practice.

Radiofrequency Volume Reduction Snoreplasty (RFVR)

The introduction of radiofrequency technology has made it possible to reduce thermal damage due to diathermocoagulation and thereby also reduce post-operative pain. The use of RF, a minimally invasive technique that can also be performed under local anesthesia, requires the use of a needle probe that is fixed in the median and paramedian palatal area in order to determine, by means of radiofrequencies, the coagulative necrosis of proteins and subsequent scarring with consequent retraction of soft tissues.

This procedure, performed in a single session or in multiple sessions, can be performed just in the median or in both the median and paramedian areas of the soft palate, we will speak respectively of "single lesion" and "multiple lesion" protocol. The most frequent complications are represented by erosion and ulceration of the lining mucosa. Although these phenomena cause greater post-operative pain, they usually do not affect the final result of the treatment when they affect the ventral aspect of the soft palate. On the other hand, excessively deep lesions should be avoided as, by causing damage to the mucosa of the dorsal aspect of the palate, they can cause an alteration of the healing dynamics.

As for the results, several scientific studies have found an efficacy of the palatal RFVR of over 80%, with better results for the "multiple lesion" protocol. The application of the palatal RFVR can therefore be considered an excellent therapeutic alternative in patients suffering from snoring of palatal origin but it can also be effective in mild OSAS, both as a single technique and in combination in a multilevel protocol. On the other hand, this technology is excessively expensive as it requires multiple interventions, radio frequency generators and expensive disposable handpieces.

Injection Snoreplasty

Injection snoreplasty was introduced for the first time in 2001 by Brietzke and coll. It exploits a mechanism similar to RFVR but, unlike this, it does not generate coagulative necrosis to induce a scar retraction but rather the sclerotic capacity of some substances injected at the level of the submucosal layer of the soft palate to induce the formation of retracting scars. These substances are mainly represented by sodium tetradecyl sulfate (STS) at 1 or 3% and by ethanol at 50%. STS is a fairly safe and widely used preparation for the treatment of varicose veins. The injection of the preparation, diluted to 1 or 3%, at the level of the soft palate induces the development of an aseptic inflammation capable of determining a scar which, by stiffening the soft palate, makes the tissues of this region less susceptible to vibrations. base of the uvula and two injections at the paramedian level. With a similar method, according to some studies, treatment with 50% ethanol would cause a similar sclerotic effect but with a higher incidence of transient palatal fistula which, however, would tend to self-repair. Injection snoreplasty is therefore a safe, simple and minimally invasive outpatient procedure that can cause only mild post-operative pain. It is useful for simple snoring and can also find application in mild forms of obstructive sleep apnea and residual snoring in patients already surgically treated for palatal moderate-severe OSAS.

Pillar® Palatal Implants

It consists in the insertion, inside the soft palate, of three millimeter polyester cylinders of 18mm in length and 2mm in diameter. The cylinders are applied under local anesthesia, thanks to a special applicator, at the junction between the soft and hard palate, in a parallel way, stimulating a fibrotic reaction that creates a capsule around the implant with the aim of stiffening the soft palate by reducing the vibration. In a meta-analysis carried out in 2013 by Choi and coll. it was found that the use of Pillar implants significantly reduces snoring, in fact, according to the visual-analogue scale (VAS) of snoring sound loudness, the VAS significantly improved in all 7 studies taken into consideration. However, this meta-analysis showed that in cases of coexistence of a sleep respiratory disorder this tended to persist. The most frequent complication is represented by the extrusion of the implant: once extruded it must be removed and replaced with a new one next to the previous one. Due to the poor clinical results found and the rare, but still detected episodes of implant expulsion with a percentage from 0 to 25%, this method is rarely applied to date.

Velo-Uvulo-Pharyngeal Lift (VUPL)

In 2008 Hur proposed a technique based on the stiffening of the soft palate through the trans-mucosal introduction of non-absorbable sutures at the level of the fibro-muscular plane of the palate. This study obtained poor results on OSAS, but highlighted the perfect tolerability of these sutures, already widely used in plastic surgery, at the palatal level, allowing to obtain the desired changes at the soft tissue level.

In 2012 Mantovani and coll. developed a new surgical technique of VUPL called "Roman blinds" which, in addition to raising and stiffening the palate, allows to widen the oropharyngeal space: this is possible through the use of anchored non-absorbable 2-0 sutures. to the posterior nasal spine and the 2 pterogoidal hamuls through three small incisions. The first suture (Mersilene, Ethicon Inc., Somerville, New Jersey, USA) is anchored laterally to the posterior nasal spine by means of a muco-periosteal incision through the fibromuscular layer of the soft palate and, by means of several passages in -and-out transmucosal according to a semicircular trajectory, it is made to come out homolaterally at the base of the uvula, the needle is then inserted horizontally through the uvular muscle and made to come out contralaterally to then reach the posterior nasal spine again. Similarly, the same procedure is performed bilaterally between the pterygoid hamulus and the postero-superior portion of the posterior palatine pillar. The three threads are finally firmly knotted, inserted in the context of the submucosal tissue and the mucosa is sutured. Patients undergoing this procedure reported a marked improvement in clinical symptoms in terms of ESS (Epworth sleepiness scale), SSS (Snoring scale score) and LAS (Linear analogue scale). During the postoperative period, oropharyngeal pain, odynophagia, and oropharyngeal foreign body sensation may occur. Compared to traditional ablative techniques, VUPL can be considered conservative and minimally invasive by carrying out a selective action on the palate-pharyngeal mucosa, on fibrous tissues and muscles. Subsequently, the technique was further refined with the use of "barbed" sutures (QUill ® Knotless Tissue Closure Device, Angiotech Pharmaceutical inc., Vancouver, CA) which do not require knots as they are self-locking and allow to obtain new geometries of suture.

Laser-Assisted Uvulo-Palatoplasty (LAUP), Cautery-Assisted Uvulo-Palatoplasty (CAUP) and Cold-Steel Uvulo-Palatoplasty (CUP)

In 1990 Kamami developed a procedure under local anesthesia called LAUP. This technique in the 90s due to its simplicity of application has quickly taken off in Europe and the USA, with the appearance of innumerable variants. The technique involves two paramedian incisions of the palate, at full thickness, from both sides of the uvula with a height of 1-2 cm. and a total or partial uvulectomy. Incision is performed with a CO_2 laser or, less frequently, with a diode or Yag laser.

Section of the soft palate is performed in several successive sessions gradually widening the incision lines.

The technique is certainly simple, quick and effective in the presence of a not excessively thick palate and a not excessively hypertrophic uvula. Moreover, the gradualness of the multistep approach reduces the risk of permanent velar insufficiency and allows to monitor clinical progress.

On the other hand, it is necessary to consider the high cost of using the CO_2 laser, the high incidence of post-operative paraesthesia and the high post-operative pain due to the presence of an exposed and unsutured incision. Multiplying everything by the 3-5 sessions on average required, it is possible to understand why about 20% of patients who undergo this treatment decide, already from the first sessions, to abandon the therapeutic path. With the aim of improving outcomes, reducing costs and post-operative pain, alternative techniques have been developed over the decades. The so-called "modified LAUP" exploit the use of variable incision geometries, the use of sutures and the combination with a submucosal debulking. Other variants could be performed in single session under general anesthesia as proposed by Dickson and Mintz.

Therefore, due to poor results and frequent side effects from the early 2000s LAUP is not recommended as surgical procedures. In 2001, the Standards of Practice Committee of the American Academy of Sleep Medicine issued some guidelines regarding the LAUP advising against its use.

Cautery-Assisted Uvulo-Palatoplasty represents a variant of the LAUP but, unlike this, it exploits the use of an electrocautery. Large databases on clinical results are not available but, unlike the LAUP, it would appear to be burdened by significant edema and greater postoperative pain.

Cold-steel Uvulo-Palatoplasty represents a further variant of the LAUP technique. This technique exploits the use of a retrograde bite forceps similar to that used in nasal-sinus endoscopic surgery. Patient preparation and anesthesia are similar to the methods described for the LAUP and CAUP procedure. Vertical cuts lateral to the uvula bilaterally are made with a back-biting endoscopic through-cut forceps, uvula is grasped with a forceps and is reshaped to a smaller size or is completely removed. Despite the CUP technique seems to be a safe and effective in treatment for snoring and mild obstructive sleep apnea, literature is poor in convincing results. As in the LAUP, CAUP and CUP are not recommended as surgical procedures.

Microdebrider-Assisted Uvulo-Palatoplasty (MAUPP)

Microdebrider is an instrument commonly used in sinus surgery that at the turn of the 1990s and 2000s it also found useful use in the treatment of snoring. MAUPP is performed under local anesthesia in fact wide infiltration of the surgical field is an essential step in vasoconstricting the vessels and preventing arterial bleeding. The uvula is resected first, then the lateral part of the palate is trimmed. The main complications of this procedure are represented by postoperative pain, intra and postoperative bleeding. Postoperative management includes pain control and patient reassurance. MAUPP compared to LAUP requires lower costs and shorter training however, both for the few clinical cases described in the literature and for the greater tendency to use non-ablative techniques, this method has now been almost abandoned.

Cautery-Assisted Palatal Stiffening Operation (CAPSO)

Cautery-Assisted Palatal Stiffening Operation (CAPSO) is a mucosal surgery that induces a midline scar on the oral surface of the soft palate with a vector tightening the palate and directed away from the nasopharynx, therefore not narrowing the nasopharyngeal aperture. It can be performed under local anesthesia. Topical anesthesia begins with oral spray followed by a 5 mL of 2% lidocaine with 1:100,000 units of epinephrine injection performed submucosally in the midline soft palate extending 1 cm laterally on each side. A sheathed needle tip cautery maps out an inverted U on the soft palate. A 2-cm strip of midline soft palate mucosa is removed in an anterior-to-posterior direction, exposing the palatopharyngeus and muscularis uvulae muscles. The midline nasal surface of the uvular mucosa is cauterized to enhance the stiffening effect. The wound is allowed to heal by secondary intention. Postoperative complications included pain, bleeding and temporary velopharyngeal incompetence. By postoperative week 2 or 3, the palate is stiffened, and snoring is either eliminated or greatly reduced with no voluntary palatal flutter. By 4 weeks postoperatively, the palate appears healed and stiffened. CAPSO success rate for snoring relief at 92% initially and then falling to 77% at 1 year, therefore its results make it an excellent surgical alternative in patients suffering from snoring or mild OSAS.

Uvulo-Palatopharingoplasty (UPPP)

This ablative technique was first described by Ikematsu in 1963, since then numerous variants have been proposed, as long as UPPP is to be considered as a group of procedures united by a circular myomucosal resection of the soft palate including a more or less variable portion of its free margin, resection of the uvula and palatine tonsils. The procedure is done under general anesthesia, supplemented by local infiltration. Tonsillectomy is performed, if not previously done, taking care not to damage the palatine pillars. Then incision lines are marked at the level of the anterior wall of the soft palate lateral to the glossopalatal arch from the inferior pole of the tonsillar fossa toward the root of the uvula. Subsequently the incision line is marked at the level of the posterior wall of the soft palate by overturning the uvula and traction cranially the palate. The mucosae of the soft palate, tonsillar fossa, and the lateral aspect of the uvula are undermined and elevated by sharp and blunt dissection and removed, including the submucosal tissues, so that the underlying muscular layer is preserved. The rim of the posterior pillar mucosa is then adequately trimmed and lifted upward and laterally. The mucosal edges are then approximated between the corresponding portions of the palatal arches and saturated with absorbable sutures with only moderate tension. This brings the palatal arch forward, resulting in a significant increase in the anteroposterior dimension of the oropharyngeal space. Finally, if a redundant posterior pharyngeal wall mucosa is detected, an additional excision of the posterior pharyngeal mucosa may be necessary and the remaining mucosa can be stretched laterally and sutured. In the late 1980's Carenfelt introduced the Laser Uvulo-Palatopharyngoplasty (LUPP), it was similar to classical UPPP under general anesthesia, but used the CO_2 laser for incisions.

The classic UPPP of Ikematsu and Fujita and its numerous technical variants less invasive introduced during the 90s, are today not more viable due to the low success rate and high rate of complications of this procedure such as sensation of a pharyngeal foreign body, feeling of pharyngeal dryness, palatine veil incompetence with nasal regurgitation, rhinooropharyngeal stenosis and high flow losses in patients with N-CPAP. In our experience uvulopalatopharyngoplasty associated with tonsillectomy made it possible to achive a complete therapeutic response in 78% of patients, however four patients had relief of symptoms but retained apnea/hypopnea index scores greater than 5. A meta-analysis on UPPP-treated patients performed by Sher and coll. revealed that only 41% achieved surgical success defined by a 50% reduction in AHI or an AHI below 20 postoperatively. Other studies in the literature also highlight the possibility of worsening of apnea-hypopnea indices after UPPP. Hassid and coll. have recently described a decrease in success rates with increasing follow-up periods therefore a polysomnographic follow-up is recommended after 1-3 years. From the data it is clear that the effectiveness of UPPP decreases over the years.

Uvulo-Palatal Flaps (UPF)

The uvulo-palatal flap, introduced by Powell and coll. in 1996, is a technique that basically consists of suturing the uvula to the anterior wall of the soft palate. Anesthetic with a vasoconstrictor is injected in the ventral surface of the soft palate and uvula, then the uvula is grasped and reflected back toward the soft-hard palate junction, the opening into the nasopharynx is examined and the uvula retracted sufficiently to allow this reflection to reveal a crease between the mucosa of the palatal edge and corresponding muscle. If further advancement is desired, relaxing incisions are made at the lateral aspect to provide greater anterior release of the UPF and increase the retro-palatal area. The ventral mucosa is then removed and a portion of the tip of the uvula is amputated to remove the excess mucosa. The palate is folded on itself, and the mucosa of the dorsal palate and uvula is sutured into position. The procedure can be done as an outpatient or under general anesthesia and the operation could be preceded by tonsillectomy. Palatal flaps are generally an interesting alternative to UPPP and are indicated for primary snoring and mild to moderate OSAS. In comparison to UPPP this procedure is potentially reversible if velopharyngeal insufficiency occurs and, because muscular tissue is not removed, the normal physiologic mobility of the palate is maintained and the likelihood of scar contracture and subsequent nasopharyngeal stenosis is decreased. An important additional benefit is a decrease in postoperative pain because there is no disruption of muscle tissue or presence of denuded surfaces. An extended uvulo-palatal flap (EUPF) was described by Li et al. and included the previous procedure but used dissection and removal of submucosal adipose tissue of the soft palate and supratonsillar area. The indications to the UPF represent the only real limit of this procedure compared to the UPPP: the rigorous selection of cases in relation to the palatal conformation allows its application only in cases of regular or thin palates with elongated but not hypertrophic uvula. There are few data in the literature regarding the treatment of snoring, while there is some study about the treatment of OSAS. From the limited data available is possible to assume that UPF and UPPP have comparable results in the treatment of mild OSAS when performed as a single step surgery, or in the treatment of moderate to severe OSAS when multilevel surgery is performed.

Anterior Pharingoplasty (AP)

It consists of a technique of palatal tightening introduced for the first time by Pang and coll. in 2008, indicated in the treatment of snoring and mild-moderate OSAS associated with tonsillectomy. Pang performed the procedure under local anesthesia if it was not associated with tonsillectomy in the case of absent or small tonsils (grade 0-2) or in general anesthesia when associated with tonsillectomy (grade 3-4 tonsils).

The technique consists in practicing a partial uvulectomy, removing only the mucosa. Followed by the removal of a rectangle of anterior mucosa of the palate about 40-50 mm long and 7-10 mm high, until the underlying musculature is uncovered. And then after haemostasis, the two upper and lower flaps are gathered together with absorbable sutures anchored at full thickness in the musculature of the palate, creating an elevation and anteriorization of the palate. The indications to perform an anterior pharyngoplasty are simple snoring, AHI <20 and BMI <32, clinical evidence of velopalatal hypertrophy, elongation of the soft palate and anteroposterior retropalatal collapse at the Mueller maneuver. Pang reported no major complications and showed improvement in snoring and sleepiness using VAS and ESS: all patients had improvement in their snoring, and the patients and their sleep partners were satisfied with the result at a mean of more than 30 months postoperatively.

Lateral Pharingoplasty (LP)

It is the first technique to pay significant attention to the role of the lateral wall of the pharynx in the determinism of the OSAS. Developed by Cahali in 2003 it has as a fundamental premise the stiffening of the lateral wall of the pharynx. Cahali in the indications inserted the presence of at least two of the following characteristics: lateral peritonsillar narrowing (defined as the size of peritonsillar tissues greater than 25% of the pharyngeal space, calculated as the internal distance of the mandible measured in the middle of the tonsillar fossa); tonsillar hypertrophy (defined as lateral bulkiness of the tonsils greater than 50% of the distance between the posterior tonsillar pillars); ptosic soft palate (which does not allow visualization of the posterior pharyngeal wall). In addition to these assumptions, the subjects had to present a narrowing or collapse in the retropalatal region without narrowing in the hypopharynx, both at rest and during the Müller maneuver. The first step of the surgical procedure is tonsillectomy with identification of the palatoglossus and palatofaingeo muscle. Then they identify and raise the fibers of the upper constrictor muscle of the pharynx at the level of the tonsillar fossa, as far as possible from the glossopharyngeal. Once detached from the lateropharyngeal space, the upper pharynx constrictor is sectioned in a cranio-caudal direction obtaining two muscular flaps. The medial flap is left in situ, while the lateral flap is sutured anterior to the palatoglossus muscle. Then a Z-plastic is made between the mucosa of the anterior aspect of the soft palate and the upper portion of the palate-pharyngeal muscle, covering the upper part of the tonsillar fossa, while the lower part of the loggia is closed by suturing the remaining part of the pharyngeal palate muscle to the anterior pillar. With the suspension to the palatoglossus muscle Cahali tries to give support to the oropharynx and the tongue. While with the Z plastic, he tries to orient the scar retraction laterally.

The technique has several side effects such as persistent pain, reflux of fluids from the nose. But the main complication due to the section of the upper pharyngeal constrictor is lasting dysphagia especially for solids.

Relocation Pharingoplasty (RP)

This technique introduced in 2009 by Li and coll. based on the increase in the volume of the pharyngeal vestibule acting on the lateral walls of the pharynx, with a technique similar to that of Cahali. After tonsillectomy with careful conservation of the mucosa of the palatine pillars. The pharyngeal palate muscle is taken near the uvula and rotated upwards and sideways making it approach the remaining part of the soft palate. The full-thickness tissue of two elliptical zones at the level of the soft palate is removed, including mucosa, submucosa, adipose tissue and muscle. The upper pharyngeal constrictor is sutured to the homolateral palatoglossus muscle with a cranio-caudal direction. The palatal-pharyngeal muscle is separated from the upper constrictor of the pharynx to facilitate tension-free approximation. The pharyngeal palate muscle with its mucous flap is then anteriorized and also sutured on the palatoglossus muscle. Finally, a partial uvulectomy is planned.

With this technique a single, rigid and anterior newly formed palatine is created, which puts the lateral walls of the pharynx in tension and increases the posterior space because the advancement of the posterior pillar also brings with it the dorsal portion of the palate.

The results show a significant reduction in snoring of daytime sleepiness and AHI. No post-operative bleeding, reflux of liquids from the nose or alterations of the voice were found.

This technique, unlike that of Cahali, does not involve a dissection of the upper pharyngeal constrictor with consequent opening of the lateropharyngeal space and the risk of damaging the important neurovascular structures contained in it.

Expansion Sphincter Pharingoplasty (ESP)

Even ESP is based on the fundamental concept that at pharyngeal level the obstruction linked to the collapse of the lateral walls of the pharynx plays a fundamental role. This technique was developed by Pang and Woodson in 2007 and it could be considered more effective and less invasive than lateral pharyngoplasty. The main indications are: predominantly lateral pharyngeal collapse, wide and thick posterior pillars and thick soft palate. It has specific contraindications, in addition to the general ones for palatal surgery, in the event of absence of lateral pharyngeal collapse, tonsillary pillars fused together, very thin soft palate and scar palate.

The first step of the surgery consists in bilateral tonsillectomy with identification of the palato-glosso and palato-pharyngeal muscle and preservation of the covering mucosa. The palato-pharyngeal muscle is then isolated from the surrounding tissues, preserving the fibers of the upper pharyngeal constrictor. At this point, two ligatures are placed at the level of the distal margin of the muscle, to keep the muscle fibers together and to ensure better hemostasis, since the muscle is sectioned downwards creating a superior hinged muscle flap, in part connected to the upper constrictor of the pharynx. At this point, the original technique involves an incision of the palato-glossus muscle fibers at the palatine arch plane and the suture of the distal portion of the flap at this level, and the subsequent suturing of the superficial mucous planes. In our experience this passage was modified by creating a tunnel with a klemmer forceps in the context of the soft palate with a 45° angle in the direction of the pterigoid hamulus, tipping the muscular flap inside the tunnel and fixing it with two resorbable stitches in position, obtaining an antero-lateral palate stretching. At this point the palatine pillars are joined with a resorbable suture. A partial uvulectomy is performed depending on the laxity of the uvular mucosa. Pang et al. do not report complications such as reflux of fluids from the nose or palatal insufficiency, palatal fistulas or oral infections. The key points of the surgery are: the increased space at the transverse level at the level of the pharynx both for the removal of the tonsils and for the dislocation of the palato-pharyngeal muscle, the incomplete isolation of the palato-pharyngeal muscle from the upper pharyngeal constrictor thanks to which it creates sufficient tension on the side walls. ESP also tends to widen further, in the anterolateral sense, the space at the level of the oropharyngeal vestibule during the healing phases, since the cicatricial retraction of the palate-pharyngeal muscle flap stretches the palate and the lateral walls of the pharynx even more in this sense by creating centrifugal healing vectors. Contrary to UPPP where the healing vectors were centripetal with a progressive worsening of the results obtained.

Pang et al. showed a significant improvement in AHI compared to UPPP, with a percentage of surgical success according to the Sher criteria of 82.6% for ESP against 68.1% for UPPP, with a significant difference in oropharyngeal transverse diameters post-operative where after ESP the residual transverse collapse with Muller maneuver was modest, while after UPPP it was still very evident.

In our experience ESP has proved to be an effective weapon in the management of palatal obstruction. In patients subjected exclusively to ESP due to the presence of a predominantly palatal obstructive site, an improvement in AHI was obtained, which on average was reduced by 63.4% with a success rate according to the Sher criteria of 65%. We have also shown in all patients subjected to ESP a notable improvement as regards the anatomical parameters at the oropharyngeal level. In fact, a notable dilatation of the transverse diameters and a progression of the palate considerably higher than the

UPPP, with a reduction of the oropharyngeal collapse to the Müller maneuver equal to 64.7%.

Sorrenti and Piccin suggested a Functional Expansion Pharyngoplasty for the treatment of lateral pharyngeal wall collapse. With this technique physiological correction can be obtained by taking advantage of the anatomical characteristics of the palatal pharyngeal muscle. But, similarly to the ESP, the technique requires dissection and relocation of mucosa-deprived muscles that are not devoid of mucosal tear and muscle trauma, weakness and/or fibrosis.

Barbed Reposition Pharyngoplasty (BRP)

This new technique developed by Vicini and coll., arises from the idea of using self-locking wires applied to a technique similar to relocation faringoplasty. It is based on the principle that the palatine pillars and the palate are considered as a tripod and weakening the posterior palatine pillar and moving it forward tends to unbalance the whole system forward increasing the mesopharynx space. The first step consists in tonsillectomy with careful preservation of the mucosa of the anterior and posterior pillars, therefore the lower portion of the palate-pharyngeal muscle is partially incised weakening it. Then a full-thickness mucosa and muscle triangle is removed at the upper lateral edge of the tonsillar loggia to obtain a wider and more squared space at the level of the pharyngeal vestibule. The needle is then introduced at the level of the posterior palatal spine, made to pass completely through the palate in a lateral direction, then around the pterigo-mandibular raphe and is taken out of the bed of the tonsillectomy and then passed through the upper part of the palate muscle pharyngeal making it come out near the mucosa of the posterior pillar, but not crossing it. Then the needle is passed again through the palatopharyngeal muscle and through the raphe by suspending the posterior pillar. By allowing the posterior pillar to be positioned in a more lateral and anterior position, this passage is repeated several times up to the most distal part of the palate-pharyngeal muscle and therefore the thread is passed through the soft palate blocking it.

This technique is currently the most used in our group with excellent results both for snoring and apnea. The only side effect was the pain and the sense of foreign body, which is reduced within a couple of weeks.

Vicini and coll. reported a success rate of 90% for BRP for patients with all grades of AHI, however, in a multicentre prospective study performed with 111 patients, Montevecchi and coll. reported that the success rate was 73% in a group of patients with a mean AHI of 33.4.

Despite the numerous techniques proposed for the treatment of retropalatal collapse there is a limited number of studies evaluating the success of recent techniques in the literature, and even less are the studies that comparing the results of Expansion Sphincter Pharyngoplasty and Barbed Pharyngoplasty. In our experience, in both techniques we made modifications that provided for the absence of palatal mucosal incisions being even more respectful of the anatomical structures than the original technique. We compared the outcomes of Modified Expansion Sphincter Pharyngoplasty (MESP) and Modified Barbed Pharyngoplasty (MBRP), two recent techniques of palatopharyngeal surgeries in patients with OSAS and we showed similar success rates for both techniques. Considering the advantages for MBRP the use of a knotless resorbable suture technology, minimal muscle manipulation and use of stable anchoring structure, like pterygomandibular raphe and posterior nasal spine as sustaining structure, and less invasiveness are the most important features that make MBRP superior to MESP. In conclusion MBRP may be considered superior to MESP in terms of less surgical time, no potential mucosal damage, absence of knots, and probably a faster recovery with less pain.

References

AAO-HNS Treatment of Obstructive Sleep Apnea http://www.entnet.org/content/treatment-obstructive-sleep-apnea#.

American Academy of Sleep Medicine. *Obstructive Sleep Apnea*. 2008.

American Sleep Apnea Association website. *OSA treatment options*. 2012.

Arens R, McDonough JM, Costarino AT, et al. Magnetic resonance imaging of the upper airway structure of children with obstructive sleep apnea syndrome. *Am J Respir Crit Care Med*. 2001;164:698–703.

Astor FC, Hanft KL, Benson C, Amaranath A. Analysis of short-term outcome after office-based laser-assisted uvulopalatoplasty. *Otolaryngol Head Neck Surg* 1998; 118: 478–480.

Baugh RF, Archer SM, Mitchell RB, Rosenfeld RM, Amin R, Burns JJ, Darrow DH, Giordano T, Litman RS, Li KK, Mannix ME, Schwartz RH, Setzen G, Wald ER, Wall E, Sandberg G, Patel MM; American Academy of Otolaryngology-Head and Neck Surgery Foundation. Clinical practice guideline: tonsillectomy in children. *Otolaryngol Head Neck Surg*. 2011 Jan;144(1 Suppl): S1-30.

Blumen MB, Dahan S, Wagner I, Dieuleveult T, Chabolle F. Radiofrequency versus LAUP for the treatment of snoring. *Otolaryngology – Head and Neck Surgery*. 2002; Volume 126 Number 1.

Brietzke S, Gallagher D, The effectiveness of tonsillectomy and adenoidectomy in the treatment of pediatric obstructive sleep apnea/hypopnea syndrome: A meta-analysis *Otolaryngol Head Neck Surg*, 134(6), 979-984, 2006.

Brietzke SE, Mair EA. Injection snoreplasty: how to treat snoring without all the pain and expense. *Otolaryngol Head Neck Surg* 2001; 124: 503–510.

Brietzke SE, Mair EA. Injection snoreplasty: Investigation of alternative sclerotherapy agents. *Otolaryngol Head Neck Surg*. 2004; 130:47-57.

Cahali MB. Lateral pharyngoplasty: a new treatment for obstructive sleep apnea hypopnea syndrome. *Laryngoscope*. 2003 Nov; 113(11):1961-8.

Carenfelt C. Laser uvulopalatopharyngoplasty in treatment of habitual snoring. *Ann Otol Rhinol Laryngol* 1991; 100: 451–454.

Casiano RR, Sheth S. Efficacy of cold-steel uvulopalatoplasty. *Otolaryngology - Head and Neck Surgery* November 1996.

Choi JH, Kim SN, Cho JH. Efficacy of the Pillar implant in the treatment of snoring and mild-to-moderate obstructive sleep apnea: a meta-analysis. *Laryngoscope*. 2013 Jan; 123(1):269-76.

Dickson RI, Mintz DR. One-stage Laser-assisted uvulopalatoplasty. *J Otolaryngol*. 1996; 25:155-161.

Franklin KA, Anttila H, Axelsson S, Gislason T, Maasilta P, Myhre KI, Rehnqvist N, Effects and Side-Effects of Surgery for Snoring and Obstructive Sleep Apnea – A Systematic Review. Surgery for Snoring and Sleep Apnea. *SLEEP,* Vol. 32, No. 1, 2009.

Fujita S, ConwayW, Zorlck F, et al. Surgical correction of anatomic abnormalities in obstructive sleep apnea syndrome: Uvulopalatopharyngoplasty. *Otolaryngol Head Neck Surg* 89:923-934 (Nov-Dec) 1981.

Gallina S, Dispenza F, Kulamarva G, Ballacchino A, Speciale R. Uvulopalatopharyngoplasty with tonsillectomy in the treatment of severe OSAS. *B-ENT* 2009; 5(04):245–250.

Hassid S, Afrapoli AH, Decaaestecker C, Cho- ufani G. UPPP for snoring: long-term results and patient satisfaction. *Acta Otorhinolaryngol Belg* 2002; 56: 157–162.

Hilton M. Tonsillectomy technique-tradition versus technology. *Lancet.* 2004; 364:642-3.

Hörmann K, Verse T. *Surgery for Sleep-Disordered Breathing.* Springer-Verlag Berlin Heidelberg 2005.

Hultcrantz E, Linder A, Markström A. Tonsillectomy or tonsillotomy? A randomized study comparing postoperative pain and long-term effects. *Int J Pediatr Otorhinolaryngol* 1999; 51: 171–176.

Hur J. A new treatment for snoring: sling snoreplasty with a permanent thread. *Acta otolaryngol* 2008; 128:1381-4.

Iseri M, Balcioglu O. Radiofrequency versus Injection Snoreplasty in Simple Snoring. *Otolaryngology–Head and Neck Surgery.* 2005; 133, 224-228.

Kamami YV. Laser CO_2 for snoring: preliminary results. *Acta Otorhinolaryngol Belg.* 1990; 44:451–456.

Kara CO, Ergin H, Kocak G, Kilic I, Yurdakul M. Prevalence of tonsillar hypertrophy and associated oropharyngeal symptoms in primary school children in Denizli, Turkey. *Int J Pediatr Otorhinolaryngol.* 2002; 66:175–9.

Lescanne E, Chiron B, Constant I, Couloigner V, Fauroux B, Hassani Y, Jouffroy L, Lesage V, Mondain M, Nowak C, Orliaguet G, Viot A; French Society of ENT (SFORL); French Association for Ambulatory Surgery (AFCA); French Society for Anaesthesia, Intensive Care (SFAR). Pediatric tonsillectomy: clinical practice guidelines. *Eur Ann Otorhinolaryngol Head Neck Dis.* 2012 Oct; 129(5):264-71.

Li H, Li K, Chen N, et al. Modified uvulopalatopharyngoplasty: the extended uvulopalatal flap. *Am J Otolaryngol* 2003; 24(5):311–6.

Li HY, Lee LA (2009) Relocation pharyngoplasty for obstructive sleep apnea. *Laryngoscope* 119:2472–2477.

Linee Guida in roncochirurgia ORL [Guidelines in ENT rhonosurgery] - Società Italiana di Otorinolaringoiatria e Chirurgia Cervico-Facciale - Argomenti Di *Acta Otorhinolaryngologica Italica* 2007.

Lorusso F, Dispenza F, Modica DM, Gallina S. The Role of Modified Expansion Sphincter Pharyngoplasty in Multilevel Obstructive Sleep Apnea Syndrome Surgery. *Int Arch Otorhinolaryngol.* 2018 Oct; 22(4):432-436.

Lorusso F, Dispenza F, Saraniti C, Sireci F, Modica DM, Gallina S. Sleep disordered breathing: evaluation of dynamic patterns of the upper airways in obese subjects. *Otorinolaringologia* 2014; 64:57–64

Lorusso F, Gallina S, Modica DM, Di Salvo N, Riggio F. Bipolar Quantum Molecular Resonance versus Blunt Dissection tonsillectomy. *B-ENT.* 2015; 11(2):101-8.

Lorusso F, Martines F, Mistretta A, Alagna E, Modica Dm, Dispenza F, Gallina S. Effects of adenotonsillectomy on neurocognitive and behavioural function in pediatric obstructive sleep apnea syndrome. *B-ENT*, 2018, 14, 113-118.

Mair EA, Day RH, Cautery-assisted palatal stiffening operation. *Otolaryngology– Head and Neck Surgery*; April 2000.

Mantovani M, Minetti A, Torretta S, Pincherle A, Tassone G, Pignataro L. The velo-uvulo-pharyngeal lift or "roman blinds" technique for treatment of snoring:a preliminary report. *Acta Otorhinolaryngol Ital.* 2012 Feb; 32(1):48-53.

Mantovani M, Minetti A, Torretta S, Pincherle A, Tassone G, Pignataro L. The "Barbed Roman Blinds" technique: a step forward. *Acta Otorhinolaryngol Ital.* 2013 Apr; 33(2):128.

Maurer JT. Update on surgical treatment for sleep apnoea. *Swiss Med Wkly.* 2009; 139(43–44):624–629.

Modica DM, Lorusso F, Presti G, Fasola S, Gallina S. Our Assessment Using Palate Postoperative Problems Score (PPOPS): Tool for the

Evaluation of Results in Palatal Surgery Techniques. *Indian J Otolaryngol Head Neck Surg.* 2019 Oct; 71(Suppl 1):766-770.

Montevecchi F, Meccariello G, Firinu E, et al. Prospective multicentre study on barbed reposition pharyngoplasty standing alone or as a part of multilevel surgery for sleep apnoea. *Clin Otolaryngol* 2018; 43: 483–488.

Mortimore IL, Bradley PA, Murray JA, Douglas NJ. Uvulopalatopharyngoplasty may compromise nasal CPAP therapy in sleep apnea syndrome. *Am J Respir Crit Care Med* 1996; 154:1759–1762.

Nelson LM. Radiofrequency treatment for obstructive tonsillar hypertrophy. *Arch Otolaryngol Head Neck Surg* 2000; 126: 736–740.

Olszewska E, Panek J, O'Day J, Rogowski M. Usefulness of snoreplasty in the treatment of simple snoring and mild obstructive sleep apnea/hypopnea syndrome – Preliminary report. *Otolaryngol Pol.* 2013; http://dx.doi.org/10.1016/j.otpol.2013.07.005.

Pang KP, Tan R, Puraviappan P, Terris DJ. Anterior palatoplasty for the treatment of OSA: three-year results. *Otolaryngol Head Neck Surg.* 2009 Aug; 141(2):253-6.

Pang KP, Woodson BT. Expansion sphincter pharyngoplasty: a new technique for the treatment of obstructive sleep apnea. *Otolaryngol Head Neck Surg.* 2007 Jul; 137(1):110-4.

Powel N, Riley R, Guilleminault C, Troell R. A Reversible Uvulopalatal *Flap for Snoring and Sleep Apnea Syndrome.* 1996 Sleep, Vol. 19, No.7.

Sher AE, Flexon PB, Hillman D, Emery B, Swieca J, Smith TL, Cartwright R, Dierks E, Nelson L. Temperature-controlled radiofrequency tissue volume reduction in the human soft palate. *Otolaryngology– Head and Neck Surgery* 2001; Volume 125 Number 4.

Sher AE, Schechtman KB, Piccirillo JR. The Efficacy of Surgical Modifications of the Upper Airway in Adults with Obstructive Sleep Apnea Syndrome. *1996 American Sleep Disorders Association and Sleep Research Society,* 19(2): 156--177.

Shintani T, Asakura K, Kataura A. Adenotonsillar hypertrophy and skeletal morphology of children with obstructive sleep apnea syndrome. *Acta Otolaryngol Suppl.* 1996; 523:222–4.

SNLG Appropriatezza e sicurezza degli interventi di tonsillectomia e/o adenoidectomia [*SNLG Appropriateness and safety of tonsillectomy and/or adenoidectomy procedures*]. 2008.http://www.snlg-iss.it/lgn

Sorrenti G. Piccin O. Functional expansion pharyngoplasty in the treatment of obstructive sleep apnea. *Laryngoscope.* 2013; 123:2905-2908.

Sundaram S, Bridgman SA, Lim J, Lasserson TJ. Surgery for obstructive sleep apnoea. *Cochrane Database Syst Rev.* 2005 Oct 19;(4):CD001004. Review.

Tarabichi M. Microdebrider-assisted uvulopalatoplasty. *Otolaryngol Head Neck Surg.* 1998; 119:131-3.

Tzifa KT, Shehab ZP, Robin PE. The relation between tonsillectomy and snoring. *Clin Otolaryngol* 1998; 23: 148–151.

Vicini C, Hendawy E, Campanini A, Eesa M, Bahgat A, AlGhamdi S, Meccariello G,DeVito A, Montevecchi F, Mantovani M. Barbed reposition pharyngoplasty (BRP) for OSAHS: a feasibility, safety, efficacy and teachability pilot study. "We are onthe giant's shoulders". *Eur Arch Otorhinolaryngol.* 2015 Apr 12.

Vicini CA. Chirurgia della roncopatia [Snoring surgery]. *Eureka editore* 2007; pag 147-163.

Wassmuth Z, Mair EA, Loube D, Leonard D. Cautery-assisted palatal stiffening operation for the treatment of obstructive sleep apnea syndrome. *Otolaryngology– Head and Neck Surgery*; July 2000.

Weingarten C. Snare Uvuloplasty. *Laryngoscope* 1995; 205: October.

Whinney DJ, Williamson PA, Bicknell PG. Punctate diathermy of the soft palate: a new approach in the surgical management of snoring. *J Laryngol Otol* 1995; 109: 849–852.

Yaremchuk K. Palatal Procedures for Obstructive Sleep Apnea. *Otolaryngol Clin N Am.* 2016; http://dx.doi.org/10.1016/j.otc.2016.07.011 oto.theclinics.com 0030-6665/16/ª 2016 Elsevier Inc.

Zinder DJ, Postma GN. Outpatient cautery-assisted uvulopalatoplasty. *Laryngoscope* 105: November 1995.

In: Advances in Sleep Apnea
Editors: F. Lorusso et al.
ISBN: 978-1-53619-758-7

Chapter 13

TRANSORAL ROBOTIC SURGERY FOR OBSTRUCTIVE SLEEP APNEA SYNDROME

Giovanni Cammaroto[1,*], Luigi Marco Stringa[2], Khai Beng Chong[3], Giuseppe Meccariello[1], Giannicola Iannella[1], Andrea De Vito[4], Stefano Pelucchi[2] and Claudio Vicini[1,2]

[1]Head and Neck Department, ENT Unit, Morgagni-Pierantoni Hospital, AUSL of Romagna, Forlì, Italy
[2]Department of Otolaryngology, Head and Neck Surgery, University of Ferrara, Ferrara, Italy
[3]Department of Otorhinolaryngology, Tan Tock Seng Hospital, Novena, Singapore
[4]Head and Neck Department, ENT Unit, Santa Maria delle Croci Hospital, AUSL of Romagna, Ravenna, Italy

[*] Corresponding Author's Email: giovanni.cammaroto@hotmail.com.

Abstract

Although most patients benefit from the use of the gold standard CPAP therapy, OSAHS patients who are unable to fit on it or patients who are non-compliant can find an effective alternative in surgery. The application of TORS in the surgical treatment of OSAHS is recent but it has shown promising results. In fact, thanks to its technology, the base of tongue (BOT) obstructions can be reached with excellent visualization, allowing selective and minimally invasive excision of redundant lingual tissue. Not all patients are suitable for this kind of surgery. For this reason, in order to reduce the rate of surgical failure and post-operative complications, attentive patient selection should be done by integrating the clinical history, physical findings, DISE and imaging data. Despite favorable results, robotic surgery in particularly TORS is encountering obstacles that prevent its widespread application. The high costs for the robotic system lack of specific instruments for surgery of the head and neck region and anatomical limitations for surgical access for robotic surgery seems to be the principal factors. On the other hand, thanks to the growing interest in this kind of surgery, several solutions have been proposed. The development of the single-port technology and application of robotic technology in multilevel surgery seems to represent promising opportunities. Further efforts will be needed to define the crucial role of this innovative surgical approach that has shown great potential in providing positive benefits in the treatment of OSAHS.

Introduction

Obstructive sleep apnea-hypopnea syndrome (OSAHS) is a widespread social health problem that affects at least 2-4% of the adult population. OSAHS is characterized by obstruction of the airflow due to structural collapse of the upper airways during sleep. OSAHS not only undermines the quality of life, but it also represents an independent risk factor for hypertension, myocardial infarction and stroke, increasing the risk of death for each patient. Due to its multifactorial pathophysiology and systemic implications, a multidisciplinary approach is recommended to manage OSAHS patients effectively. Although continuous positive airway pressure (CPAP) is considered the gold standard treatment, surgery represents one of the therapeutic options but it has been criticized due to a lack of evidence supporting its efficacy as well as heterogeneity of published outcomes. Considering the frequent multilevel airflow obstruction identified by sleep endoscopy, different surgical techniques have been developed to restore normal patency of the upper airways. Although oncological surgery represents the most described field of application, transoral robotic surgery (TORS) has been shown to be a well-documented and effective surgical option for the treatment of base of tongue (BOT) obstruction in patients affected by OSAHS.

In the present chapter, we will try to give an overview of the use of TORS for the treatment of OSAHS, describing its application at present, limitations and possible future challenges.

PRINCIPLES

The BOT is one of the possible sites of upper airway obstruction in OSAHS and its obstructive role in sleep apnea may be assessed directly by awake endoscopy, Drug Induced Sleep Endoscopy (DISE), as well as by imaging. The first surgical approach treating OSAHS as a consequence of lingual hypertrophy was proposed by Chabolle in 1999 (open transcervical Tongue Base Reduction Hyoepiglottoplasty, TBRHE). Due to its technical difficulties and potential associated morbidities, the experience in this surgical option remains limited to the literature. Thanks to technological advancement and growing interest in minimally invasive procedures, the first transoral robotic surgery (TORS) for OSAHS was presented by Vicini et al. in 2010, as a robotic evolution of the previous technique. After showing very promising results, many authors started to look in depth and further refined this technique. TORS is now widely applied in sleep surgery and allows a selective therapeutic approach. Depending on patient characteristics, in particularly the histology and geometry of the obstructive tissue, different surgical choices can be considered. If the lymphoid tissue of the tongue is the main obstructive component, lingual tonsillectomy will be the most suitable choice. More frequently both lymphoid and muscular tissue are responsible for the enlarged BOT and will require tongue base debulking including removal of a midline wedge of oral tongue. The total volume of lingual tissue removed and the percentages of lymphoid and/or muscular component of the tongue does not influence the clinical outcomes 1 year after surgery. Moreover it has been shown that lymphoid tissue removal may not be permanent and 8.8% of patients with BOT excision by TORS may present with lymphoid tissue regrowth. For these cases, no correlation between the grade of regrowth, time interval from surgery and volume of lymphoid tissue removal has been found. The epiglottis can be involved in obstruction of upper airways, generally from primary collapse and in some cases, secondary collapse. For these cases, a concomitant supraglottoplasty can be performed with TORS. Many OSAHS patients present with multilevel obstruction. Due to the substantial cost of robotic surgery, BOT surgery is often performed concomitant with other surgical approaches like nasal surgery such as septoplasty and turbinoplasty, and soft palate surgery such as expansion sphincter pharyngoplasty (ESP), barbed relocation pharyngoplasty (BRP) and uvulopalatopharyngoplasty (UPPP). When comparing the association of TORS with various palatal techniques, it has been demonstrated that combined TORS-ESP and TORS-BRP are more effective than TORS-UPPP, with surgical success of 90% for the former and 50% for the latter, with "surgical success" being defined as 50% reduction of pre-operative AHI and AHI < 20. Due to the complexity of OSAHS presentation and highly variable therapeutic options, meticulous assessment of patients should be done to reduce the incidence of therapeutic failures. Most essential information can be assessed using DISE during TORS work-up, allowing better localization of the sites of upper airway collapse and to capture additional details about the dynamic behavior of the base of tongue and supraglottic region. Some unfavourable conditions for surgery of the base of the tongue can be preventively detected, such as significant lateral pharyngeal wall collapse and a small mouth opening with interincisive distance of less than 25 mm. Another condition that must be taken into account is the high risk of TORS failure for patients with body mass index (BMI) >30 kg/m^2. All these conditions have been demonstrated to increase the rate of surgical failure. OSAHS is not only a pathology of adults, but children can also present with obstructive problems. In the pediatric population, OSAHS is primarily a consequence of adenotonsillar hypertrophy that can be treated with standard adenotonsillectomy. In some cases, children may present with BOT hypertrophy and/or epiglottis collapse as a cofactor of the OSAHS pathology. In these cases TORS it has been demonstrated as a safe and effective approach.

TECHNIQUE

Up to now, the most commonly described robotic system is the Da Vinci system, in which the primary surgeon maneuvers the console with the information being translated by an executor system comprising different arms which can be loaded with camera and specific instruments. The patient is positioned in supine on the operating table, with neck flexed and head extended (sniffing position). To better reveal hidden areas during dissection, external compression can be applied by the surgical assistant positioned at the head of the patient. Whenever possible, nasotracheal intubation is the preferred choice to allow best exposure of the surgical area and widest range of motion for the robotic arms. Oropharyngeal intubation can still be done but it may cause some difficulties for the operators. Prophylactic tracheotomy is recommended to better manage post-operative complications, especially for multilevel surgery and for patients who had prior difficult intubation. Usually either a Davis-Meyer or Crowe-Davis mouth-gag is applied to obtain the best exposure of the surgical field. For the same reason a suture is passed through the tongue body to pull out the BOT. No teeth or soft tissue protecting devices are used, as they may cause reduction of the baseline narrow mouth opening. In order to provide endoscopic vision for the primary surgeon, a 3D scope is positioned in the center, usually 30° up-facing. Following scope insertion, the other robot arms are connected to a couple of 5 mm instruments such as a round tip cautery and a Maryland forceps. The position of the instruments can be changed depending on the side of surgery.

Based on the structural and histological features of lingual obstruction, variable techniques can be performed by TORS:

– Lingual Tonsillectomy

When airflow obstruction is a consequence of exclusive lingual tonsil hypertrophy, selective removal of lymphoid tissue is recommended. Lingual tonsillectomy represents a group of procedures in which the hypertrophic lymphoid tissue is excised while preserving the underlying muscle. This group of surgical approaches is generally easy and safe to perform as the lymphoid tissue is devoid of critical blood vessels and/or nerves.

– Posterior Midline Glossectomy

If other than the lymphoid there is additional lingual muscular tissue responsible for the obstruction, a variable amount of the different lingual components needs to be removed. In posterior midline glossectomy both muscular fibers and lymphoid tissue are resected around the midline, with several possible shapes of resection: "V" or "U" or "Δ" shape. Tissue removal around midline reduces the risk of complications such as injury to the lingual blood vessels and nerves that run along the lateral side of the base of the tongue. Careful dissection under magnification may allow identification and preservation of blood vessels and nerves if encountered.

– Tongue Base Reduction

In this approach, a variable amount of lymphoid and muscular tissue of the tongue base is progressively removed, deeper around the midline, with a final "T" or "mushroom" shaped resection. Careful dissection under magnification may allow identification and preservation of blood vessels and nerves if encountered. The rationale for this approach is to optimize the volume of tissue removed, working in safe superficial and deep areas, resulting in more tissue resected.

- Supraglottoplasty

In addition to previous approaches, modification to the shape of the epiglottis can be performed as an optional step following the main tongue base procedure. Other than hypertrophic lingual tissue, floppy and/or redundant epiglottis, aryepiglottic fold, and/or arytenoid mucosa may be responsible for airway collapse during inspiratory phases. During supraglottoplasty, the plane of resection should be above the pharyngo-epiglottic folds to minimize the risk of aspiration and to prevent bleeding from branches of the superior laryngeal vessels. In addition to stabilizing the supraglottic tissue, healing by secondary intention in the vallecula and adjacent areas from this procedure results in anterior advancement of the epiglottis.

Complications

Although the use of TORS for the treatment of OSAHS is relatively recent, with its wide application in the last few years, it is now possible to appreciate not only its advantages but also the associated complications encountered. TORS has been proven to be a safe technique with a low rate of post-surgical problems. The most common post-operative complication is transient dysphagia with a rate of 7.2%, although it appears not to be related to the volume of tissue removed from the base of tongue. Post-operative bleeding has been reported in 4.2% of cases. Transient hypogeusia, pharyngeal edema and globus have been described as a consequence of tongue blade compression on the lingual nerves and pharyngeal wall or following exposure to high temperature from the monopolar cautery. No major complication has been reported.

Alternatives

Since the beginning of the application of TORS for the treatment of airway obstruction in OSAHS, this innovative technique has shown encouraging results. Some factors are preventing it from becoming a gold standard procedure. First of all, economic limitations play a key role in preventing the widespread use of TORS. For this reason, alternative techniques have been proposed and Coblation has been shown to be a reliable and well-documented technique. Coblation technology allows low temperature, less traumatic ablation of the lingual soft tissue. Coblation is generally used under direct vision or with 2D camera system, limiting its accuracy. Lots of effort has been made to compare these two different approaches, analyzing their similarities and differences. Both techniques seem to be effective with some differences in failure rates: 34.4% and 38.5% for TORS and Coblation respectively. This can be explained by the ability to perform both BOT tissue excision and supraglottoplasty using TORS but not with Coblation surgery. On the other hand, post-operative complication rate is consistently lower with Coblation surgery (8.4%) compared to TORS (21.3%). However, major complications, such as neurovascular injuries are low for both techniques. Another important factor that must be taken into account is the difference in cost, which is estimated to be 730$ per robotic procedure versus 250$ per coblation procedure, on top of the cost for each surgical system: 2,000,000$ for the Robotic system against 20,000$ for Coblation system. The key point to take note is that both technologies can be applied to a wide range of procedures, presumably with different effectiveness for each procedure.

Conclusion

The application of TORS in the treatment of upper airway obstruction is a recent development in the surgical approaches for OSAHS. Its effectiveness is widely documented with clear standardized settings especially with regard to the treatment of BOT obstruction. Different procedures can be performed using robotic system, depending on the characteristics of the obstructive tissue, and multilevel surgery is commonly done with robotic BOT reduction. Despite the undeniable advantages such as the robotic system's magnification and high-definition three dimensional camera system, ability to perform four-handed surgery, motion scaling and tremor filtration technology, some obstacles are preventing TORS from becoming a standard surgical solution for tongue base obstruction. Some effective alternatives like Coblation technology has been elaborated, but thanks to its incomparable qualities, TORS seems to still give better results. Further efforts are needed to confirm previous results and clarify the increasingly crucial role of robotic surgery in the treatment of OSAHS.

References

Cammaroto, G., Meccariello, G., Costantini, M., Stomeo, F., Hoff, P., Montevecchi, F., Vicini, C. Trans-Oral Robotic Tongue Reduction for OSA- Does Lingual Anatomy Influence the Surgical Outcome? *J. Clin. Sleep Med.* 2018 Aug 15; 14(8):1347-1351.

Cammaroto, G., Montevecchi, F., D'Agostino, G., Zaccardo, E., Bellini, C., Meccariello, G., Vivini, C. Palatal surgery in a transoral robotic setting (TORS): preliminary results of a retrospective comparison between uvulopalatopharyngoplasty (UPPP), expansion sphincter pharyngoplasty (ESP) and barbed repositioning pharyngoplasty (BRP). *Acta Otorhinolaryngol. Ital.* 2017 Oct; 37(5):406-409.

Cammaroto, G., Montevecchi, F., D'Agostino, G., Zeccardo, E., Bellini, C., Galletti, B., Shams, M., Negm, H., Vicini, C. Tongue reduction for OSAHS: TORSs vs coblations, technologies vs techniques, apples vs oranges. *Eur. Arch. Otorhinolaryngol.* 2017; 274(2):637-45.

Cammaroto, G., Stringa, L. M., Zhang, H., Capaccio, P., Galletti, F., Galletti, B., Meccariello, G., Iannella, G., Pelucchi, S., Baghat, A. and Vicini, C. Alternative Applications of Trans-Oral Robotic Surgery (TORS): A Systematic Review. *J. Clin. Med.* 2020 Jan 11; 9(1):201.

Chabolle, F., Wagner, I., Blumen, M. B., Se'quert, C., Fleury, B., De Dieuleveult, T. Tongue base reduction with hyoepiglottoplasty: a treatment for severe obstructive sleep apnea. *Laryngoscope* 1999; 109:1273-1280.

Friedman, M., Hamilton, C., Samuelson, C. G., Kelley, K., Taylor, D., Pearson-Chauhan, K., Maley, A., Taylor, R., Venkatesan, T. K. (2012) Transoral robotic glossectomy for the treatment of obstructive sleep apnea-hypopnea syndrome. *Otolaryngol. Head Neck Surg.* 146(5):854-862.

Hoff, P. T., Glazer, T. A., Spector, M. E. (2014) Body mass index predicts success in patients undergoing transoral robotic surgery for obstructive sleep apnea. *ORL J. Otorhinolaryngol. Relat. Spec.* 76: 266-272.

Iannella, G., Magliulo, G., Montevecchi, F., De Vito, A., Polimeni, A., De Vincentiis, M., Meccariello, G., D'Agostino, G., Gobbi, R., Cammaroto, G., Stomeo, F. P., Pang, K., Rotenberg, B., Vicini, C. Lingual Tonsil Lymphatic Tissue Regrowth in Patients Undergoing Transoral Robotic Surgery. *Laryngoscope* 2019 Nov; 129(11):2652-2657.

Lin, A. C., Koltai, P. J. (2009) Persistent pediatric obstructive sleep apnea and lingual tonsillectomy. *Otolaryngol. Head Neck Surg.* 141:81-85.

Lorusso, F., Dispenza, F., Modica, D. M., Gallina, S. The Role of Modified Expansion Sphincter Pharyngoplasty in Multilevel Obstructive Sleep Apnea Syndrome Surgery. *Int. Arch. Otorhinolaryngol.* 2018 Oct; 22(4):432-436.

Lorusso, F., Gallina, S., Modica, D. M., Di Salvo, N., Riggio, F. Bipolar Quantum Molecular Resonance versus Blunt Dissection tonsillectomy. *B-ENT* 2015; 11(02):101-108.

Lorusso, F., Martines, F., Mistretta, A., Dispenza, F., Gallina, S. Effects of adenotonsillectomy on neurocognitive and behavioural function in pediatric obstructive sleep apnea syndrome. *B-ENT* 2018; 14:113-118.

Marin, J. M., Carrizo, S. J., Vicente, E., Agusti, A. G. Long-term cardio-vascular outcomes in men with obstructive sleep apnoea-hypopnoea with or without treatment with continuous positive airway pressure: an observational study. *Lancet* 2005; 365: 1046-1053.

Meccariello, G., Cammaroto, G., Montevecchi, F., Hoff, P. T., Spector, M. E., Negm, H., Shams, M., Bellini, C., Zeccardo, E., Vicini, C. Transoral robotic surgery for the management of obstructive sleep apnea: a systematic review and meta-analysis. *Eur. Arch. Otorhinolaryngol.* 2017 Feb; 274(2):647-653.

Vicini, C., Dallan, I., Canzi, P., Frassineti, S., La Pietra, M. G., Montevecchi, F. Transoral robotic tongue base resection in obstructive sleep apnoea-hypopnoea syndrome: a preliminary report. *ORL J. Otorhinolaryngol. Relat. Spec.* 2010; 72:22-27.

Vicini, C., Montevecchi, F. Transoral Robotic Surgery for Obstructive Sleep Apnea: Past, Present, and Future. *Sleep Med. Clin.* 2019 Mar; 14(1):67-72.

Yaggi, H. K., Concato, J., Kernan, W. N., Lichtman, J. H., Brass, L. M., Mohsenin, V. Obstructive sleep apnea as a risk factor for stroke and death. *N Engl. J. Med.* 2005; 353:2034-2041.

In: Advances in Sleep Apnea
Editors: F. Lorusso et al.
ISBN: 978-1-53619-758-7

Chapter 14

ADVANCES IN THE ROLE OF BARIATRIC SURGERY IN THE TREATMENT OF OSAS

Stefania Martorana[1], Giuseppina Guercio[1] and Gianni Pantuso[1,*]
[1]Endocrine and Obesity Surgery Unit,
Policlinico Universitario "P. Giaccone",
Palermo, Italy

ABSTRACT

Obstructive sleep apnea-hypopnea syndrome (OSAHS) is characterized by the complete or partial collapse of the upper airway during sleep, resulting in successive episodes of cessation or decrease in respiratory airflow, in which obesity is an important risk factor. The prevalence of the disease in morbidly obese patients is about 70%. Continuous positive airway pressure (CPAP) and weight loss represent the treatment of choice for obese patients with OSAHS. However, weight loss by dieting often produces unsatisfactory results, and long-term adherence to CPAP is also poor. Thus, bariatric surgery has emerged as the treatment for morbid obesity and various associated co-morbidities.

* Corresponding Author's Email: gianni.pantuso@unipa.it.

All bariatric patients should be screened for OSAHS to reduce the risk of perioperative complications.

Multiple intraoperative strategies exist to minimize the risk of cardiopulmonary complications.

CPAP therapy is recommended in the early postoperative period.

INTRODUCTION

Obesity is a chronic disease that has become epidemic in the United States and worldwide; the progressively escalating rates of overweight and obesity worldwide have led to an introduction of a new term "globesity". The more severe form of obesity, known as grade III or morbid obesity is associated with multiple co-morbidities, like dyslipidemia, hypertension, diabetes, arthritis and OSAHS.

OSAHS is a sleep-related breathing disorder, characterized by recurrent upper-airway obstruction during sleep, resulting in a cycle of hypoxemia, increased respiratory effort, and frequent arousals.

The etiology of OSAHS is complex, and obesity is one of the most important causes. According to obesity guidelines in adults, a body mass index (BMI) between 25.0kg/m2 and 29.9kg/m2 is defined as overweight, grade I obesity as BMI > 30kg/m2, grade II obesity as BMI > 35kg/m2, grade III or morbid obesity as BMI > 40kg/m2 or >35kg/m2 in combination with obesity related co-morbidities. OSAHS is associated with overweight and obesity. About 60% – 90% adult patients with OSAHS are overweight, and the prevalence of OSAHS in obese or severely obese population is almost twice that in normal-weight adults. In morbid obese patients, the prevalence of OSAHS is about 70%.

PHYSIOPATHOLOGY

Although the mechanisms are still poorly understood, OSAHS is associated with deposition of fat about the upper airways, causing their collapse. Obesity-related adipose tissue accumulates around the upper airway and increases in neck circumference. These changes reduce intraluminal airway caliber and increase extraluminal tissue pressure resulting in elevated mechanical loading of pharyngeal structures. As obese patients have more severe upper airway collapsibility, fat deposition in the abdomen and thorax decreases chest wall compliance and thus leads to a further decrease in lung capacity, resulting in obese patients being at risk for increased severity of OSAHS.

Evidence also suggests that there is interference in endocrinological regulation of leptin, the hormone that suppresses appetite and alters energy expenditure. Patients with morbid obesity have higher levels of leptin, indicating that they are resistant to the effects of this hormone. This could be the cause of obesity, i.e., they cannot get satiated. Individuals with OSAHS have 50% higher leptin levels than healthy controls and also do not show satiety. Thus, there appears to be potentiation of resistence to leptin in OSAHS, predisposing the patient to a cycle of weight gain and worsening apnea.

TREATMENT

The treatment of choice for OSAS is the use of CPAP during sleep associated with a long-term weight loss strategy. However, significant weight loss is often difficult, and its maintenance is even more challenging for many people. At the same time, the use of CPAP does not show good adherence because of being long-term and uncomfortable.

Thus, bariatric surgery has now been utilized in morbidly obese patients who have failed conservative therapy or have significant comorbidities.

At present, there are no OSAHS guidelines specific to bariatric surgery. OSAHS has been mentioned as an obesity-related co-morbidity in the guidelines for surgical treatment of obesity and T2D.

Worldwide, the accepted criteria for bariatric surgery include the following: being 18-65 years of age and having a BMI ≥ 40kg/m2 or ≥ 35kg/m2 with OSAHS or other obesity-related comorbidities.

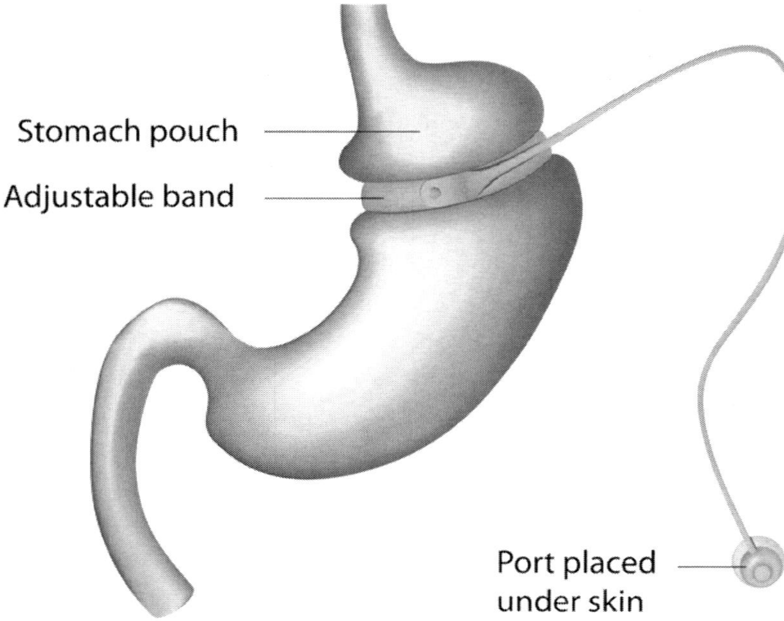

Figure 1. Laparoscopic adjustable gastric banding.

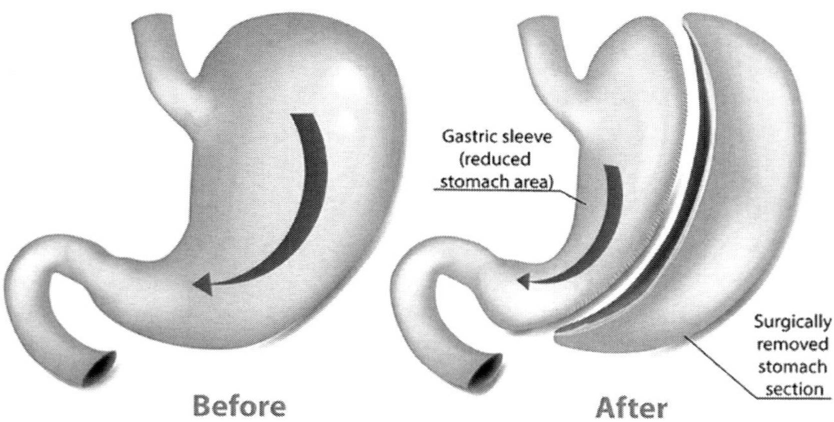

Figure 2. Sleeve Gastrectomy.

Bariatric surgery procedures are divided into 3 categories: laparoscopic adjustable gastric banding (LAGB) (Figure 1) and laparoscopic sleeve gastrectomy (LSG) (Figure 2) that reduce gastric pouch size; biliopancreatic diversion (BPD) (Figure 3) with or without duodenal switch (BPD-DS) (Figure 4) surgeries that results in body malabsorption; Roux-en-Y gastric bypass (RYGB) (Figure 5) that results in a combination of restrictive and malabsorptive components.

All these different surgeries have shown a significant effect on OSAHS, including resolution or improvement in the majority of cases. However, the most frequent weight loss surgical methods include nowadays LSG and RYGB. LAGB and BPD were abandoned due to the rate of reoperations and associated malnutrition, respectively.

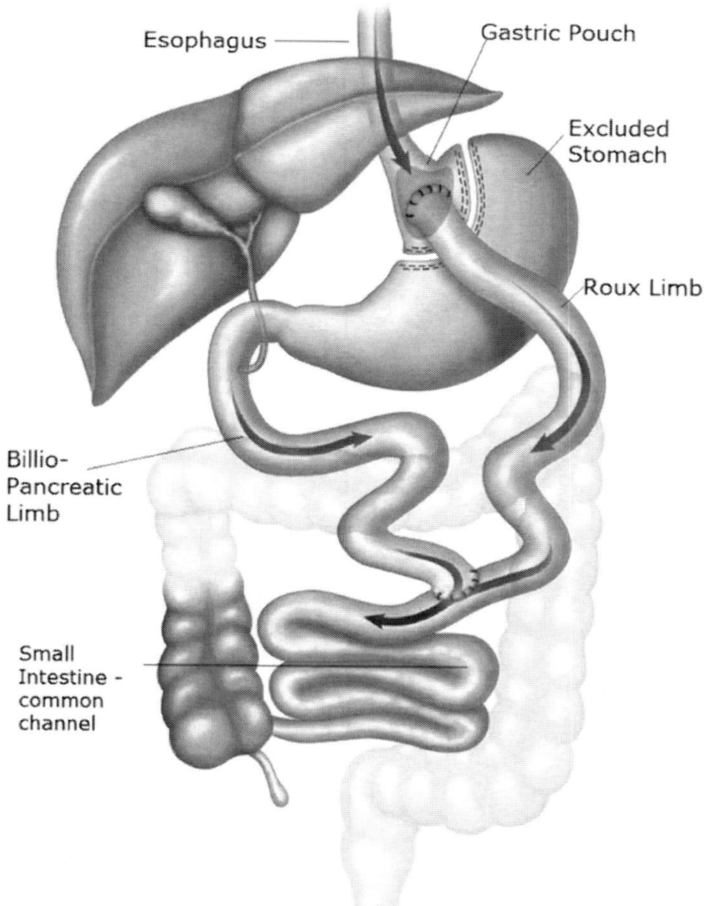

Figure 3. Biliopancreatic diversion.

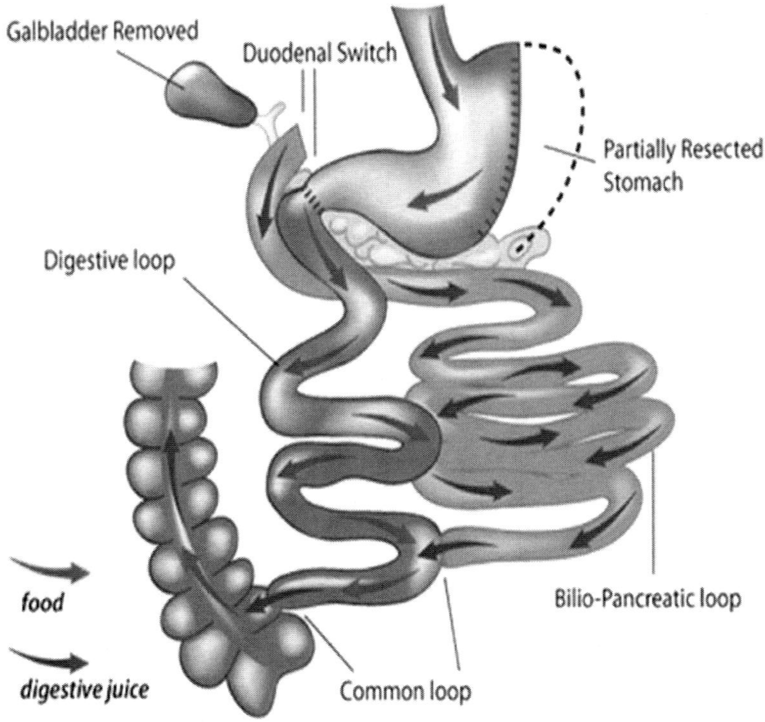

Figure 4. Biliopancreatic diversion with duodenal switch.

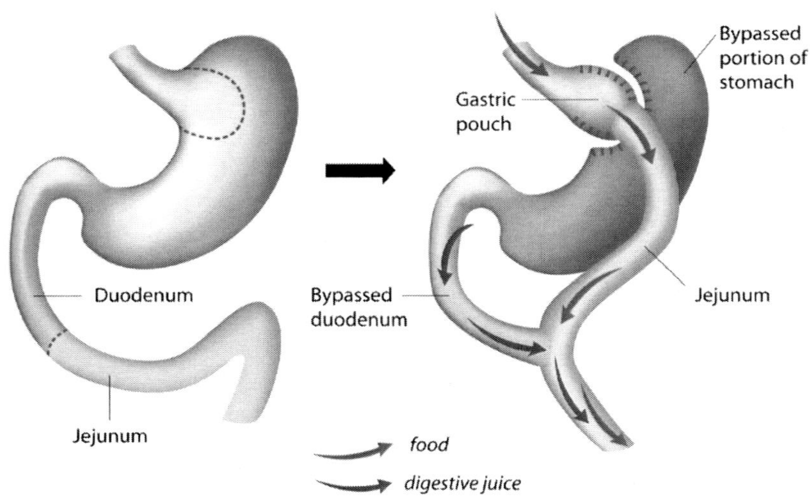

Figure 5. Roux-en-Y gastric bypass.

Anyway, in most cases, bariatric surgery results in significant weight loss and improvement in the indices of sleep-disordered breathing. In addition, OSA is underdiagnosed in a significant proportion of obese patients undergoing bariatric surgery.

Therefore, recognizing OSAHS is an important aspect of the perioperative care of bariatric patients. Both morbid obesity and OSAHS are risk factors for intraoperative difficulties.

Most bariatric surgery programs now employ routine screening for OSAHS in all patients, regardless of whether or not they have sleep complaints, because most cases of OSAHS were previously not being diagnosed before the surgical procedure.

Currently, the gold standard for diagnosis of OSA is an overnight laboratory polysomnography, that verify and quantify the occurrence of episodes of respiratory airflow cessation, accompanied by loud intermittent snoring and associated or not with nocturnal awakening and episodes of desaturation, measured by the *apnea-hypopnea index* (AHI).

CPAP is recommended in all bariatric patients with moderately or severe OSA (AHI > 15/h).

As a certain time period is necessary to get used to CPAP, patients should get acclimated to its use prior to surgery if possible. This may take up to several weeks. When admitted to the hospital, patients should use their own CPAP mask and machine for optimal mask fit and pressure requirements.

Other intraoperative ventilation precautions include preoxygenation, positive end-expiratory pressure (PEEP) and low tidal volume. Optimal preoxygenation is achieved by placing patients in sitting position (90°). This extends time to apnea with 1min when compared with supine position. The ramped position is the preferred position for induction, intubation and ventilation as this improves oxygenation and the laryngoscopic view.

Providing CPAP and PEEP during induction avoids airway collapse and increases end-expiratory lung volume. This combination extends time to hypoxic apnea by 1 min, prolonging time for intubation. Extubation is considered well tolerated when a patient is fully awake and should directly be followed by CPAP treatment. Continuous monitoring is recommended for all OSA patients in the early postoperative period.

OSA patients using CPAP should be re-evaluated with a formal sleep study prior to the decision of discontinuing CPAP. Optimal timing of this re-evaluation is unknown.

Conclusion

Obesity is a well-known risk factor for OSAHS. The treatment of choice is the use of CPAP, combined with a long-term weight loss strategy. However, weight loss by dieting often produces unsatisfactory results. Thus, bariatric surgery has now been utilized in morbidly obese patients who have failed conservative therapy or have significant comorbidities. The most frequent weight loss surgical methods include LSG and RYGB. All bariatric patients should be screened for OSAHS to reduce the risk of perioperative complications. Multiple strategies exist to minimize the risk of cardiopulmonary complications: correct positioning of the patient, preoxygenation, positive end-expiratory pressure (PEEP) during induction, maintenance of low tidal volume during surgery and performance of multimodal anesthesia and analgesia with avoidance of opioids. Bariatric surgery results in significant weight loss and improvement in the indices of sleep-disordered breathing.

References

Bruno, A., Di Sano, C., Lorusso, F., Dino, P., Russo, D., Ballacchino, A., Gallina, S., Modica, D. M., Chiappara, G., Simon, H. U., Pace, E. Notch-1 decreased expression contributes to leptin receptor downregulation in nasal epithelium from allergic turbinates. *Biochim. Biophys. Acta Mol. Basis Dis.*, 2019 Jun. 1; 1865(6):1642 - 1650.

Buchwald, H., Oien, D. M. (2013). Metabolic/bariatric surgery worldwide 2011. *Obes. Surg.*, 23(4):427 - 36.

Carneiro, G., Flório, R. T., Zanella, M. T., Pradella-Hallinan, M., Ribeiro-Filho, F. F., Tufik, S. et al. (2012). Is mandatory screening for obstructive sleep apnea with polysomnography in all severely obese patients indicated? *Sleep Breath*, 16(1):163 - 8.

Castriotta, R. J., Chung, P. (2019). Cutting for cures: Bariatric surgery and obstructive sleep apnea. *J. Clin. Sleep Med.,* 15(10): 1391 - 1392.

de Raaff, C., Gorter-Stam, M., de Vries, N. et al. (2017). Perioperative management of obstructive sleep apnea in bariatric surgery: A consensus guideline. *Surg. Obes. Relat. Dis.,* 13(7):1095 - 1109.

De Stefano, A., Di Giovanni, P., Kulamarva, G., Gennachi, S., Di Fonzo, F., Sallustio, V., Patrocinio, D., Candido, S., Lamarca, G., Dispenza, F. Oropharyngeal dysphagia in elderly population suffering from mild cognitive impairment and mild dementia: Understanding the link (2020). *American Journal of Otolaryngology - Head and Neck Medicine and Surgery,* 41 (4), art. no. 102501.

De Stefano, A., Dispenza, F., Kulamarva, G., Lamarca, G., Faita, A., Merico, A., Sardanelli, G., Gabellone, S., Antonaci, A. *Predictive Factors of Severity and Persistence of Oropharyngeal Dysphagia in Sub-Acute Stroke.*

Dixon, J. B., Schachter, L. M., O'Brien, A. E. (2003). Predicting sleep apnea and excessive day sleepiness in the severely obese – indicators for polysomnography. *Chest,* 123: 1134 - 41.

Farinholt, G. N., Carr, A. D., Chang, E. J., Ali, M. R. (2013). A call to arms: obese men with more severe comorbid disease and underutilization of bariatric operations. *Surg. Endosc.*, 27(12): 4556 - 63.

Frey, W. C., Pilcher, J. (2003). Obstructive sleep-related breathing disorders in patients evaluated for bariatric surgery. *Obes. Surg.,* 13: 676 - 83.

Gami, A. S., Caples, S. M., Somers, V. K. (2003). Obesity and obstructive sleep apnea. *Endocrinol. Metab. Clin. North Am.,* 32(4):869 - 94.

Ibrahim, A. M., Thumma, J. R., Dimick, J. B. (2017). Reoperation and medicare expenditures after laparoscopic gastric band surgery. *JAMA Surg.,* 152(9):835 - 42.

Jensen, M. D., Ryan, D. H., Apovian, C. M. et al. (2014). 2013 AHA/ACC/TOS guideline for the management of overweight and obesity in adults: A report of the American College of Cardiology/American Heart Association Task Force on Practice Guidelines and The Obesity Society. *Circulation,* 129:S102 - 38 (25 Suppl. 2).

Lorusso, F., Dispenza, F., Modica, D. M., Gallina, S. The Role of Modified Expansion Sphincter Pharyngoplasty in Multilevel Obstructive Sleep Apnea Syndrome Surgery. *Int. Arch. Otorhinolaryngol.*, 2018 Oct.; 22(4):432 - 436.

Lorusso, F., Dispenza, F., Saraniti, C., Sireci, F., Modica, D. M., Gallina, S. Sleep disordered breathing: Evaluation of dynamic patterns of the upper airways in obese subjects. *Otorinolaringologia,* 2014; 64:57 - 64.

Lorusso, F., Gallina, S., Modica, D. M., Di Salvo, N., Riggio, F. Bipolar Quantum Molecular Resonance versus Blunt Dissection tonsillectomy. *B-ENT,* 2015; 11(02):101 - 108.

Lorusso, F., Dispenza, F., Martinciglio, G., Battaglia, A., Gallina, S. Postural changes in patients undergoing hyoid surgery for OSAS. *EuroMediterranean Biomedical Journal,* 2017; 12(29):140 - 143.

Lorusso, F., Martines, F., Mistretta, A., Dispenza, F., Gallina, S. Effects of adenotonsillectomy on neurocognitive and behavioural function in pediatric obstructive sleep apnea syndrome. *B-ENT*, 2018; 14:113 - 118.

Marik, P. (2000). Leptin, obesity, and obstructive sleep apnea. *Chest,* 118: 569 - 71.

Modica, D. M., Lorusso, F., Presti, G., Fasola, S., Gallina, S. Our Assessment Using Palate Postoperative Problems Score (PPOPS): Tool for the Evaluation of Results in Palatal Surgery Techniques. *Indian J. Otolaryngol. Head Neck Surg.,* 2019 Oct.; 71(Suppl. 1):766 -.770.

Modica, D. M., Marchese, D., Lorusso, F., Speciale, R., Saraniti, C., Gallina, S. Functional Nasal Surgery and Use of CPAP in OSAS Patients: Our Experience. *Indian J. Otolaryngol. Head Neck Surg.,* 2018 Dec.; 70(4):559 - 565.

Naimark, A., Cherniack, R. M. (1960). Compliance of the respiratory system and its components in health and obesity. *J. Appl. Physiol.,* 15:377 - 82.

Nepomnayshy, D., Hesham, W., Erikson, B., MacDonald, J., Iorio, R., Brams, D. (2013). Sleep apnea: Is routine preoperative screening necessary? *Obes. Surg.,* 23(3):287 - 91.

NIH conference. (1991). Gastrointestinal surgery for severe obesity. Consensus Development Conference Panel. *Ann. Intern. Med.,* 115 (12):956 - 61.

O'Keeffe, T., Patterson, E. J. (2004). Evidence supporting routine polysomnography before bariatric surgery. *Obes. Surg.,* 14: 23 - 6.

O'Keeffe, T., Patterson, E. J. (2004). Evidence supporting routine polysomnography before bariatric surgery. *Obes. Surg.,* 14(1):23 - 6.

Peppard, P. E., Young, T., Palta, M., Dempsey, J., Skatrud, J. (2000). Longitudinal study of moderate weight change and sleep-disordered breathing. *JAMA,* 284(23):3015 - 21.

Rasmussen, J. J., Fuller, W. D., Ali, M. R. (2012). Sleep apnea syndrome is significantly underdiagnosed in bariatric surgical patients. *Surg. Obes. Relat. Dis.,* 8(5):569 - 73.

Romero-Corral, A., Caples, S. M., Lopez-Jimenez, F., Somers, V. K. (2010). Interactions between obesity and obstructive sleep apnea: Implications for treatment. *Chest,* 137(3):711 - 9.

Schwartz, A. R., Patil, S. P., Squier, S., Schneider, H., Kirkness, J. P., Smith, P. L. (2010). Obesity and upper airway control during sleep. *J. Appl. Physiol.,* (1985), 108(2):430 - 5.

Shah, N., Roux, F. (2009). The relationship of obesity and obstructive sleep apnea. *Clin. Chest Med.,* 30(3):455 - 65.

Shah, N., Roux, F. (2009). The relationship of obesity and obstructive sleep apnea. *Clin. Chest Med.,* 30(3):455 - 65.

Shah, U., Wong, J., Wong, D. T., Chung, F. (2016). Preoxygenation and intraoperative ventilation strategies in obese patients: A comprehensive review. *Curr. Opin. Anaesthesiol.,* 29: 109 - 118.

White, D. P. (2005). Pathogenesis of obstructive and central sleep apnea. *Am. J. Respir. Crit. Care Med.,* 172(11):1363 - 70.

Wolk, R., Ahamsuzzaman, A., Somers, V. K. (2003). Obesity, sleep apnea, and hypertension. *Hypertension,* 42: 1067 - 74.

Xiaoping Ming, M. D. et al. (2021). *Surgery for Obesity and Related Diseases,* 17, 215 - 220.

Yeh, P. S., Lee, Y. C., Lee, W. J., Chen, S. B., Ho, S. J., Peng, W. B. et al. (2010). Clinical predictors of obstructive sleep apnea in Asian bariatric patients. *Obes. Surg.,* 20(1):30 - 5.

In: Advances in Sleep Apnea
Editors: F. Lorusso et al.
ISBN: 978-1-53619-758-7

Chapter 15

EFFECT OF OSAS ON INNER EAR

Onofrio Guzzo, Francesco Dispenza*, Salvatore Gallina and Francesco Lorusso
Department of Otolaryngology, Head and Neck Surgery,
Policlinico Paolo Giaccone University of Palermo, Palermo, Italy

ABSTRACT

Obstructive sleep apnea syndrome (OSAS) is a common breathing disorder that occurs during sleep. OSAS is associated with cardiologic, neurologic and metabolic comorbidity, but it's also responsible of a sensorineural hearing loss. In this chapter we will focus on the state of the art on the pathophysiological mechanisms that correlate OSAS with hearing loss and his effects on audiological diagnostic tests.

Continuous Positive Airway Pressure (CPAP) is the main non-surgical therapy of OSAS, can it be used in the treatment of hearing loss-OSAS related?

---

* Corresponding Author's Email: francesco.dispenza@gmail.com.

INTRODUCTION

Over the past decade, interest in sleep and sleep disorders has increased substantially. Most of this renewed interest within the otolaryngology community has been focused on obstructive sleep apnea (OSA), a sleep-related breathing disorder. As the waistline of the average American has grown, so too has the incidence of OSA. Population-based estimates published in 1997 suggested that 2% of women and 4% of men over age 50 have symptomatic OSA, but more recent estimates have demonstrated an increasing prevalence with estimates of moderate-to-severe OSA in 13% to 50% of middle-aged men and 6% to 23% of middle-aged women.

Obstructive sleep-related breathing disorders include snoring, upper airway resistance syndrome (UARS) and Obstructive Sleep Apnea (OSA).

Diagnostic criteria for OSA in adults requires a polysomnogram or home sleep apnea test (HSAT) that demonstrates either (1) 5 or more predominately obstructive respiratory events (obstructive and/or mixed apneas, hypopneas, or Respiratory Effort Related Arousals RERAs) per hour of sleep, in association with symptoms or comorbidities, or (2) 15 or more predominately respiratory events per hour of sleep regardless of symptoms or comorbidities.

Symptoms related to OSA include excessive daytime somnolence, waking with gasping, choking, or breath holding; or witnessed reports of apneas, loud snoring, or both. Comorbidities include hypertension, a mood disorder, cognitive dysfunction, coronary artery disease, stroke, congestive heart failure, atrial fibrillation, or type 2 diabetes mellitus. Diagnosis may be made on in-lab Polysomnography (PSG) or by Home Sleep Apnea Testing (HSAT).

Each episode of apnea or hypopnea must last a minimum of 10 seconds, is commonly accompanied by reductions in blood oxygen saturation of at least 3% to 4%, and is usually terminated by brief, unconscious arousals from sleep. Thus OSA causes fragmentation and disruption of the normal sleep cycle, resulting in symptoms of Excessive Daytime Sleepiness (EDS) and difficulty with concentration and alertness. Snoring between apneas is a frequent complaint of bed partners and is often the symptom that prompts these patients to seek medical attention, although excessive daytime somnolence is a common initial complaint. Many OSA sufferers complain of awakening from sleep with morning headache, sore throat, and fatigue or a feeling of being unrefreshed regardless of the duration of sleep.

According to AASM's (American Academy of Sleep Medicine) 2007 criteria, this classifies mild OSA as 5 to 15 events per hour, moderate as 15 to 30 events, and severe as 30 events or more.

A number of negative health effects have been attributed to untreated OSA, including increased mortality, increased the risk of fatal and nonfatal motor vehicle accidents by 2.5-fold.

In addition, untreated OSA is reported to a significant proportion of the mortality and morbidity related to OSA occurs through its effects on the cardiovascular system, which can result in hypertension, coronary heart disease, congestive heart failure, arrhythmias, pulmonary hypertension, stroke, and sudden death. Untreated moderate and severe OSA has been reported to result in a threefold increase in fatal and nonfatal cardiovascular events, compared with both healthy men without OSA and men with CPAP-treated OSA.

Untreated OSA has been demonstrated to be an independent risk factor for insulin resistance. Recently it has been suggested that OSA may contribute to the development of diabetes and *metabolic syndrome.* However, further research is needed to determine whether there is an independent link between OSA and metabolic abnormalities.

The prevalence of gastroesophageal reflux disease in OSA patients is significantly higher than in the general population. Even though these disorders commonly occur together, no temporal or causal relationship has ever been demonstrated between the two. This may reflect the fact that they share similar risk factors. Treatment of OSA with CPAP has been demonstrated to decrease the occurrence of gastroesophageal reflux disease.

Neurocognitive deficits have also been associated with OSA. Untreated OSA has been documented to cause EDS, impaired mood, problems with attention, working memory, and executive function, all of which are improved with CPAP treatment.

In this chapter we will focus on consequences of OSAS on vestibular system and mostly on the auditory pathway.

EFFECTS ON THE VESTIBULAR SYSTEM

The recurrent apnoic episode, which is so characteristic of OSAS, results in a continuous reduction in the haemoglobin oxygen saturation.

Based on the evidence that the vestibular nuclei are more sensitive to hypoxia than other cerebral nuclei, as demonstrated in animal experiments, Gallina et al. hypothesis is that the functional alteration of the vestibular nuclei may be an index of abnormal activity of the respiratory nuclei considering the anatomical contiguity of this centre. The hypoxic damage could also be the cause of a deficit of the peripheral vestibular system.

The susceptibility of the posterior labyrinth to a hypoxic state was proven by the high percentage of vestibular reflex alterations observed during caloric stimulation. The test results were found to be worse in patients with a severe grade of OSAS.

If the peripheral vestibular system becomes asymmetric due to hypoxic damage, the central vestibular system corrects this disequilibrium between the two sides. S. Gallina et al. results can also indicate that the central vestibular system is more resistant to the hypoxic state. Because of this, a unilateral peripheral vestibular deficit may be well compensated by the central vestibular system and the equilibrium may be restored.

PATHOPHYSIOLOGY OF THE HEARING LOSS

Before going in to the pathophysiology theories correlating OSAS to hearing loss, it is necessary to deepen in the vascular supply of inner ear.

Vascular Supply of Inner Ear

The inner ear is supplied by only one end artery which it named the labyrinthine artery (LA).

The LA mostly derives from the anterior inferior cerebellar artery and most often has three branches within the internal acoustic canal (IAC), namely:

1. the anterior vestibular artery (AVA)
2. the vestibulo-cochlear artery (VCA)
3. the cochlear artery (CA).

The VCA divides into cochlear and vestibular branches which run in opposite directions. The vestibular branch supplies the vestibule and semicircular canals, while the cochlear branch runs spirally along the Scala Vestibuli to anastomose with the CA. The cochlear branch mostly supplies the second quarter of the basal turn, but it sometimes supplies the entire cochlea. The CA is said to be the dominating vessel for the cochlea and can be replaced by the cochlear branch of the VCA. Siebenmann defines this as the 'tractus spiralis arteriosus'. Various descriptions of the venous drainage exist, but there is no general consensus about the descriptions. The venous routes go along the cochlear and vestibular aqueducts with the inferior cochlear vein and vein of the vestibular aqueduct (VA), respectively. Some authors have described a vein in the IAC, but others have denied it.

Several studies have shown a higher prevalence of hearing loss in apneic and snoring patients. The mechanisms underlying this relationship are still to be fully clarified.

There are many physiopathological theories that correlate OSAS to hearing loss, here are the most accredited in the literature.

Oxidative Stress by ROS

The repeated episodes of hypoxia and normoxia are considered the main factors influencing the production of reactive oxygen species (ROS) and the promotion of oxidative stress, endothelial dysregulation, activation and propagation of inflammatory cascades with vascular dysfunction, reduced basal and functional capillarity rarefaction with an additional risk of impaired peripheral perfusion.

Therefore, OSAS may lead to cerebral vascular insufficiency resulting in hypoxia, acute hemodynamic change, decreased cerebral blood flow during episodes of apnea and ischemic injury to the cochlea. Both inner ear and acoustic nerve are highly dependent on the oxygen supply; specifically the cochlea is sensitive to circulatory alterations because of its single terminal artery supply and insufficient collateral circulation. Particularly the cochlear outer hair cells of the basal turn suffer from the free-radical damage, probably because of their significant lower activity of glutathione-related antioxidant enzymes.

Casale et al. reported that the adverse effect of OSAS on the hearing system may be due to intermittent hypoxia and ischemia associated with repeated obstruction of the airways.

Increased Plasma Viscosity

Steiner et al. reported that blood plasma viscosity increases in patients with OSAS and that this compromises microcirculation.

Bernand et al. also reported that this hyperviscosity can lead to impairment of the hearing system.

Acoustic Trauma

On the other hand, hearing impairment could be attributable to chronic noise to which snoring patients are exposed (acoustic trauma).

Ekin et al. suggested that hearing loss was the result of exposure to constant noise from snoring rather than the occurrence of hypoxia.

This hypothesis are still to be proven, and studies have not yet shown definite clinical and auxiliary evidence.

Studies performed by Hoffestein et al., which analyzed the correlation between snoring and presbycusis, based on an analysis of audiometry tests in snoring patients, have not demonstrated a significant impact on hearing and have shown that snoring is not a factor that influences hearing.

M. C. Spinosi et al. results show distribution of hearing loss in different groups that appear to be independent from the presence or absence of snoring, either complicated or uncomplicated by mild OSAS. No correlation between auditory performance in snoring patients with particular alterations or audiological pattern was detected.

Based on M. C. Spinosi et al. study, chronic exposure to noise in simple snoring patients and patients with mild OSAS does not seem to be a predisposing or causative factor of hearing loss.

Decreased Oxyhemoglobin Saturation

In Y.J. See et al. study Oxyhemoglobin saturation, especially the lowest oxyhemoglobin saturation level, showed lower thresholds in the hearing impairment group than in the control group ($p = 0.039$ at NREM stage; $p = 0.029$ at REM stage; $p = 0.001$ at total sleep stage). After adjusting for other risk factors, the sole variable that remained significant was lowest oxyhemoglobin saturation (total; $p = 0.046$). In the correlation analysis, a decreasing lowest oxyhemoglobin saturation (from all subjects, $n = 41$) correlated with a greater mean hearing threshold ($R(2) = 0.297$; $p < 0.001$).

Their results indicated that lowest oxyhemoglobin saturation in polysomnography is the only variable correlated with the hearing threshold. This finding could be predictive of possible hearing alternation in patients with severe OSAS.

A Role Played by Hair-Cell Mitochondria: A Mouse-Based Study

Investigating the exact pathophysiology of OSAS comorbidities and the genes related to them is critical. However, patients with OSAS commonly display a variety of confounding factors that may result in a misinterpretation of results, even after meticulous analysis. These factors limit the potential of determining causal associations between OSAS and its consequences. To overcome this obstacle, animals exposed to Chronic Intermittent Hypoxia (CIH) have been established as models of OSAS and are widely utilized to study possible phenotypes and provide insights into the pathophysiology of various OSAS-induced complications.

In Y.J. See et al. study of a mouse model of OSAS, they observed that CIH had an adverse effect on auditory function as well as of mitochondria being part of the pathophysiology of hearing impairment. They observed that hair-cell mitochondria in CIH mice were fewer compared to that in Sham and also displayed an aberrant morphology. The mRNA levels of PGC-1α and Tfam were higher in the CIH group than in the Sham group. Moreover, the expression of Voltage-Dependent Anion Channel (VDAC) was increased in the tectorial membrane, the basilar membrane, and especially in the inner hair cells of CIH mice. Further investigation is required to determine whether mitochondria could serve as a valid target for preventive or therapeutic purposes.

Effects on Diagnostic Tests

Scientific literature is full of results concerning the impact of OSAS on auditory pathway studied by audiological diagnostic tests, like audiometric, speech discrimination, Transient Evoked Otoacoustic Emissions (TEOAE), auditory processing, sequencing tests (Duration Pattern Test DPT, Frequency Pattern Test FPT) and Auditory Brainstem Response (ABR).

M.S. Gozeler et al. determined a mild sensorineural hearing loss in patients with OSAS, indeed, hearing threshold values in the patients with OSAS were significantly higher compared to the control group at 500, 1000, 2000, 4000, and 8000 Hz in both ears. No statistically significant difference was observed in TEOAE test results between the patient and control groups in terms of Signal Noise Ratio (SNR) or amplitude values. However, test reproducibility values in both ears were significantly lower in the study group compared to the control group.

In the A. İriz et al. study, the auditory pathways were tested via speech discrimination rates, central processing, and sequencing tests in moderate-to-severe OSAS patients and control subjects with normal hearing thresholds. A significant loss in speech discrimination was found in the OSAS patients compared to the control group. Likewise, significant deterioration was found in both auditory processing and sequencing tests (DPT, FPT) in OSAS patients compared to the control group. As a result, it was found that cochlear processing and central auditory damage could occur before the presentation of apparent hearing loss in OSAS patients.

Martines et al. reported that the hearing thresholds of OSAS patients at extended high frequencies were significantly higher than those of patients with simple snoring. However, they also reported that mean hearing thresholds between the frequencies of 250 and 8000 Hz did not differ between individuals with OSAS and simple snoring. At the TEOAE test, significantly lower SNR values were determined only at frequencies of 3000 and 4000 Hz between the severe OSAS and simple snoring groups.

Casale et al. reported that mean hearing thresholds were within normal limits in patients with OSAS, but that these were significantly higher than those of the control group. Additionally, when individual frequencies were analyzed, hearing thresholds at 4000 Hz were significantly higher than those of the control group. In the TEOAE test, they observed significantly lower reproducibility and SNR values in patients with OSAS compared with the control group. Similarly, Matsumura et al. observed no significant difference between groups in terms of mean hearing thresholds but determined significantly higher hearing thresholds at high frequencies of the OSAS group as compared to the control group. Ballaccihino et al. determined significantly high hearing loss in individuals at risk of OSAS with the STOP-BANG questionnaire and significantly low SNR values using the TEOAE test.

Ekin et al. reported that hearing thresholds were not affected at low and high frequencies in individuals with OSAS and/or simple snoring compared to the control group, but observed significantly high hearing thresholds at extended high frequencies. When subjects with simple snoring and the OSAS were compared, however, they determined no difference in hearing thresholds at any frequencies.

Auditory Brainstem Response (ABR) and OSAS

In clinic, the integrity of auditory neural pathway is generally examined by ABR elicited by a series of impulse sounds via airor bone-conduction ways. The ABR reflects the synaptic activity of auditory brainstem neurons, and makes it a useful tool in studying the functional integrity for OSAS. Some studies reported prolonged peak latencies and latencies in wave intervals such as I–V and III–V of the click-evoked auditory brainstem response (click-ABR) in OSAS patients.

The pathophysiologic mechanism may be accounted for by the neurotransmitter synthesis disorders and the abnormal conduction of the nerve impulse in the auditory pathway, which is due to hyperlipidemia caused by respiratory disturbances. However, other studies claimed that no abnormal click-ABR found in the OSAS patients, suggesting no acute or chronic injury in the auditory brainstem caused by repeated nocturnal hypoxemia. These conflicting findings inspire the need of new methods and more sophisticated studies in this regard.

Speech-Evoked Auditory Brainstem Response (Speech-ABR) and OSAS

Speech-evoked Auditory Brainstem Response (speech-ABR) is a new technique of auditory evoked brainstem response in recent years. A commonly used stimulus is a 40-ms synthesized syllable /*da*/. The speech-ABR elicited by/*da*/contains seven feature peaks termed waves V-A-C-D-E-F-O, which are commonly analyzed in both time and frequency domains.

It was reported that the transient components of speech-ABR showed significant abnormalities for some patients, such as learning problem children (LPC) and persistent developmental stuttering (PDS) population, while these patients are with normal click-ABR. These findings suggest that speech-ABR may be a more effective method for detecting auditory function than click-ABR. Therefore, speech-ABR may play a role in the study of neurological status of auditory system, and may be a useful tool to detect the early impairments of neurological functions in patients with OSAS.

By comparing the latency of these waves, we found that OSAS patients appeared to have longer latency values than the control group for the transient portion of the speech-ABR (except for peak A).

Statistical analysis results show that there are significant latency differences between OSAS and control groups for peak V, peak C, and peak O ($P<0.05$). No significant latency differences are founded for peak A, peak D, peak E and peak F ($P>0.05$).

CONCLUSION

Obstructive sleep apnea syndrome (OSAS) is a common breathing disorder that occurs during sleep.

Recent estimates have demonstrated an increasing prevalence with estimates of moderate-to-severe OSA in 13% to 50% of middle-aged men and 6% to 23% of middle-aged women.

The targets of OSAS are innumerable, and the auditory path is one of them. The damage of the auditory pathway is manifested by sensorineural hearing loss. There are many physiopathological theories set out that try to explain the mechanisms of OSAS that determine hearing loss like oxidative stress by ROS, decreased oxyhemoglobin saturation, increased plasma viscosity, acoustic trauma mediated by snoring.

Cause of OSAS is the cause of hearing loss in some patients, in the M. Deniz et al. study, they evaluated whether patients using a continuous positive airway pressure (CPAP) device for obstructive sleep apnea syndrome (OSAS) have improvement or deterioration in their auditory systems.

No improvement in the hearing system on the patients using a CPAP device was detected. Deterioration in hearing was detected in 13.63% and 9.09% of the patients with and without CPAP use, respectively. No statistically significant difference was found between the two groups.

Q. Fu et al. reported that the transient components of speech-ABR were significantly and positively correlated with the AHI in mild and moderate OSAS patients, while the change in conventional click-ABR is not detectable. As these components reflect the coding of temporal information in speech syllable, this finding suggests that OSAS may be responsible for the deficits of temporal information processing which can be represented by the speech-ABR. Thus speech-ABR can be a potential biomarker in the diagnosis and evaluation at early stage of OSAS.

Further investigation of its mechanisms could assist in establishing a detailed pathophysiology of OSAS-induced hearing disturbance and related therapy.

References

Ballacchino A, Salvago P, Cannizzaro E, et al. Association between sleep-disordered breathing and hearing disorders; clinical observation insicilian patients. *Acta Med Mediterr.* 2015; 31:607–14.

Bernáth I, McNamara P, Szternák N, Szakács Z, Köves P, Terray-Horváth A, Vida Z. Hyperviscosity as a possible cause of positive acoustic evoked potential findings in patients with sleep apnea: a dual electrophysiological and hemorheological study. *Sleep Med.* 2009 Mar; 10(3):361-7. doi: 10.1016/j.sleep.2008.03.012. Epub 2008 Jul 24. PMID: 18656422.

Bruno A, Di Sano C, Lorusso F, Dino P, Russo D, Ballacchino A, Gallina S, Modica DM, Chiappara G, Simon HU, Pace E. Notch-1 decreased expression contributes to leptin receptor downregulation in nasal epithelium from allergic turbinates. *Biochim Biophys Acta Mol Basis Dis.* 2019 Jun 1; 1865(6):1642-1650.

Cadby, et al: Severity of OSA is an independent predictor of incident atrial fibrillation hospitalization in a large sleep-clinic cohort, *Chest* 148:945–952, 2015.

Casale M, Vesperini E, Potena M, Pappacena M, Bressi F, Baptista PJ, Salvinelli F. Is obstructive sleep apnea syndrome a risk factor for auditory pathway? *Sleep Breath.* 2012 Jun; 16(2):413-7. doi: 10. 1007/s11325-011-0517-x. Epub 2011 Apr 9. PMID: 21479758.

Deniz M, Ersözlü T. Evaluation of the changes in the hearing system over the years among patients with OSAS using a CPAP device. *Cranio.* 2020 Jun 28:1-4. doi: 10.1080/08869634.2020.1783050. Epub ahead of print. PMID: 32597382.

Dispenza F, Mazzucco W, Mazzola S, Martines F. Observational study on risk factors determining residual dizziness after successful benign paroxysmal positional vertigo treatment: The role of subclinical BPPV. *Acta Otorhinolaryngol Ital,* 2019; 347-352.

Ekin S, Turan M, Arısoy A, Gunbatar H, Sunnetcioglu A, Asker S, Yıldız H. Is There a Relationship Between Obstructive Sleep Apnea (OSA) and Hearing Loss? *Med Sci Monit.* 2016 Sep 2; 22:3124-8. doi: 10.12659/msm.897347. PMID: 27588548; PMCID: PMC5019138.

Fu Q, Wang T, Liang Y, Lin Y, Zhao X, Wan J, Fan S. Auditory Deficits in Patients With Mild and Moderate Obstructive Sleep Apnea Syndrome: A Speech Syllable Evoked Auditory Brainstem Response Study. *Clin Exp Otorhinolaryngol.* 2019 Feb; 12(1):58-65. doi: 10.21053/ceo.2018.00017. Epub 2018 Aug 24. PMID: 30134647; PMCID: PMC6315215.

Gallina S, Dispenza F, Kulamarva G, Riggio F, Speciale R. Obstructive sleep apnoea syndrome (OSAS): effects on the vestibular system. *Acta Otorhinolaryngol Ital.* 2010 Dec; 30(6):281-4. PMID: 21808447; PMCID: PMC3146317.

Gozeler MS, Sengoz F. Auditory Function of Patients with Obstructive Sleep Apnea Syndrome: A Study. *Eurasian J Med.* 2020 Jun; 52(2):176-179. doi: 10.5152/eurasianjmed.2019.18373. Epub 2020 Jun 4. PMID: 32612427; PMCID: PMC7311141.

Graf KI, Karaus M, Heinemann S, et al: Gastroesophageal reflux in patients with sleep apnea syndrome, *Z Gastroenterol* 33(12):689–693, 1995.

He J, Kryger MH, Zorick FJ, et al: Mortality and apnea index in obstructive sleep apnea. Experience in 385 male patients, *Chest* 94(1):9–14, 1988.

Heinemann S, Graf KI, Karaus M, et al: Occurrence of obstructive sleep related respiratory disorder in conjunction with gastroesophageal reflux, *Pneumologie* 49(Suppl 1):139–141, 1995.

Heinzer, et al: Prevalence of sleep-disordered breathing in the general population: the HypnoLaus study, *Lancet Respir Med* 3:310–318, 2015.

Hoffstein V., Haight J., Cole P., Zamel N.: Does snoring contribute to presbycusis? *Am J Respir. Crit. Care Med.* 1999; 159: 1351–1354.

Hung, et al: Association of sleep apnoea with myocardial infarction in men, *Lancet* 336:261–264, 1990.

Ip MS, Lam B, Ng MM, et al: Obstructive sleep apnea is independently associated with insulin resistance, *Am J Respir Crit Care Med* 165(5):670–676, 2002.

İriz A, Düzlü M, Köktürk O, Kemaloğlu YK, Eravcı FC, Küükünal IS, Karamert R. The effect of obstructive sleep apnea syndrome on the central auditory system. *Turk J Med Sci.* 2018 Feb 23; 48(1):5-9. doi: 10.3906/sag-1705-66. PMID: 29479935.

Johnson, et al: Frequency of sleep apnea in stroke and TIA patients: a meta-analysis, *J Clin Sleep Med* 6:131–137, 2010.

Loke, et al: Association of obstructive sleep apnea with risk of serious cardiovascular events: a systematic review and meta-analysis, *Circ Cardiovasc Qual Outcomes* 5:720–728, 2012.

Lorusso F, Dispenza F, Modica DM, Gallina S. The Role of Modified Expansion Sphincter Pharyngoplasty in Multilevel Obstructive Sleep Apnea Syndrome Surgery. *Int Arch Otorhinolaryngol.* 2018 Oct; 22(4):432-436.

Lorusso F, Dispenza F, Saraniti C, Sireci F, Modica DM, Gallina S. Sleep disordered breathing: evaluation of dynamic patterns of the upper airways in obese subjects. *Otorinolaringologia* 2014; 64:57–64.

Lorusso F, Gallina S, Modica DM, Di Salvo N, Riggio F. Bipolar Quantum Molecular Resonance versus *Blunt Dissection tonsillectomy. B-ENT* 2015; 11(02):101–108.

Lorusso, F., Dispenza, F., Martinciglio, G., ...Battaglia, A., Gallina, S. Postural changes in patients undergoing hyoid surgery for OSAS. EuroMediterranean *Biomedical Journal,* 2017; 12(29):140-143.

Lorusso, F., Martines, F., Mistretta, A., ...Dispenza, F., Gallina, S.Effects of adenotonsillectomy on neurocognitive and behavioural function in pediatric obstructive sleep apnea syndrome. *B-ENT* 2018; 14:113-118.

Marin JM, Carrizo SJ, Vicente E, et al: Long-term cardiovascular outcomes in men with obstructive sleep apnoea-hypopnoea with or without treatment with continuous positive airway pressure: an observational study, *Lancet* 365(9464):1046–1053, 2005.

Martines F, Ballacchino A, Sireci F, Mucia M, La Mattina E, Rizzo S, Salvago P. Audiologic profile of OSAS and simple snoring patients: the effect of chronic nocturnal intermittent hypoxia on auditory function. *Eur Arch Otorhinolaryngol.* 2016 Jun; 273(6):1419-24. doi: 10.1007/s00405-015-3714-6. Epub 2015 Jul 12. PMID: 26164293.

Martines F, Dispenza F, Montlbano C, Priola R, Torrente A, La Gumina R, Brighina F, Galletti F, Salvago P. Comparison of electrocochleography and video head impulse test findings in vestibular migraine and ménière disease: A preliminary study. *J Int Adv Otol* 2020; 183-189.

Matsumura E, Matas CG, Magliaro FCL, Pedreño RM, Lorenzi-Filho G, Sanches SGG, Carvallo RMM. Evaluation of peripheral auditory pathways and brainstem in obstructive sleep apnea. *Braz J Otorhinolaryngol.* 2016 Nov 25:S1808-8694(16)30233-6. doi: 10. 1016/j.bjorl.2016.10.014. Epub ahead of print. PMID: 28024827.

Mei X, Atturo F, Wadin K, Larsson S, Agrawal S, Ladak HM, Li H, Rask-Andersen H. Human inner ear blood supply revisited: the Uppsala collection of temporal bone-an international resource of education and collaboration. *Ups J Med Sci.* 2018 Sep;123(3):131-142. doi: 10.1080/03009734.2018.1492654. Epub 2018 Sep 11. PMID: 30204028; PMCID: PMC6198224.

Modica DM, Lorusso F, Presti G, Fasola S, Gallina S. Our Assessment Using Palate Postoperative Problems Score (PPOPS): Tool for the Evaluation of Results in Palatal Surgery Techniques. *Indian J Otolaryngol Head Neck Surg.* 2019 Oct; 71(Suppl 1):766-770.

Modica DM, Marchese D, Lorusso F, Speciale R, Saraniti C, Gallina S. Functional Nasal Surgery and Use of CPAP in OSAS Patients: Our Experience. *Indian J Otolaryngol Head Neck Surg.* 2018 Dec; 70(4):559-565.

Peppard, et al.: Increased prevalence of sleep-disordered breathing in adults, *Am J Epidemiol* 177(9):1006–1014, 2013.

Peppard, et al.: Prospective study of the association between sleep-disordered breathing and hypertension, *N Engl J Med* 342:1378–1384, 2000.

Quan SF, Wright R, Baldwin CM, et al: Obstructive sleep apnea-hypopnea and neurocognitive functioning in the sleep heart health study, *Sleep Med* 7(6):498–507, 2006.

Redline, et al: Obstructive sleep apnea–hypopnea and incident stroke, *Am J Respir Crit Care Med* 182: 269–277, 2010.

Sardesai M.G., Tan A.K., Fitzpatrick M.: Noise-induced hearing loss in snorers and their bed partners. *J. Otolaryngol.* 2003; 32: 141–145.

Sassani A, Findley LJ, Kryger M, et al: Reducing motor-vehicle collisions, costs, and fatalities by treating obstructive sleep apnea syndrome, *Sleep* 27(3):453–458, 2004.

Seo YJ, Chung HJ, Park SY, Kim CH, Lee JG, Kim SH, Cho HJ. Lowest Oxyhemoglobin Saturation May Be an Independent Factor Influencing Auditory Function in Severe Obstructive Sleep Apnea. *J Clin Sleep Med.* 2016 May 15;12(5):653-8. doi: 10.5664/jcsm.5786. PMID: 26857050; PMCID: PMC4865550.

Seo YJ, Ju HM, Lee SH, Kwak SH, Kang MJ, Yoon JH, Kim CH, Cho HJ. Damage of Inner Ear Sensory Hair Cells via Mitochondrial Loss in a Murine Model of Sleep Apnea With Chronic Intermittent Hypoxia. *Sleep.* 2017 Sep 1; 40(9). doi: 10.1093/sleep/zsx106. PMID: 28934520.

Sha SH, Taylor R, Forge A, Schacht J (2001) Differential vulnerability of basal and apical hair cells is based on intrinsic susceptibility to free radicals. *Hear Res* 155:1–8.

Siebenmann F. *Die Blutgefässa des Labyrinthes des menschlichen Ohres* [*The blood vessels of the labyrinth of the human ear*]. Wiesbaden, Germany: C. F. Bergmann; 1894.

Spinosi MC, D'Amico F, Passali G, Cingi C, Rodriguez H, Passali D. Hearing loss in mild OSAS and simple snoring patients. *Otolaryngol Pol.* 2017 Apr 30; 71(2):11-15. doi: 10.5604/01.3001.0009.8409. PMID: 28485295.

Steiner S, Jax T, Evers S, Hennersdorf M, Schwalen A, Strauer BE. Altered blood rheology in obstructive sleep apnea as a mediator of cardiovascular risk. *Cardiology.* 2005; 104(2):92-6. doi: 10.1159/000086729. Epub 2005 Jul 7. PMID: 16015032.

Tawk M, Goodrich S, Kinasewitz G, et al: The effect of 1 week of continuous positive airway pressure treatment in obstructive sleep apnea patients with concomitant gastroesophageal reflux, *Chest* 130(4):1003–1008, 2006.

Teramoto S, Ohga E, Matsui H, et al: Obstructive sleep apnea syndrome may be a significant cause of gastroesophageal reflux disease in older people, *J Am Geriatr Soc* 47(10):1273–1274, 1999.

Yoshida S, Sasa M, Takaori S. Different sensitivity to hypoxia in neuronal activities of lateral vestibular and spinal trigemi- nal nuclei. *Stroke* 1988;19:357-64.

Young T, Evans L, Finn L, et al: Estimation of the clinically diagnosed proportion of sleep apnea syndrome in middle-aged men and women, *Sleep* 20(9):705–706, 1997.

In: Advances in Sleep Apnea
Editors: F. Lorusso et al.
ISBN: 978-1-53619-758-7

Chapter 16

ADVANCES IN REHABILITATION IN OSAS

Roberta Priola, Salvatore Gallina, Angelo Torrente and Francesco Lorusso**
Department of Otolaryngology, Head and Neck Surgery,
Policlinico Paolo Giaccone University of Palermo, Palermo, Italy

ABSTRACT

The treatment of obstructive sleep apnea syndrome (OSAS) is focused on increasing airway patency during sleep and, to date, continuous positive airway pressure (CPAP) represents the treatment of choice to improve upper airway obstruction. Unfortunately, such technique is poor tolerated and nonadherent patients range between 29 and 83%. In some cases, other therapeutical approaches to consider are constituted by oral appliance or surgical treatment, but they may be not sufficient too. Recently, new methods for OSAS rehabilitation have been investigated to customize the treatment for each patient. Positional therapy (PT), myofunctional therapy (MT), body exercises training and upper-airway stimulation of the hypoglossal nerve are some examples of OSAS rehabilitative approaches to use alone or in association with other different techniques. Such rehabilitative approaches for OSAS patients will be discussed in this chapter.

* Corresponding Author's Email: dott.francescolorusso@gmail.com.

INTRODUCTION

Obstructive sleep apnea syndrome (OSAS) is a sleep disorder characterized by episodes of partial or complete upper-airway collapse, with reduction or interruption of airflow. Prevalence in general adult population ranges from 13% to 33% in men and from 6% to 19% in women.

There are several risk factors that increase the prevalence of such disease and obesity is the most important one. Pathogenetically, increased adipose tissue within the tongue and pharynx compromises upper-airways diameters and makes them more prone to collapse during sleep. However, it is likely that both elevated mechanical load and impaired neuromuscular response are required for the development of OSA. The mechanical load may be even due to a restricted lung expansion caused both by abdominal and chest wall fat accumulation, impairing diaphragmatic excursion and rib cage expansion, respectively. Functional residual capacity and residual volume are, therefore, reduced in obese individuals and this dysfunction reduces tracheal caudal traction, increasing upper airways collapsibility. Moreover, imaging of the upper airways has consistently shown a reduction of their size, predominantly in the lateral dimensions; this alteration has been variously attributed to an increased size of the lateral pharyngeal fat pads or to an increased muscle thickness in the lateral pharyngeal wall. Moreover, another mechanism pointed out is that obesity causes elevated levels of inflammatory cytokines, including tumor necrosis factor-α, and such alteration increases daytime sleepiness.

Other important risk factors for this syndrome include male sex, increased tonsillar and adenoid tissue and certain craniofacial abnormalities (e.g., retrognathia and maxillary insufficiency). Above all the predisposing conditions, adenotonsillar hypertrophy, obesity, and hypotonic neuromuscular disease are the most common causes of OSA in children.

Four main pathogenetic factors may be found in OSAS: ventilatory response to disturbances (loop gain), pharyngeal anatomy/collapsibility, upper airways recruitment threshold and arousal threshold. There are several dilator muscles that behave in a complex and coordinated manner to maintain airway patency. The genioglossus, an inspiratory phasic muscle, is the major upper airway dilator muscle, which is important for the protrusion and retraction of the tongue. The genioglossus is a typically inspiratory phasic muscle with tonic activity during expiration.

A patient with OSAS shows both nocturnal and daytime symptoms: nocturnal symptoms include snoring, apneas, sudden awakenings with a feeling of suffocation (gasping or choking) and nocturia; daytime symptoms can include awakening headache, excessive sleepiness, dry mouth feeling, concentration difficulties and memory issues. Moreover, OSAS patients show a higher risk of congestive heart failure, atrial fibrillation, treatment refractory hypertension, type 2 diabetes, stroke, pulmonary hypertension and, moreover, they represent a dangerous driving population.

The diagnosis of the patient with suspected OSAS includes an evaluation of sleep, clinical tools and questionnaires. In particular, OSAS diagnosis is based on sleep study and polysomnography (PSG) is the gold standard test in adult patients. The third edition of the International Classification of Sleep Disorders (ICSD-3) defines the diagnosis of OSA as the presence of an obstructive respiratory disturbance index (RDI) ≥ 5 events/h at the PSG associated with the typical symptoms of OSA or an obstructive RDI ≥ 15 events/h, even in the absence of symptoms. As far as clinical questionnaires are concerned, the most used are the Epworth Sleepiness Scale (ESS), Berlin Questionnaire, STOP-BANG questionnaire, STOP questionnaire and OSA50 questionnaire,

The gold standard for OSAS therapy is the use of Continuous Positive Airway Pressure (C-PAP) devices, that determine the opening of the upper airway and have been shown to normalize sleep architecture, reducing daily and nightly symptoms and the related complications. Unfortunately, due to several factors, such as mask discomfort, nasal congestion, local irritation, and claustrophobia, C-PAP devices are hardly tolerated. Consequently, adherence to C-PAP, defined as the use of the device for at least 4 hours per night, is very variable and some studies show how nonadherent patients range from 29 to 83%.

There are several surgical procedures able to reduce Pcrit and to enlarge the diameter of upper airway and there are a lot of different techniques used in OSA patient. Some examples are constituted by functional nose surgery, tonsillectomy and soft palate surgery. Other surgical procedures are hyoid bone suspension, maxillomandibular osteotomy, mandibular distraction osteogenesis and transoral robotic surgery (TORS). Furthermore, patients with mild or moderate OSA or patients with severe OSA that refuse C-PAP therapy may benefit from oral appliances such as mandibular advancement devices (MAD).

In addition to the already widely used therapies described above, possible treatment options have been developed as a method to treat OSA and they have shown promising in feasibility trials. Positional therapy, myofunctional therapy (MT), body exercises training and upper-airway stimulation of the hypoglossal nerve (HGN) are some of these therapies. More than 50% of cases of OSA are worse or exist solely in certain positions, which is typically the supine position in most cases. Positional therapy (PT) aims at preventing sleep in the supine position. Since the dilator muscles of the upper airway play a critical role in maintaining an open airway during sleep and weight is the first risk factor of OSA, researchers have explored body exercises and other airway training that target oral cavity and oropharyngeal structures as a method to treat OSA.

1. Positional Therapy

There are certain patients who present apneas just in some sleeping positions, notably in the supine position (i.e., Positional OSA – POSA). Although several definitions have been utilized in literature, currently there are no universal criteria for the diagnosis of POSA. Cartwright defined POSA as a difference of 50% or more in the apnea index between supine and non-supine position. It has been demonstrated that P-Crit is higher in the supine position when compared with the lateral position, indicating a higher collapsibility of the upper airway in the first case. Markund et al. defined POSA as supine AHI ≥ 10/h with lateral AHI < 10/h. Mador et al. and Permut et al. added to Cartwright's definition that non-supine AHI should be < 5/h to qualify as POSA. Bignold et al. excluded mild OSA from their definition of POSA. They defined POSA as an overall AHI ≥ 15/h, with supine AHI twice the non-supine AHI, ≥ 20 min of sleep in supine and non-supine postures and a non-supine AHI < 15/h. Frank et al. proposed a new classification called Amsterdam Positional OSA Classification (APOC). The diagnostic criteria to diagnose POSA are:

1. Diagnosis of OSA according to the American Academy of Sleep Medicine (AASM) criteria
2. More than 10% of the total sleep time (TST) recorded both in the best sleeping position (BSP) and in the worst sleeping position (WSP)
3. APOC I: have a BSP AHI <5/h
   APOC II: have a BSP AHI in a lower OSA severity category than in WSP
   APOC III: have an overall AHI of at least 40/h with a reduction of 25% or more in BSP AHI.

APOC I may be treated with just Positional Therapy (PT) resulting in an AHI < 5, patients in APOC II and III can benefit from PT resulting in a less invasive primary treatment.

The APOC system showed a sensitivity of 98%, a specificity of 88%, a positive predictive value of 89% and a negative predictive value of 98% compared to other classifications.

Usually, 70% to 80% of patients with POSA have mild or moderate OSA.

The patients with POSA show an inverse relationship between POSA and body mass index (BMI). Moreover, when compared with non-POSA patients, they show to have a smaller neck circumference, a more backward positioning of the lower jaw, lower facial height, longer posterior airway space measurements, and a smaller volume of lateral pharyngeal wall tissue.

As already mentioned, in this particular group of patients, there is indication for a specific therapy, called positional therapy (PT), used to avoid the worst sleeping position causing POSA. Various devices have been tested, such as positional alarms. The tennis ball technique (TBT) represents the traditional PT: TBT works causing discomfort when sleeping supine, forcing the patient to roll into a non-supine position. Although it reduces AHI, it provokes backache, discomfort, and a deterioration of sleep quality or daytime alertness and this implies a reduction in compliance and in long-term results.

Recent technological advances have renewed the interest in PT for the treatment of POSA. Some new devices used are represented by chest-worn and neck-worn devices.

The chest-worn devices are two and they are the "position monitoring and supine alarm device" and the Sleep Position Trainer (SPT); both devices are fastened to the chest with a strap, so that the device is located on the sternum and provide a vibrating stimulus if the supine position is identified through an internal position-sensitive tilt switch or a 3-dimensional digital accelerometer.

The original neck-worn device was described by van Maanen et al. and consisted of a small vibrating apparatus powered by 3 small batteries. The position sensor provided a vibrating stimulus with a delay of 10s after the supine position was assumed and until a different sleeping position was detected. Anyway, the use of this system has been abandoned. Levendowski et al. described the Neck Position Therapy Device (Night Shift Sleep Positioner, Advanced Brain Monitoring, Carlsbad, CA), a small battery-powered device fixed on the back of the neck with an adjustable non-latex silicone rubber strap secured by a magnetic clasp. Using a 3-dimensional digital accelerometer, a vibrating stimulus is provided if the patient assumes the supine sleeping position.

A lightweight semirigid synthetic foam (Zzoma Positional Device) device was studied by Permut et al. The Zzoma Positional Device is worn on the back, with the elastic belts brought around each side of the patient and secured anteriorly. The device, with its particular shape, keeps the patients positioned on their side and prevents the supine position.

A triangular pillow with space to place arms (SONA Pillow, Kissimmee, Florida) was used by Zuberi et al. to promote persistent lateral positioning and downward positioning of the jaw during sleep.

Among the devices described above, the Night Shift, the Zzoma Positional Device and the SONA Pillow are the ones approved by the US Food and Drug Administration for the treatment of POSA.

Permut et al. compared PT with CPAP therapy in patients with mild-to-moderate OSA. They found no difference between the two therapeutical approaches in reduction of AHI to less than 5 events per hour (92% and 97%, respectively), in sleep quality, in nocturnal oxygenation, and in the increase of the lowest SaO_2. Moreover, 50% of patients preferred PT, 34% preferred CPAP therapy, and 16% had no preference.

Additionally, Benoist et al. compared PT versus oral appliance therapy (OAT) and showed an equal result at short-term in reducing the median AHI in patients with mild to moderate POSA.

Van Maanen et al. investigated the influence of sleeping position in palatal surgery. They showed that, in patients who previously underwent uvulopalatopharyngoplasty (UPPP) or Z-palatoplasty with or without radiofrequency ablation of the tongue base, the reduction in AHI was significantly higher in non-positional OSA patients compared to POSA ones. They suggested to apply PT after surgery or even to start with PT as monotherapy prior to surgery. Benoist et al. performed another study to treat residual POSA in patients who underwent partial effective upper airway surgery with additional PT. They obtained a positive effect of additional treatment with PT in about one third of the patients. The overall treatment response was 37.5% and the compliance rate with PT was 89.0%.

Finally, a 12 months follow-up of PT was performed by de Ruiter et al. They demonstrated that a significant decrease in AHI and ODI compared to baseline was maintained and no changes in sleep efficiency was found. Moreover, the adherence to therapy per night was high (5.2/h) even after 12 months.

2. Orofacial Myofunctional Therapy and Body Exercises

2.1. Orofacial Myofunctional Therapy

The site of primary collapse typically lies within a small segment of the oropharynx, where the collapse is a consequence of the sleep state-dependent tone reduction of the upper airway dilator muscles. In particular, genioglossus is the largest and the most powerful upper airway dilator, even if its activation alone may be insufficient to reduce pharyngeal collapsibility.

Generally, orofacial and pharyngeal muscles dysfunction and impaired oropharyngeal control are possible contributing factors to airway collapse, mainly when associated with an anatomical predisposition. Patients with OSA are classified in four pathophysiological traits based on: the passive critical closing pressure of the upper airway (P-Crit), arousal threshold, loop gain, and muscle responsiveness (following PALM classification, 1,2a,2b,3). It has been demonstrated that patients in three of the four PALM categories will benefit from anatomic interventions. Among these, therapeutic procedures of muscle training are used to improve OSA. There is proof that muscle training during wakefulness is able reduce upper airway collapsibility during sleep in patients with OSAS. Orofacial myofunctional therapy (OMT), or oropharyngeal exercises, with the promotion of changes in dysfunctional upper airway muscles, is believed to reduce consistently OSA severity and its associated symptoms in adults. In particular, such exercises are derived from speech therapy and consist of isometric and isotonic exercises involving the tongue, the soft palate and the lateral pharyngeal walls and the epiglottis. The basic exercises include functions such as suction, swallowing, chewing, breathing, and speech.

Guimaraes et al. proposed several exercises to improve upper oropharyngeal muscles tone. They proposed precise exercises for each group of muscles:

- **Soft palate.** Pronouncing an oral vowel intermittently (isotonic exercise) and continuously (isometric exercise). These exercises recruit the palatopharyngeus, palatoglossus, uvula, tensor veli palatini, and levator veli palatini muscles. These exercises have to be repeated daily for 3 minutes.
- **Tongue.** (1) Brushing the superior and lateral surfaces of the tongue while the tongue is positioned in the floor of the mouth (five times each movement, three times a day); (2) placing the tip of the tongue against the front of the palate and sliding the

tongue backward (a total of 3 minutes throughout the day); (3) forced tongue sucking upward against the palate, pressing the entire tongue against the palate (a total of 3 minutes throughout the day); (4) forcing the back of the tongue against the floor of the mouth while keeping the tip of the tongue in contact with the inferior incisive teeth (a total of 3 minutes throughout the day). The dimensions of the tongue (area and volume) are significantly associated with upper airway collapsibility and AHI. Furthermore, in patients with OSA, the tongue fat (in mm^3) is more represented than in control patients. The increased tongue volume leads to a reduction of the air space in the retroglossal region, thus increasing the risk of obstructive sleep apnea. The suprahyoid muscles, such as the geniohyoid, stylohyoid, mylohyoid, anterior digastric and posterior digastric muscles, together with the styloglossus and genioglossus muscles, participate in the tongue positioning during rest, sleep and deglutition. During some OMT exercises (2 and 3) it is stimulated also an increase in resistance and fatigue threshold of these muscles. Moreover, suprahyoid muscles determine the elevation of the tongue and displace the hyoid bone in an anterior and upper direction. Therefore, another result of OMT may be a higher positioning of the hyoid bone, which appears to be positioned lower in patients with OSA.

- **Facial.** These exercises recruit the orbicularis oris, buccinator, major zygomaticus, minor zygomaticus, levator labii superioris, levator anguli oris, lateral pterygoid, and medial pterygoid muscles. The volume and flaccidity of the cheeks may be an additional predictor of OSA risk corresponding on fat deposition also affecting the tongue and pharynx. The exercises include: (1) Orbicularis oris muscle pressure with mouth closed (isometric exercise). Recruited to close with pressure for 30 seconds, and right after, requested to realize the posterior exercise. (2) Suction movements contracting only the buccinator; performed with repetitions (isotonic) and holding position (isometric). (3) Recruitment of the buccinator muscle against the finger that is introduced in the oral cavity, pressing the buccinator muscle outward. (4) Alternated elevation of the mouth angle muscle (isometric exercise) and after, with repetitions (isotonic exercise). Patients are requested to complete 10 intermittent elevations three times. (5) Lateral jaw movements with alternating elevation of the mouth angle muscle (isometric exercise).

Guimaraes et al. proposed, moreover, OMT for stomatognathic functions. In these cases, OMT consists of habits elimination and behavioral modifications, jaw stabilization exercises, repatterning the oral facial muscles and changing their function for optimal nasal breathing, oral rest position, chewing, and swallowing.

1. **Breathing and Speech:** (1) Forced nasal inspiration and oral expiration in conjunction with phonation of open vowels, while sitting; (2) Balloon inflation with prolonged nasal inspiration and then forced blowing, repeated five times without taking the balloon out of the mouth.
2. **Swallowing and Chewing:** Alternate bilateral chewing and deglutition, using the tongue in the palate, closed teeth, without perioral contraction, whenever feeding. This exercise aims to educate for the correct position of the tongue while eating and targets the appropriate functionality and movement of the tongue and jaw.

There is evidence that OMT produces several benefits in OSAS patients; specifically, we can assist to an AHI reduction in adults with moderate OSA, to an increased percentage of lowest oxygen saturation (SaO_2), to a reduction of the arousal index, to an improvement of quality of sleep scores, to a reduction of daytime sleepiness with a significant improvement of ESS and even of quality of life and morning headache. Moreover, several studies demonstrated the efficacy of oropharyngeal muscles training in significantly reducing snoring frequency and intensity. In addition, despite no significant changes in body habitus, patients who undergo OMT show a significant reduction in neck circumference, suggesting that such training is able to induce upper airway remodeling.

Another possibility is training the upper airway by didgeridoo playing. This musical technique reduces upper airway collapsibility and, consequently, even daytime sleepiness in moderate OSAS patients, as evaluated by AHI and Epworth Sleepiness Scale, respectively.

2.2. Body Exercises

Exercise program is another management option to improve OSA that is associated with a reduced incidence of sleep-disordered breathing. As pointed out in a recent review, the different programs include aerobic exercises with or without breathing exercises and resistance training with light walking. Anyway, the best option resulted to be the combination of aerobic exercises and resistance training. Several hypotheses have been proposed to explain the beneficial effects of physical exercise on patients with OSA:

- *Increased upper airway dilator muscle tone:* During physical activity the respiratory muscles, particularly the diaphragm, work at an increased rate. Since exercise increases respiratory muscle recruitment, it seems plausible that endurance exercise might result in increased upper airway muscle activation; such effect increases upper airway diameter, reduces airway resistance, and opposes to pharyngeal collapse during sleep.
- *Reduced fluid accumulation within the neck:* Sedentary lifestyle and reduced ambulation are associated with fluid retention in the legs, given the central role of leg muscles in venous fluid dynamics. During sleep, the lying down position contributes to fluid repositioning and to an accumulation of them in the neck, with an increased laryngeal compression. This mechanism can increase the severity of OSA, given that most OSA patients have a sedentary lifestyle.
- *Increased slow-wave sleep:* Long-term exercise may also be responsible for positive effects on sleep architecture such as increased total sleep time and delayed REM sleep onset, increased slow-wave sleep (SWS) and reduced REM sleep, with a decrease in AHI as a consequence.

- *Reduced body weight:* Studies showed that a 10% decrease in body weight is associated with a 30% improvement in AHI. Exercise can lead to weight loss and reduction in BMI and studies indeed suggest that a reduction in BMI is associated with a reduction in the adipose tissue volume in the pharyngeal airway. Moreover, A study showed how exercise program, in association with diet, is able to induce a significant weight loss and improvement in clinically important neurobehavioral, cardiometabolic outcomes and day-time sleepiness, even in absence of a significant improvement in AHI. Such important result supports the concept that obesity itself contributes to daytime somnolence regardless of OSA.
- *Reduced systemic inflammatory response:* Visceral fat deposits represent a rich source of humoral mediators and inflammatory cytokines and this may impact negatively on neural pathways associated with respiratory control. Leptin, an adipocyte-derived factor affecting respiratory control, act as a respiratory stimulant, and an impairment in leptin signaling, as occurs in leptin-resistant or leptin-deficient states of obesity, is associated with obesity hypoventilation syndrome in humans. So, exercise program can reverse low grade inflammation markers and leptin levels in patients with an altered metabolism.

2.3. OMT in Children

Oral breathing and lip hypotonia are peculiar characteristics in children with OSA. They are associated with increased nasal resistance and malposition of the tongue, thereby exacerbating the impaired development and further hampering the growth of the maxilla and mandible. Moreover, deficits in orofacial muscles are caused by mouth breathing during sleep and this directly affects the position and strength of the tongue, causing abnormal airway development and obstruction.

Adenotonsillectomy (AT) remains the first-line treatment in children with adenotonsillar hypertrophy, even if recent evidence suggests that the outcome of this surgical procedure may not be as favorable as expected and that residual OSA persists in some cases. This treatment produces changes in the oropharyngeal structure but may have no effect on either functionality or neuromuscular disorders.

Villa et al. proposed three groups of oropharyngeal exercises (i.e., nasal breathing rehabilitation, labial seal and lip tone exercises, and tongue posture exercises) and showed how such exercises may be used as additional treatment to improve the oropharyngeal muscles hypotonia, nasal obstruction, nasal patency, and a proper closure of the mouth in children with residual OSA after adenotonsillectomy.

When used as first line therapy, OMT had positive effects on tongue behavior, restoring the normal tongue resting position after two months of treatment and enhancing tongue strength, maximum peak pressure, and endurance. These aspects are associated with the restoration of nasal breathing and a reduction in mouth breathing, which in turn improve nocturnal breathing. Furthermore, these changes are related to nocturnal symptom reduction and result in a higher oxygen saturation.

Children oropharyngeal reeducation may be initiated when they reach the age of 5–6 years old. The duration of the treatment is variable, but it typically consists of 3–6 months of active therapy, followed by a maintenance period of the same duration. The duration of the treatment is largely related to the degree of effort parents make in reinforcing their child to perform his/her exercises.

3. Hypoglossal Nerve Stimulation

For individuals with moderate-to-severe OSAS who are intolerant to C-PAP, upper airway stimulation (UAS) surgery with implantable hypoglossal nerve stimulation (HGNS) devices has emerged as an effective alternative therapy.

UAS uses electrical stimulation to activate the intrinsic and extrinsic muscles of the tongue in order to open the pharynx. A substantial benefit for patients is that there is no tissue removal or alteration of airway anatomy from this type of surgery. The electrical stimulation of the genioglossus (GG) muscle, the largest upper airway dilator muscle, causes tongue protrusion and stiffening of the anterior pharyngeal wall, and is therefore a potential therapeutic target for OSAS. Significant decreases in the activity of GG have been observed during sleep in patients with OSAS when compared with controls. Such finding led to early attempts to treat the disorder by electrical stimulation of the pharyngeal muscles with transcutaneous intraoral, and intramuscular electrodes. The major limitation with such electrical stimulation techniques is their tendency to induce arousal, presumably due to sensory stimulation, which limited their potential application as a long-term therapy for OSAS.

Several subsequent projects since then attempted to prove the usefulness of chronic HGNS as a novel therapeutic approach to sleep apnea. During HGNS, breathing acts are detected by an implanted sensor lead in the intercostal space, which subsequently delivers input to an implanted pulse generator (IPG) in the infraclavicular space. The IPG ultimately delivers an electrical stimulus to HGN fibers via a precisely placed stimulation cuff. The net result of this stimulation is the protrusion of a stiffened tongue synchronized with inspiration, which leads to a reduction in upper airway collapse during sleep. It was observed that HGN stimulation resulted in a lower risk of arousal than direct intramuscular stimulation. Indeed, the branches of the HGN that innervate the GG predominantly contain efferent motor fibers, so that stimulation activates just the GG muscle with minimal sensory feedback.

Moreover, it is worth to note that the effects of HGNS depend on which branches are stimulated. The proximal truncular segment of HGN innerves both intrinsic and extrinsic tongue musculature. If this segment is stimulated, it will produce a nonselective, and thus less effective, result. A more distal stimulation of the protrusive muscles has been demonstrated to be more efficient. HGN splits into medial (m-HGN) and lateral (l-HGN) contingents. The m-HGN branches are preferentially distributed to the GG and to the transverse and vertical intrinsic tongue muscles, which stiffen the tongue body, whereas the l-HGN branch is distributed predominantly to the styloglossus and hyoglossus muscles, which provide tongue retraction. Sturm et al. showed the strongest GG responses are elicited by stimulating the HGN superior medial branches which innerve more strongly the horizontal fibers of GG.

The GG is a fan-shaped muscle that originates from the mandibular symphysis and comprises two major functional components with differing effects on pharyngeal patency: horizontal fibers and vertical fibers. The former ones protrude the tongue and their contraction leads to symmetric pharyngeal enlargement and reductions in pharyngeal collapsibility; the latter ones depress the tongue and compromise the posterior airspace without decreasing pharyngeal collapsibility. Reductions in airway collapsibility have been most attributed to the dilating action of horizontal fibers.

Stimulation of HGN produces also a retropalatal effect. The palatoglossus muscle forms the anterior palatal pillars and connects the soft palate to the tongue base, inserting into the latter one. Normally, when the tongue protrudes forward, the palatoglossus muscle moves in an anterior direction thereby causing the increase in the retropalatal cross-sectional area.

The feasibility of HGNS and its potential as a therapeutic approach for the treatment of OSAS was initially described by Eisele et al. and Schwartz et al. who showed that HGNS could decrease the frequency of obstructive apneic and hypopneic events and improve the severity of oxyhemoglobin desaturation without arousing patients from sleep. The STAR trial, the initial multicenter trial with follow-up at 12 months, found a decrease of 68% in AHI score and 70% in ODI score after implantation of the upper-airway stimulation system. Moreover, Functional Outcomes of Sleep Questionnaire (FOSQ) and ESS indicated a significant improvement at 12 months. This study showed that the group of patients with BMI ≤32 or AHI score ≤ 50 events per hour treated with HGNS obtained a more consistent improvement than the ones with BMI >32 or AHI >50, even if the current BMI upper limit per FDA stimulation is 35. On the contrary, Huntley et al. treated with HGNS patients with BMI >32 and they found no differences between elevated and non-elevated BMI (≤32) cohorts in postoperative AHI, O_2 desaturation nadir, daytime sleepiness, rate of surgical success, or rate of cure. The ADHERE registry, a large multicenter prospective and retrospective observational registry that represents the follow-up of the STAR trial, showed a significant and stable improvement in PSG measures and subjective ESS and FOSQ scores at 18, 24, 36, and 48 months after HGNS. Even after 3 and 5 years authors obtained a persistent response to HGNS therapy.

There are several types of stimulator available on the market.

The Inspire I system is composed of an IPG placed subcutaneously in the region of pectoralis muscles, that is connected to the respiratory sensor implanted in the midline of the manubrium by means of a sensor lead. A stimulation lead connects the stimulator to the half-cuff electrode around the HGN. The device is placed unilaterally (generally on the right-side) on a peripheral branch of the HGN that innervates the genioglossus muscle and distal to the anterior branch of the ansa hypoglossi.

The Inspire II Upper Airway Stimulation device (Inspire Medical Systems, Inc., Maple Grove, MN) is made of stimulation lead, a sensing lead and an IPG. The IPG is implanted in a subcutaneous pocket in the right mid-infraclavicular region and it is connected to the stimulation lead, incorporates a cuff section that includes 3 electrodes, placed in m-HGN branch and to the sensory lead that is planted between the internal and external intercostal muscles at the superior border of the fourth to sixth rib.

The Aura6000 system (ImThera Medical, Inc., San Diego, CA) stimulate selectively the proximal trunk of the HGN. It is characterized by continuous nerve stimulation without a respiratory sensing lead, but alternates electrical stimulation impulses through different electrode configurations to rest some neuromuscular groups while others are stimulated.

Finally, the Nyxoah system (Nyxoah S.A. Brussels, Belgium) is a device composed of two main different parts: the Genio™ Implantable Stimulator (Nyxoah S.A. Brussels, Belgium), an implanted device placed in the submental area adjacent to the GG muscle through a surgical procedure, and an external activation chip attached to the skin with a disposable patch, which contains batteries and activates the implantable stimulator through radio frequencies. It is implanted over both GG muscles with the stimulating paddle electrodes facing the medial branches of the HGN on each muscle bilaterally.

There are several possible adverse events following HGNS surgery. These include:

- Damage to blood vessels in the proximity of the implant
- Excessive bleeding
- Nerve trauma or damage
- Allergic and/or rejection response to the implanted materials
- Infections
- Local irritation, seroma, hematoma, erosion, or swelling
- Persistent pain, numbness, or inflammation at the implant site
- Discomfort form the stimulation
- Tongue movement restrictions, irritation resulting from tongue abrasions on preexisting sharp or broken teeth
- Tongue soreness or weakness
- Problems with swallowing or speaking
- Undesirable change in stimulation over time, possibly related to tissue changes around electrodes, shifts in electrode position, loose electrical connections, or lead fractures
- Fibrosis to the extent that makes difficult to remove the system without damaging the surrounding structures
- Dry mouth
- Other acute symptoms (e.g., headaches, coughing, choking, dysphasia, and speech-related events)
- Insomnia

STAR trial reported that the most common procedure-related events were numbness/pain at the incision sites, and the common therapy-related events were some discomfort associated with stimulation (40%), tongue soreness, including abrasion on the lower side of the tongue abrasions caused by movement of the tongue over the lower incisors (21%) and temporary tongue weakness after surgery (18%).

The compliance in patients who undergo to HGNS is high, approximately 6.5h per night.

Therapeutic effectiveness of HGNS is dependent on the obstruction site. Predominant retro-lingual obstruction is a considered success criterium, since the direct effect of HGNS is tongue protrusion. Patients who have obstruction at multiple levels may not obtain as much benefit from this approach unless they have good mechanical coupling between movement of the oro- and velopharyngeal airways.

REFERENCES

Aiello, KD; Caughey, WG; Nelluri, B; Sharma, A; Mookadam, F; Mookadam, M. Effect of exercise training on sleep apnea: A systematic review and meta-analysis. *Respir Med.*, 2016, 116, 85-92. doi: 10.1016/j.rmed.2016.05.015.

American Academy of Sleep Medicine. *International Classification of Sleep Disorders*. 3rd ed. Darien, IL: American Academy of Sleep Medicine, 2014.

Andrade, FM; Pedrosa, RP. The role of physical exercise in obstructive sleep apnea. *J Bras Pneumol.*, 2016, 42(6), 457-464. doi: 10.1590/S1806-37562016000000156.

Baltzan, MA; Elkholi, O; Wolkove, N. Evidence of interrelated side effects with reduced compliance in patients treated with nasal CPAP. *Sleep Med*, (2009), 10, 198–205.

Barnes, M; Goldsworthy, UR; Cary, BA; Hill, CJ. A diet and exercise program to improve clinical outcomes in patients with obstructive sleep apnea--a feasibility study. *J Clin Sleep Med.*, 2009, 5(5), 409-415.

Benoist, L; de Ruiter, M; de Lange, J; de Vries, N. A randomized, controlled trial of positional therapy versus oral appliance therapy for position-dependent sleep apnea. *Sleep Med*, (2017), 34, 109–117. https://doi.org/10.1016/j.sleep.2017.01.024.

Benoist, LBL; Verhagen, M; Torensma, B; van Maanen, JP; de Vries, N. Positional therapy in patients with residual positional obstructive sleep apnea after upper airway surgery. *Sleep Breath.*, 2017 May, 21(2), 279-288. doi: 10.1007/s11325-016-1397-x. Epub 2016 Aug 17. PMID: 27535072.

Bignold, JJ; Mercer, JD; Antic, NA; McEvoy, RD; Catcheside, PG. Accurate position monitoring and improved supinedependent obstructive sleep apnea with a new position recording and supine avoidance device. *J Clin Sleep Med*, (2011), 7, 376–383.

Bisogni, V; Pengo, MF; De Vito, A; Maiolino, G; Rossi, GP; Moxham, J; Steier, J. Electrical stimulation for the treatment of obstructive sleep apnoea: a review of the evidence. *Expert Rev Respir Med.*, 2017 Sep, 11(9), 711-720. doi: 10.1080/17476348.2017.1358619. Epub 2017 Jul 27. PMID: 28730908.

Bollens, B; Reychler, G. Efficacy of exercise as a treatment for Obstructive Sleep Apnea Syndrome: A systematic review. *Complement Ther Med.*, 2018, 41, 208-214. doi: 10.1016/j.ctim.2018.10.002.

Boon, M; et al. Upper airway stimulation for obstructive sleep apnea: results from the ADHERE registry. *Otolaryngol Head Neck Surg.*, 2018, 159, 379–85.

Boyd, SB; Walters, AS; Waite, P; Harding, SM; Song, Y. Long-Term Effectiveness and Safety of Maxillomandibular Advancement for Treatment of Obstructive Sleep Apnea. *J Clin Sleep Med.*, 2015, 11(7), 699-708. Published 2015 Jul 15. doi: 10.5664/jcsm.4838.

Bruno, A; Di Sano, C; Lorusso, F; Dino, P; Russo, D; Ballacchino, A; Gallina, S; Modica, DM; Chiappara, G; Simon, HU; Pace, E. Notch-1 decreased expression contributes to leptin receptor downregulation in nasal epithelium from allergic turbinates. *Biochim Biophys Acta Mol Basis Dis.*, 2019, Jun 1, 1865(6), 1642-1650.

Camacho, M; Certal, V; Abdullatif, J; Zaghi, S; Ruoff, CM; Capasso, R; Kushida, CA. Myofunctional therapy to treat obstructive sleep apnea: a systematic review and meta-analysis. *SLEEP*, 2015, 38(5), 669–675.

Camacho, M; Guilleminault, C; Wei, JM; et al. Oropharyngeal and tongue exercises (myofunctional therapy) for snoring: a systematic review and meta-analysis. *Eur Arch Otorhinolaryngol.*, 2018, 275(4), 849-855. doi: 10.1007/s00405-017-4848-5.

Cartwright, RD. Effect of sleep position on sleep apnea severity. *Sleep*, (1984), 7, 110–114.

Certal, VF; Zaghi, S; Riaz, M; Vieira, AS; Pinheiro, CT; Kushida, C; Capasso, R; Camacho, M. Hypoglossal nerve stimulation in the treatment of obstructive sleep apnea: A systematic review and meta-analysis. *Laryngoscope.*, 2015 May, 125(5), 1254-64. doi: 10.1002/lary.25032. Epub 2014 Nov 12. PMID: 25389029.

Chai-Coetzer, CL; Antic, NA; Rowland, LS; et al. A simplified model of screening questionnaire and home monitoring for obstructive sleep apnoea in primary care. *Thorax.*, 2011, 66(3), 213–219.

Chan, AS; Lee, RW; Cistulli, PA. Dental appliance treatment for obstructive sleep apnea. *Chest.*, 2007, 132(2), 693-699. doi: 10.1378/chest.06-2038.

Chung, F; Subramanyam, R; Liao, P; Sasaki, E; Shapiro, C; Sun, Y. High STOPBang score indicates a high probability of obstructive sleep apnoea. *Br J Anaesth.*, 2012, 108(5), 768–775.

de Ruiter, MHT; Benoist, LBL; de Vries, N; de Lange, J. Durability of treatment effects of the Sleep Position Trainer versus oral appliance therapy in positional OSA: 12-month follow-up of a randomized controlled trial [published correction appears in Sleep Breath., 2018 May, 22(2), 451]. *Sleep Breath.*, 2018, 22(2), 441-450. doi: 10.1007/s11325-017-1568-4.

Decker, MJ; Haaga, J; Arnold, JL; Atzberger, D; Strohl, KP. Functional electrical stimulation and respiration during sleep. *J Appl Physiol*, 1993, 75, 1053-61.

Delaey, P; Duisit, J; Behets, C; Duprez, T; Gianello, P; Lengelé, B. Specific branches of hypoglossal nerve to genioglossus muscle as a potential target of selective neurostimulation in obstructive sleep apnea: anatomical and morphometric study. *Surg Radiol Anat.*, 2017, 39(5), 507-515. doi: 10.1007/s00276-016-1778-7.

Dempsey, JA; Veasey, SC; Morgan, BJ; O'Donnell, CP. *Pathophysiology of sleep apnea. Physiol Rev*, 2010, 90, 47-112

Driver, HS; Taylor, SR. Exercise and sleep. *Sleep Med Rev.*, 2000, 4(4), 387-402. doi: 10.1053/smrv.2000.0110.

Eastwood, PR; Barnes, M; Walsh, JH; et al. Treating obstructive sleep apnea with hypoglossal nerve stimulation. *Sleep.*, 2011, 34(11), 1479-1486. Published 2011 Nov 1. doi: 10.5665/sleep.1380.

Eckert, DJ; White, DP; Jordan, AS; Malhotra, A; Wellman, A. Defining phenotypic causes of obstructive sleep apnea. Identification of novel therapeutic targets. *Am J Crit Care Med*, 2013, 188, 996–1004.

Eijsvogel, MM; Ubbink, R; Dekker, J; Oppersma, E; de Jongh, FH; van der Palen, J; et al. Sleep position trainer versus tennis ball technique in positional obstructive sleep apnea syndrome. *J Clin Sleep Med*, 2015, 11, 139–147.

Eisele, DW; Smith, PL; Alam, DS; Schwartz, AR. Direct hypoglossal nerve stimulation in obstructive sleep apnea. *Arch Otolaryngol Head Neck Surg*, 1997, 123, 57-61.

Elmorsy, Shawky. The role of oral myofunctional therapy in managing patients with mild to moderate obstructive sleep apnea. *PAN Arab*

Journal of Rhinology, (2012), Vol. 2, No. 1, March, 2012. Vol. 2, No. 1, March, 2012.

Epstein, LJ; Kristo, D; Strollo, PJ; Jr. et al. Clinical guideline for the evaluation; management and long-term care of obstructive sleep apnea in adults. *J Clin Sleep Med.*, 2009, 5(3), 263-276.

Ertekin, C; Aydogdu, I. Neurophysiology of swallowing. *Clin Neurophysiol.*, 2003, 114(12), 2226–44.

Fleury Curado, T; Oliven, A; Sennes, LU; Polotsky, VY; Eisele, D; Schwartz AR. Neurostimulation Treatment of OSA. *Chest.*, 2018, 154(6), 1435-1447. doi: 10.1016/j.chest.2018.08.1070.

Frank, MH; Ravesloot, MJ; van Maanen, JP; Verhagen, E; de Lange, J; de Vries, N. Positional OSA part 1: Towards a clinical classification system for position-dependent obstructive sleep apnoea. *Sleep Breath.*, 2015 May, 19(2), 473-80. doi: 10.1007/s11325-014-1022-9. Epub 2014 Jun 19. PMID: 24943728.

Guilleminault, C; Powell, N; Bowman, B; Stoohs, R. The effect of electrical stimulation on obstructive sleep apnea syndrome. *Chest*, 1995, 107, 67-73.

Guimarães, KC; Drager, LF; Genta, PR; Marcondes, BF; Lorenzi-Filho, G. Effects of oropharyngeal exercises on patients with moderate obstructive sleep apnea syndrome. *Am J Respir Crit Care Med.*, 2009, 179(10), 962-966. doi: 10.1164/rccm.200806-981OC.

Heiser, C; Thaler, E; Boon, M; Soose, RJ; Woodson, BT. Updates of operative techniques for upper airway stimulation. *Laryngoscope*, 2016, 126, S12–S16.

Hirata, RP; Schorr, F; Kayamori, F; et al. Upper airway collapsibility assessed by negative expiratory pressure while awake is associated with upper airway anatomy. *J Clin Sleep Med.*, 2016, 12, 1339–1346.

Huntley, C; et al. Upper airway stimulation in patients with obstructive sleep apnea and an elevated body mass index: a multi-institutional review. *Laryngoscope.*, 2018, 128(10), 2425–8.

Johns, MW. A new method for measuring daytime sleepiness: the Epworth sleepiness scale. *Sleep.*, 1991, 14(6), 540–545.

Kezirian, EJ; Boudewyns, A; Eisele, DW; et al. Electrical stimulation of the hypoglossal nerve in the treatment of obstructive sleep apnea.

Sleep Med Rev., 2010, 14(5), 299-305. doi: 10.1016/j.smrv.2009.10.009.

Kim, EJ; Choi, JH; Kim, KW; et al. The impacts of open-mouth breathing on upper airway space in obstructive sleep apnea: 3-D MDCT analysis. *Eur Arch Otorhinolaryngol.*, 2011, 268, 533–539.

Leto, V; Kayamori, F; Montes, MI; et al. Effects of Oropharyngeal Exercises on Snoring: A Randomized Trial. *Chest.*, 2015, 148(3), 683-691. doi: 10.1378/chest.14-2953.

Levendowski, DJ; Seagraves, S; Popovic, D; Westbrook, PR. Assessment of a neckbased treatment and monitoring device for positional obstructive sleep apnea. *J Clin Sleep Med*, 2014, 10, 863–871.

Lewis, R; Pételle, B; Campbell, MC; et al. Implantation of the nyxoah bilateral hypoglossal nerve stimulator for obstructive sleep apnea. *Laryngoscope Investig Otolaryngol.*, 2019, 4(6), 703-707. Published 2019 Nov 22. doi: 10.1002/lio2.312.

Lorusso, F; Dispenza, F; Modica, DM; Gallina, S. The Role of Modified Expansion Sphincter Pharyngoplasty in Multilevel Obstructive Sleep Apnea Syndrome Surgery. *Int Arch Otorhinolaryngol.*, 2018 Oct, 22(4), 432-436.

Lorusso, F; Dispenza, F; Saraniti, C; Sireci, F; Modica, DM; Gallina, S. Sleep disordered breathing: evaluation of dynamic patterns of the upper airways in obese subjects. *Otorinolaringologia*, 2014, 64, 57–64.

Lorusso, F; Gallina, S; Modica, DM; Di Salvo, N; Riggio, F. Bipolar Quantum Molecular Resonance versus Blunt Dissection tonsillectomy. *B-ENT*, 2015, 11(02), 101–108

Lorusso, F; Dispenza, F; Martinciglio, G; Battaglia, A; Gallina, S. Postural changes in patients undergoing hyoid surgery for OSAS. *EuroMediterranean Biomedical Journal*, 2017, 12(29), 140-143.

Lorusso, F; Martines, F; Mistretta, A; Dispenza, F; Gallina, S. Effects of adenotonsillectomy on neurocognitive and behavioural function in pediatric obstructive sleep apnea syndrome. *B-ENT*, 2018, 14, 113-118

Mador, MJ; Kufel, TJ; Magalang, UJ; Rajesh, SK; Watwe, V; Grant, BJ. Prevalence of positional sleep apnea in patients undergoing polysomnography. *Chest*, (2005), 128, 2130–2137.

Malhotra, A; Huang, Y; Fogel, RB; Pillar, G; Edwards, JK; Kikinis, R; Loring, SH; White, DP. The male predisposition to pharyngeal collapse: importance of airway length. *Am J Respir Crit Care Med*, 166, 1388–1395, 2002.

Marklund, M; Persson, M; Franklin, KA. Treatment success with a mandibular advancement device is related to supinedependent sleep apnea. *Chest*, (1998), 114, 1630–1635.

Maurer, Joachim T; et al. "Operative technique of upper airway stimulation: an implantable treatment of obstructive sleep apnea." *Operative Techniques in Otolaryngology-Head and Neck Surgery*, 23.3, (2012), 227-233.

Mezzanotte, WS; Tangel, DJ; White, SC. Influence of sleep onset on upper-airway muscle activity in apnea patients versus normal controls. *Am J Respir Crit Care Med*, 1996, 153, 1880-7.

Modica, DM; Marchese, D; Lorusso, F; Speciale, R; Saraniti, C; Gallina, S. Functional Nasal Surgery and Use of CPAP in OSAS Patients: Our Experience. *Indian J Otolaryngol Head Neck Surg.*, 2018 Dec, 70(4), 559-565.

Nemati, S; Gerami, H; Soltanipour, S; Saberi, A; Moghadam, SK; Setva, F. The effects of oropharyngeal-lingual exercises in patients with primary snoring. *Eur Arch Otorhinolaryngol.*, 2015, 272(4), 1027-1031. doi: 10.1007/s00405-014-3382-y.

Netzer, NC; Stoohs, RA; Netzer, CM; Clark, K; Strohl, KP. Using the Berlin Questionnaire to identify patients at risk for the sleep apnea syndrome. *AnnIntern Med.*, 1999, 131(7), 485–491.

Newman, AB; Foster, G; Givelber, R; et al. Progression and regression of sleep-disordered breathing with changes in weight: the Sleep Heart Health Study. *Arch Intern Med*, 2005, 165, 2408- 2413.

Oksenberg, A; Silverberg, DS; Arons, E; Radwan, H. Positional vs nonpositional obstructive sleep apnea patients: anthropomorphic, nocturnal polysomnographic, and multiple sleep latency test data. *Chest.*, 1997, 112(3), 629–639.

Oliven, A; Odeh, M; Geitini, L; et al. Effect of coactivation of tongue protrusor and retractor muscles on pharyngeal lumen and airflow in sleep apnea patients. *J Appl Physiol*, (1985), 2007, 103(5), 1662-1668. doi: 10.1152/japplphysiol.00620.2007.

Omobomi, O; Quan, SF. Positional therapy in the management of positional obstructive sleep apnea-a review of the current literature. *Sleep Breath.*, 2018 May, 22(2), 297-304. doi: 10.1007/s11325-017-1561-y. Epub 2017 Aug 29. PMID: 28852945.

Ow, AT; Cheung, LK. Meta-analysis of mandibular distraction osteogenesis: clinical applications and functional outcomes. *Plast Reconstr Surg*, 2008, 121, 54e–69e.

Pataka, A; Daskalopoulou, E; Kalamaras, G; Fekete Passa, K; Argyropoulou, P. Evaluation of five different questionnaires for assessing sleep apnea syndrome in a sleep clinic. *Sleep Med.*, 2014, 15(7), 776–781.

Pearson, WG; Jr. Langmore, SE; Zumwalt, AC. Evaluating the structural properties of suprahyoid muscles and their potential for moving the hyoid. *Dysphagia.*, 2011, 26, 345–351.

Penzel, T; Moller, M; Becker, HF; et al. Effect of sleep position and sleep stage on the collapsibility of the upper airways in patients with sleep apnea. *Sleep*, 2001, 24(1), 90–5.

Permut, I; Diaz-Abad, M; Chatila, W; Crocetti, J; Gaughan, JP; D'Alonzo, GE; Krachman SL. Comparison of positional therapy to CPAP in patients with positional obstructive sleep apnea. *J Clin Sleep Med*, (2010), 6, 238–243.

Piccin, O; Scaramuzzino, G; Martone, C; Marra, F; Gobbi, R; Sorrenti, G. Modified hyoid suspension technique in the treatment of multilevel related obstructive sleep apnea. *Otolaryngol Head Neck Surg.*, 2014, 150(02), 321–324.

Prikladnicki, A; Martinez, D; Brunetto, MG; Fiori, CZ; Lenz, MDCS; Gomes, E. Diagnostic performance of cheeks appearance in sleep apnea. *Cranio.*, 201, 21, 1–8.

Puhan, MA; Suarez, A; Lo Cascio, C; Zahn, A; Heitz, M; Braendli, O. Didgeridoo playing as alternative treatment for obstructive sleep apnoea syndrome: randomised controlled trial. *BMJ.*, 2006, 332(7536), 266-270. doi: 10.1136/bmj.38705.470590.55.

Randerath, WJ; Galetke, W; Domanski, U; Weitkunat, R; Ruhle, KH. Tonguemuscle training by intraoral electrical neurostimulation in patients with obstructive sleep apnea. *Sleep*, 2004, 27, 254–259.

Ravesloot, MJ; Frank, MH; van Maanen, JP; Verhagen, EA; de Lange, J; de Vries, N. Positional OSA part 2: retrospective cohort analysis with a new classification system (APOC). *Sleep Breath.*, 2016, 20(2), 881–888.

Ravesloot, MJ; van Maanen, JP; Dun, L; de Vries, N. The undervalued potential of positional therapy in position-dependent snoring and obstructive sleep apnea – a review of the literature. *Sleep Breath*, 2013, 17, 39–49.

Ravesloot, MJL; Benoist, L; van Maanen, P; de Vries, N. Novel Positional Devices for the Treatment of Positional Obstructive Sleep Apnea, and How This Relates to Sleep Surgery. *Adv Otorhinolaryngol.*, 2017, 80, 28-36. doi: 10.1159/000470819. Epub 2017 Jul 17. PMID: 28738340.

Ravesloot, MJL; White, D; Heinzer, R; Oksenberg, A; Pépin, JL. Efficacy of the New Generation of Devices for Positional Therapy for Patients With Positional Obstructive Sleep Apnea: A Systematic Review of the Literature and Meta-Analysis. *J Clin Sleep Med.*, 2017 Jun 15, 13(6), 813-824. doi: 10.5664/jcsm.6622. PMID: 28212691, PMCID: PMC5443742.

Salman, Salam O. ed. *Modern Management of Obstructive Sleep Apnea*. Springer, 2019.

Schwartz, AR; Bennett, ML; Smith, PL; et al. Therapeutic electrical stimulation of the hypoglossal nerve in obstructive sleep apnea. *Arch Otolaryngol Head Neck Surg*, 2001, 127, 1216-23.

Senaratna, CV; et al., Prevalence of obstructive sleep apnea in the general population: A systematic review, *Sleep Medicine Reviews* (2016), http://dx.doi.org/10.1016/j.smrv.2016.07.00.

Steffen, A; Kilic, A; Inke, KR; et al. Tongue motion variability with changes of upper airway stimulation electrode configuration and effects on treatment outcomes. *Laryngoscope*, 2017, 128, 1970–1976.

Steier, J; Seymour, J; Rafferty, GF; et al. Continuous transcutaneous submental electrical stimulation in obstructive sleep apnea: a feasibility study. *Chest*, 2011, 140, 998–1007.

Strollo, PJ; Jr. Soose, RJ; Maurer, JT; et al. Upper-airway stimulation for obstructive sleep apnea. *N Engl J Med*, 2014, 370, 139–149.

Sturm, JJ; Modik, O; Suurna, MV. Neurophysiological monitoring of tongue muscle activation during hypoglossal nerve stimulation. *Laryngoscope.*, 2019, 10.1002/lary.28341. doi: 10.1002/lary.28341.

Van de Graaff, WB; Gottfried, SB; Mitra, J; van Lunteren, E; Cherniack, NS; Strohl, KP. Respiratory function of hyoid muscles and hyoid arch. *J Appl Physiol Respir Environ Exerc Physiol*, (1984), 57(1), 197–204.

van Maanen, JP; Meester, KA; Dun, LN; Koutsourelakis, I; Witte, BI; Laman, DM; et al. The sleep position trainer: a new treatment for positional obstructive sleep apnoea. *Sleep Breath*, 2013, 17, 771–779.

van Maanen, JP; Richard, W; van Kesteren, ER; Ravesloot, MJ; Laman, DM; Hilgevoord, AA; et al. Evaluation of a new simple treatment for positional sleep apnoea patients. *J Sleep Res*, 2012, 21, 322–329.

van Maanen, JP; Witte, BI; de Vries, N. Positional therapy and palatal surgery; in de Vries N, Ravesloot MJL, van Maanen JP (eds): *Positional Therapy in Obstructive Sleep Apnea*. Cham, Springer, 2015, pp. 297–310.

Vgontzas, AN; Papanicolaou, DA; Bixler, EO; et al. Elevation of plasma cytokines in disorders of excessive daytime sleepiness: role of sleep disturbance and obesity. *J Clin Endocrinol Metab*, 1997, 82, 1313-1316.

Vicini, C; Montevecchi, F; Tenti, G; et al., Transoral robotic surgery: tongue base reduction and supraglottoplasty for obstructive sleep apnea. *Operative Technique in Otolaryngology.*, 2012, 23, 45–47.

Villa, MP; Brasili, L; Ferretti, A; et al. Oropharyngeal exercises to reduce symptoms of OSA after AT. *Sleep Breath.*, 2015, 19(1), 281-289. doi: 10.1007/s11325-014-1011-z.

Villa, MP; Evangelisti, M; Martella, S; Barreto, M; Del Pozzo, M. Can myofunctional therapy increase tongue tone and reduce symptoms in children with sleep-disordered breathing?. *Sleep Breath.*, 2017, 21(4), 1025-1032. doi: 10.1007/s11325-017-1489-2.

Villa, Maria Pia; Melania Evangelisti. "Oropharyngeal Exercises for Treatment of Pediatric Obstructive Sleep-Disordered Breathing." *Current Sleep Medicine Reports*, 5.2, (2019), 33-40.

Weaver, TE; Grunstein, RR. Adherence to continuous positive airway pressure therapy: the challenge to effective treatment. *Proc Am Thorac Soc*, 2008, 5, 173–178.

Wellman, A; Eckert, DJ; Jordan, AS; Edwards, BA; Passaglia, CL; Jackson, AC; Gautam, S; Owens, RL; Malhotra, A; White, DP. A method for measuring and modeling the physiological traits causing obstructive sleep apnea. *J Appl Physiol*, 110, 1627–1637, 2011.

Woodson, BT; et al. Three-year outcomes of cranial nerve stimulation for obstructive sleep apnea: the STAR trial. *Otolaryngol Head Neck Surg.*, 2016, 154, 181–8.

Woodson, BT; et al. Upper airway stimulation for obstructive sleep apnea: 5-year outcomes. *Otolaryngol Head Neck Surg.*, 2018, 159, 194–202.

Zuberi, NA; Rekab, K; Nguyen, HV. Sleep apnea avoidance pillow effects on obstructive sleep apnea syndrome and snoring. *Sleep Breath.*, 2004 Dec, 8(4), 201-7. doi: 10.1007/s11325-004-0201-5. PMID: 15611895.

Editors' Contact Information

Francesco Lorusso, MD
UOC Otorinolaringoiatria,
Azienda Ospedaliera universitaria Policlinico
"P.Giaccone", Palermo, Italy

Salvatore Gallina
Associate Professor of Otolaryngology
UOC Otorinolaringoiatria,
Azienda Ospedaliera universitaria Policlinico
"P.Giaccone", Palermo, Italy

INDEX

A

B

C

D

L

M

N

O

P

R

S